D1259330

Second Edition

Evidence-Based Management in Healthcare

PRINCIPLES, CASES, AND PERSPECTIVES

Anthony R. Kovner | Thomas D'Aunno | Editors

AUPHA

Health Administration Press, Chicago, Illinois

Association of University Programs in Health Administration, Washington, DC

Your board, staff, or clients may also benefit from this book's insight. For more information on quantity discounts, contact the Health Administration Press Marketing Manager at (312) 424-9450.

This publication is intended to provide accurate and authoritative information in regard to the subject matter covered. It is sold, or otherwise provided, with the understanding that the publisher is not engaged in rendering professional services. If professional advice or other expert assistance is required, the services of a competent professional should be sought.

The statements and opinions contained in this book are strictly those of the authors and do not represent the official positions of the American College of Healthcare Executives, the Foundation of the American College of Healthcare Executives, or the Association of University Programs in Health Administration.

21 20 19 18 17   5 4 3 2 1

Library of Congress Cataloging-in-Publication Data
Names: Kovner, Anthony R., editors. | D'Aunno, Thomas A., editors.
Title: Evidence-based management in healthcare : principles, cases, and perspectives /
    Anthony R. Kovner and Thomas D'Aunno, editors.
Description: Second edition. | Chicago, Illinois : Health Administration Press (HAP) ;
    Arlington, Virginia : Association of University Programs in Health Administration (AUPHA),
    [2017] | Includes bibliographical references.
Identifiers: LCCN 2016039581 (print) | LCCN 2016039938 (ebook) | ISBN
    9781567938715 (print : alk. paper) | ISBN 9781567938739 (xml) | ISBN
    9781567938746 (epub) | ISBN 9781567938753 (mobi) | ISBN 9781567938722 (Ebook)
Subjects: LCSH: Health services administration—Decision making. | Evidence-based medicine.
Classification: LCC RA971 .E983 2017 (print) | LCC RA971 (ebook) | DDC 362.1068—dc23
LC record available at https://lccn.loc.gov/2016039581

The paper used in this publication meets the minimum requirements of American National Standard for Information Sciences—Permanence of Paper for Printed Library Materials, ANSI Z39.48-1984. ∞™

Acquisitions editor: Janet Davis; Project manager: Michael Noren; Cover designer: James Slate; Layout: PerfecType

Found an error or a typo? We want to know! Please e-mail it to hapbooks@ache.org, mentioning the book's title and putting "Book Error" in the subject line.

For photocopying and copyright information, please contact Copyright Clearance Center at www.copyright.com or at (978) 750-8400.

Health Administration Press
A division of the Foundation of the American
    College of Healthcare Executives
One North Franklin Street, Suite 1700
Chicago, IL 60606-3529
(312) 424-2800

Association of University Programs
    in Health Administration
1730 M Street, NW
Suite 407
Washington, DC 20036
(202) 763-7283

Dedication

To Eric Barends, a fountainhead of energy whose contribution
to this book cannot be overestimated.

BRIEF CONTENTS

Part III   Scientific Evidence—Examples of Practice

Part IV   Organizational Evidence

DETAILED CONTENTS

FOREWORD

by David Blumenthal, President of the Commonwealth Fund

When I was doing my medical residency, my fellow residents and I could always identify the few master clinicians on the attending staff in our teaching hospital.

They focused intently on their patients. Their questions were respectful, artful, and precise, often eliciting that elusive historical fact that unlocked a diagnostic puzzle. Their physical exams were incredibly skillful, as though their fingers, eyes, and ears had extra dimensions of sensation. They marshalled data from the patient's history, the physical exam, laboratory results, the scientific literature, their own personal experience, and something else—intuition and wisdom—to reach an elegant synthesis and to formulate a diagnostic and therapeutic plan.

As physicians in training, our (then hand-written) notes in the medical records went on for pages. The master clinicians' were only a paragraph or two—yet they said more.

Are there the equivalent of master clinicians—*master managers*—on the administrative side of the healthcare house? I hope and believe there are. If so, one thing is absolutely clear: Among the skills they bring to their craft is the ability to find and use the evidence that is relevant to the decisions they must make. That evidence might come from a wide variety of sources: their personal experiences and observations, the information systems in their organizations, the academic literature, and the teachings of the clinical and nonclinical colleagues with whom they interact. But whatever the evidence is, and wherever it is found, the master manager must be able to master it.

Skeptics may point out that in the real world of management—at the point of the spear—objective evidence is scarce and rarely sufficient to identify a correct course of action. What's more, the ability to marshal such evidence is only one of many skills required for managerial excellence and success. However, the same could be said of master clinicians, who rarely have all the data they need when they must act. What master clinicians have acquired is the ability to milk whatever data are available for everything they're worth.

If this volume is successful, it will help aspiring master managers to perfect the equivalent skill in their own chosen role in our complex health-care system. At a minimum, it will launch readers on a life-long quest to use all the evidence available to make the very best of the copious resources we deploy for the benefit of patients in the United States and around the world.

ACKNOWLEDGMENTS

Thanks to all the chapter authors and interviewees and the staff of Health Administration Press—in particular Tulie O'Connor, who was invaluable in the editing process, and Michael Noren, for his added value to the production process.

AN INTRODUCTION

by Anthony R. Kovner and Thomas D'Aunno

Why Should Managers Read This Book?

This book is written for current and future healthcare managers, with the aim of helping them reflect about whether they or their organizations are carrying out their mission. Are the leaders asking appropriate questions? Are managers learning which stakeholders to serve and how to serve those stakeholders better? Asking the right questions is at the foundation of evidence-based management, or EBMgmt. Taking ownership of the evidence-based management process adds value to any manager's organizational contribution.

Analysis should always start with a truthful examination of how the organization is functioning now and what problems or difficulties exist with current operations. For example, what are our current hours of operation? How many patients do we see in the ambulatory center each day we are open, and each hour we are open? How many patients are on the waiting list, and how much time do our providers spend with each patient? What activities does the organization measure? What are the hours of operation of competitors? What data do we collect, and how do we collect them? Who collects the data? What would happen if we stayed open an hour later and started an hour earlier, or if we opened during an evening or a Saturday or closed half a day on another day? What is the cost of data analysis? What are the barriers to intervention of a proposed implementation?

Why Do We Care Passionately About Evidence-Based Management?

We have worked in organizations in which managers have not given sufficient value to customers for the costs of services. Our students and alumni have also worked in such organizations. We want to improve the way things operate. We have made suggestions both as managers and as workers, and we have asked difficult questions of our school: Do we attract and admit the "right" students, do we measure how we add value with students, can graduates do what employers pay them to do, do graduates get good jobs, do students enjoy the educational experience, and so on and so forth? What do we measure (what are the main things of importance to the school?), and how are we accountable for our performance? One way of addressing all these concerns is to practice evidence-based management.

Organizations do not have to use the term *evidence-based*, as long as they practice according to good EBMgmt principles. If an employer does not practice evidence-based management, managers can work elsewhere; otherwise, they can stay loyal to the employer and try to encourage evidence-based practice in their own corner, and they can introduce their colleagues to the concepts in this text.

What Did the First Edition Accomplish?

The first edition of this book, published in 2009, had four main accomplishments. First, it reviewed the movement from evidence-based medicine, which was fairly well developed at the time, to the yet-to-be-fully-developed application of evidence-based practice (EBP) to management. The coeditors knew that, even though not all physicians practiced evidence-based medicine, the evidence for what was best practice in management was scanty compared to that in medicine.

Second, the book discussed then-current theories and definitions of evidence-based management. Since the preparation of the first edition, the terminology in the field has changed somewhat, with the phrase *evidence-based practice* increasingly being used instead of *evidence-based management*. A distinction between the two terms is that evidence-based management is evidence-based practice carried out by managers rather than by clinicians, lawyers, or policymakers.

Third, the book presented ten case studies of interventions using evidence-based practice to respond to management challenges. In some instances, EBP steps were used from the outset on a project; in other instances, the EBP framework was applied retrospectively to interventions already under way or completed. Some of the ten cases explicitly followed the steps of the evidence-based process; others followed only some of the steps, or did not report certain steps. Still, all of the cases illustrated how the basic principles of evidence-based management were applied to a set of management challenges.

Fourth, the book presented research findings and conveyed what the coeditors had learned about evidence-based management as of 2009, and it discussed where the field could go from there. Richard D'Aquila observed that the most important element was that management decisions be grounded in a process whereby managers ask the right questions and assemble the right information for a decision. This point may seem simple and logical, but the process is not universally practiced. As a result, managers make many decisions based on low-quality evidence, sometimes even when evidence of higher quality is available at a reasonable cost. We believe that managers who base their actions on better evidence make better decisions and continuously improve the decision-making process in their organizations.

Why don't more managers adopt an evidence-based approach? As Kovner suggested, managers and consultants are not generally rewarded for basing their interventions on the best available evidence. The business case examining return on investment has not yet been reliably made for evidence-based management, and governing boards do not regularly review the quality of the managerial decision-making process. Increased use of evidence-based management would likely shift power in organizations away from older, traditional executives to younger, more data-driven types.

What Do We Intend to Accomplish in the Second Edition?

This second edition presents a thoroughly updated and expanded examination of evidence-based management, organized into six parts.

Part I: Overview

Part I includes chapters about the basic principles of evidence-based management, rapid evidence assessments for managers, and award-winning hospitals that use EBMgmt principles.

In chapter 1, Eric Barends, Denise M. Rousseau, and Rob B. Briner clearly define what evidence-based management is and what it is not, and they describe the four key sources of evidence. The authors highlight the need to include organizational and experiential evidence and evidence of stakeholders' values and concerns, in addition to scientific evidence.

In chapter 2, Barends, Karen Plum, and Andrew Mawson discuss the use of rapid evidence assessments, and they provide a detailed example involving a specific management issue.

In chapter 3, John R. Griffith summarizes what we've learned from the most rigorous EBMgmt process used in healthcare organizations—the Malcolm Baldrige National Quality Award. Griffith suggests how new ways to disseminate the Baldrige innovations can effectively transform hospitals.

Part II: Scientific Evidence—Doing the Work

Part II includes chapters about research opportunities and examples, ways of acquiring evidence, uptake issues for evidence-based management in healthcare, and what evidence-based management in healthcare can learn from evidence-based practice in other domains.

In chapter 4, Thomas Rundall and Terese Otte-Trojel identify research opportunities and examples pertaining to each of the four sources of evidence.

In chapter 5, Susan Kaplan Jacobs focuses on framing research questions and originating literature and information searches, drawing from her experience as a senior health sciences librarian working with Capstone teams.

In chapter 6, Thomas D'Aunno identifies barriers to the uptake of EBMgmt initiatives and suggests ways of overcoming those barriers.

In chapter 7, Rousseau and Brian C. Gunia describe lessons learned from other disciplines and domains—such as medicine, nursing, police work, and government—where evidence-based initiatives are proceeding apace.

Part III: Scientific Evidence—Examples of Practice

Part III presents examples of evidence-based management being carried out and being judged worthy of investment. Though details may be lacking about dollars invested and specific financial and other benefits received, the aim of many of these organizational initiatives was not to justify evidence-based management but rather to improve organizational and management performance.

In chapter 8, Lawrence Prybil and Michael Slubowski extend analysis of the case study from the first edition about transforming CEO evaluation at SCL Health in Denver, Colorado.

In chapter 9, Sofia Agoritsas, Steven Fishbane, and Candice Halinski discuss the Healthy Transitions Program in Late Stage Kidney Disease, carried out at Northwell Health in New York.

In chapter 10, K. Joanne McGlown, Stephen J. O'Connor, and Richard M. Shewchuk update their previous case study about hospital evacuation after Hurricane Katrina, and they comment on evidence-based criteria ten years later.

In chapter 11, Kyle L. Grazier updates her case study about integrating chronic care management and primary care. She ends her discussion with a letter from a CEO to the senior leadership team. The letter deals with an organization's quest for integration of critical behavioral health and primary care services across a network of services for patients and families.

Part IV: Organizational Evidence

The chapters of Part IV are rich in organizational data related to performance improvement efforts, management challenges, and the teaching of evidence-based competencies.

In chapter 12, Jed Weissberg and Patrick Courneya, the former and present medical directors of Kaiser Permanente, describe how that organization's leadership values research in improving organizational performance.

They also provide examples of key initiatives that have taken an evidence-based approach.

In chapter 13, Jessie L. Tucker III describes how Lyndon B. Johnson (LBJ) General Hospital in Houston, Texas, was forced to change its behavior in response to serious reimbursement challenges. Managers used benchmarked performance data to show colleagues that change was necessary, and they showed that evidence-based analysis led to improved performance.

In chapter 14, Andrew N. Garman and colleagues describe the Rush University Medical Center model for teaching evidence-based practice. Rush is an unusual educational program in healthcare because it is integrated with a medical center. Practicing managers are on the program faculty, and managers are responsible for student acquisition of required management competencies.

In chapter 15, John Donnellan describes the Capstone model at New York University's Robert F. Wagner Graduate School of Public Service, where a program for nurse leaders was codeveloped by NYU Wagner faculty and senior managers in the New York-Presbyterian health system. NY-Presbyterian's leadership realized that problems in nursing turnover were caused in no small part by nurse managers' lack of management skills. The Capstone course, which uses evidence-based management, has been a distinctive feature of the NYU/NY-Presbyterian model, with teams of students performing as consultants for senior nurse managers at NY-Presbyterian and other hospitals, notably the Hospital for Special Surgery.

In chapter 16, Kim Carlin speaks to the role that consultants play in influencing major change and transforming management practice. Carpedia, a worldwide consulting firm, emphasizes the need for managers to manage using EBP methods, with attention to developing metrics and focusing on accountability for results.

Part V: Experiential Evidence

Part V includes a chapter about a hospital manager's experience in responding to a management challenge, a demonstration of an evidence-based Capstone project as part of a program in healthcare management, and insightful interviews with three senior executives.

In chapter 17, Lynn McVey and Eric Slotsve respond to the situation of an executive manager (McVey) in dire circumstances, facing a quality and financial crisis similar to that faced by Tucker and LBJ Hospital in chapter 13. The chapter details an impressive transition from traditional management to a standardized, evidence-based approach.

In chapter 18, Bryce Clark, a former Capstone student at NYU Wagner now working in quality control at Children's Hospital Colorado, details an academic year's project focused on reducing length of stay for elective surgery patients. This process led to some notable outcomes and recommendations not directly related to the original question.

Chapters 19 through 21 present interviews with David Fine, former CEO of St. Luke's Episcopal Hospital in Houston and current president and CEO at the Catholic Health Initiatives Institute for Research and Innovation; Richard D'Aquila, president of Yale New Haven Hospital; and Michael Dowling, CEO of Northwell Health. These experienced senior managers set out to dramatically improve health system performance, and because of their outstanding results, some of their methods have been widely copied. Keep in mind, however, that part of the evidence-based management decision-making process indeed is asking, "If this intervention works in Akron, will it necessarily work in Brooklyn?"

These interviews are included in the text because they embody, with the individuals' vast energy and highest integrity, many of the key elements of evidence-based practice in daily behavior. These senior managers learn principally from studying their own organizational data and those of other organizations in the health field and in other sectors. They are familiar with the relevant scientific literature, and they know what makes for valid and reliable studies. When responding to management challenges, they ask questions that are focused and answerable. They continuously look for interventions initiated by successful innovators in other fields and geographic markets. These leaders develop teams that are rewarded for trusting one another and extending the leadership vision, and they develop successful managers to whom they give autonomy and whom they hold accountable for performance. They develop managers who want to learn and use research science to confront political opposition—usually, but not always, successfully. These senior managers are also able to cut losses from failed interventions and to learn from failures.

Part VI: Stakeholder Concerns

Stakeholder values and concerns are the focus of Part VI. Chapters 22 through 26 present interviews with five individuals reflecting a variety of stakeholder groups, and chapter 27 concludes the section with a look to the future of evidence-based management in healthcare.

In chapter 22, Ethan Basch, an oncologist, draws on his experiences in applying evidence-based medicine to cancer care, as well as on his experiences with evidence-based management in his practice of oncology.

In chapter 23, Maja Djukic, a professor of nursing management, discusses her experiences studying nurse managers. She observes that evidence-based practice is being implemented within clinical nursing but not within the management and organization of nursing services.

In chapter 24, professor and consultant John Billings discusses *big data*—defined simply as "lots of data"—which can include many millions of records, often gathered for one purpose and used for another. Using an example of Medicaid data, Billings explains how managers are coming to realize that large data sets exist and that analysis of these data can lead to improved operations. He also points out limits to the current use of big data with regard to social, housing, and transportation factors.

In chapter 25, Eric Barends relates some of his experiences as an international management consultant in evidence-based practice. He observes that EBP produces better outcomes in two different ways—first, by asking questions and, second, through critical appraisal. An appropriate organizational culture promotes asking such questions as, "How do you know this will work?" and "Do we really have that much of a problem?" Critical appraisal enables managers to distinguish trustworthy from untrustworthy evidence.

In chapter 26, Quint Studer, a successful consultant and author of numerous healthcare management books, states that people get "hung up" on the idea that the CEO needs perfect evidence. Studer observes that "it's not evidence that counts so much as accountability." He concludes that aligning goals is most important in improving performance, changing how the organization evaluates its managers going forward.

In chapter 27, Kovner and D'Aunno identify six key questions (with subquestions) about the future of evidence-based management. The questions are organized by source of evidence and consist of the following:

1. How do we identify the field of evidence-based management?
2. How can we get teams to work together?
3. How can we facilitate organizational ownership of evidence-based management?
4. How can we prepare managers to engage in evidence-based management?
5. How can we originate, standardize, and disseminate data on evidence-based management?
6. How can we get funders and regulators to behave as partners?

The book concludes with two appendixes. Appendix A presents a guide to resources that Barends suggested to students in a course in evidence-based management at NYU Wagner in 2016. Appendix B offers a starter set of further readings, based on the chapters of this book and incorporating suggestions from the Center for Evidence-Based Management (www.cebma.org).

What Have We Not Yet Been Able to Accomplish?

As of 2016, we are unable to specify the ranges of what evidence-based management will cost, in both time and money, for the organization and the manager. Much work also remains to be done in calculating the benefits of using an evidence-based process; developing a guide for managers to use in setting priorities for answerable questions; specifying the organizational capacity needed to carry out evidence-based practice; and examining how accountability is designed and works for evidence-based management in organizations.

In creating this book, we have stood on other people's shoulders. Hopefully more people will stand on ours as evidence-based management practices continue to develop, deepen, and become more widespread.

Instructor Resources

This book is accompanied by an Instructor's Manual.

For the most up-to-date information about this book and its Instructor Resources, go to ache.org/HAP and browse for the book's title or author names.

This book's Instructor Resources are available to instructors who adopt this book for use in their course. For access information, please e-mail hapbooks@ache.org.

OVERVIEW

1

EVIDENCE-BASED MANAGEMENT: THE BASIC PRINCIPLES

by Eric Barends, Denise M. Rousseau, and Rob B. Briner

Introduction

Consider this hypothetical situation: You pay a visit to a dietitian after gaining a bit of weight over the holiday season. The dietitian advises you to try diet X. It's very expensive and demands a radical change in lifestyle, but the prospect of having a slim and healthy body motivates you to stick to the diet. After a few weeks, however, you have gained five pounds and suffer serious side effects that require medical treatment. After searching the Internet, you learn that most scientific studies find diet X to be ineffective and fraught with such side effects. When you confront the diet consultant with these findings, he replies, "Why should I pay attention to scientific studies? I have 20 years of experience. Besides, the diet was developed by a famous American nutritionist whose book sold more than a million copies."[1]

Does that sound like malpractice? It probably does. Unfortunately, in management, disregarding sound evidence, relying on personal experience, and following the ideas of popular management gurus are all too common. Such tendencies are especially troubling when you consider that managerial decisions affect the working lives and well-being of people around the world. Henry Mintzberg (1990, 60) once said:

> No job is more vital to our society than that of a manager. It is the manager who determines whether our social institutions serve us well or whether they squander our talents and resources.

In this chapter, we will explain what evidence-based practice is and how it can help you and your organization make better decisions. Whether we work in a bank, hospital, large consulting firm, or small start-up company, we, as practitioners affecting the lives of so many, have a moral obligation to use the best available evidence when making decisions. We can do this by learning how to distinguish science from folklore, data from assertions, and evidence from beliefs, anecdotes, and personal opinions.

What Is Evidence-Based Practice?

The basic idea of evidence-based practice, or EBP, is that good-quality decisions should be based on a combination of critical thinking and the best available evidence. Although all management practitioners use evidence in their decisions, many pay little attention to the quality of that evidence. As a result, they make bad decisions based on unfounded beliefs and fads, leading to poor outcomes and limited understanding of why things go wrong. Evidence-based practice seeks to improve the way decisions are made. It is an approach to decision making and day-to-day work practice that helps practitioners to critically evaluate the extent to which they can trust the evidence they have at hand. It also helps practitioners to identify, find, and evaluate additional evidence relevant to their decisions.

In this chapter, we use a definition of evidence-based practice that also describes the main skills required. The definition, partly adapted from Dawes and colleagues (2005), is as follows:

> Evidence-based practice is about making decisions through the conscientious, explicit, and judicious use of the best available evidence from multiple sources by
>
> - asking (translating a practical issue or problem into an answerable question),
> - acquiring (systematically searching for and retrieving the evidence),
> - appraising (critically judging the trustworthiness and relevance of the evidence),
> - aggregating (weighing and pulling together the evidence),
> - applying (incorporating the evidence into the decision-making process), and
> - assessing (evaluating the outcome of the decision taken) to increase the likelihood of a favorable outcome.

What Counts as Evidence?

When we say *evidence*, we basically mean information. It may be based on numbers, or it may be qualitative or descriptive. Evidence may come from scientific research suggesting generally applicable facts about the world, people, or organizational practices. Evidence may also come from local organizational or business indicators, such as company metrics or observations of practice conditions. Professional experience can also be an important source of evidence—for example, an entrepreneur's past experience in setting up businesses may suggest the approach that is most likely to be successful.

Think of it in legal terms. In a court of law, evidence is presented in a variety of forms, from eyewitness testimonies and witness statements to forensic evidence and security-camera images. All this evidence helps the judge or jury decide whether a person is innocent or guilty. The same is true for management decisions. Regardless of its source, all evidence should be included if it is judged to be trustworthy and relevant.

Why Do We Need Evidence-Based Practice?

Often, practitioners prefer to make decisions rooted solely in their personal experience. However, personal judgment alone is not a highly reliable source of evidence, because it is susceptible to systematic errors. Cognitive and information-processing limits make us prone to biases that have negative effects on the quality of decisions (Bazerman 2009; Clements 2002; Kahneman 2011; Simon 1997). Even practitioners and industry experts with many years of experience are poor at making forecasts or calculating risks when relying solely on their personal judgment. Such shortcomings have been found across a variety of areas, from the credit rating of bonds (Barnett-Hart 2009), to the growth of the economy (Loungani 2000), to political developments (Tetlock 2006), to medical diagnoses (Choudhry, Fletcher, and Soumerai 2005).

Practitioners also frequently take the work practices of other organizations as evidence. Through benchmarking and so-called "best practices," practitioners may copy what other organizations are doing without critically evaluating whether these practices are actually effective and, if they are, whether they are likely to work in a different context. Benchmarking can be useful in demonstrating alternate ways of doing things, but it is not necessarily a good indicator in itself of what will work in a particular setting.

Although the shortcomings we describe are well documented, many barriers still exist to evidence-based practice. First, few practitioners have been trained in the skills required to critically evaluate the trustworthiness and relevance of information. In addition, important organizational information may be difficult to access, and the information that is available may be of poor quality. Finally, practitioners are often not aware of the current scientific evidence concerning key issues in the field.

For example, a survey of 950 human resources practitioners in the United States showed large discrepancies between what practitioners think is effective and what the current scientific research shows (Rynes, Colbert, and Brown 2002)[2]. This study has been repeated in other countries with similar findings. The results suggest that most practitioners pay little or no attention to scientific or organizational evidence, instead placing too much trust in personal judgment and experience, "best practices," and the beliefs of corporate leaders. As a result, billions of dollars are spent on management practices that are ineffective or even harmful to organizations, their members, and their clients.

Case Example

Attributes Valued in a Manager

An American information technology company believed for years that technical expertise was the most important management capability. The company thought the best managers were those who left their staff to work independently and intervened only when people got stuck with a technical problem. However, when the company asked employees what they valued most in a manager, technical expertise ranked last. Attributes that employees considered more valuable included asking good questions, taking time to meet, and caring about employees' careers and lives. Managers who did these things led top-performing teams, had the happiest employees, and experienced the lowest turnover of staff. These attributes of effective managers have been well established in scientific studies, so the company's improvement efforts could have been put in place years earlier.

What Sources of Evidence Should Be Considered?

Before making an important decision, an evidence-based practitioner first asks, "What is the available evidence?" Instead of basing a decision on personal judgment alone, an evidence-based practitioner finds out what is known by looking at multiple sources for evidence. According to the principles of evidence-based practice, four types of evidence should be taken into account:

1. Scientific evidence—findings from published scientific research
2. Organizational evidence—data, facts, and figures gathered from the organization
3. Experiential evidence—the professional experience and judgment of practitioners
4. Stakeholder evidence—the values and concerns of people who may be affected by the decision

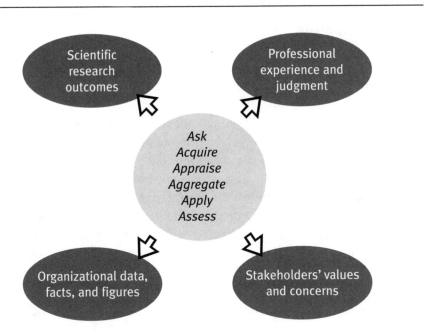

EXHIBIT 1.1
Sources of
Evidence

The sources of these types of evidence are shown in exhibit 1.1 and discussed in the sections that follow.

Scientific Evidence

The first source of evidence is scientific research published in academic journals. Over the past few decades, the volume of management research has escalated dramatically, with topics ranging from evaluating merger success and the effects of financial incentives on performance to improving employee commitment and recruitment.

Much relevant research also comes from outside the management discipline, because many of the typical problems that managers face—such as how to make better decisions, how to communicate more effectively, and how to deal with conflict—are similar across a wide range of contexts. Many practitioners learn about research findings as students or through professional courses. However, new research is always being produced, and new findings often change our understanding. To ensure that up-to-date scientific evidence is properly included in decisions, a practitioner must know how to search for studies and judge how trustworthy and relevant they are.

Case Example

A Merger of Canadian Law Firms

The board of directors of a large Canadian law firm had plans for a merger with a smaller firm nearby. The merger's objective was to integrate the back office of the two firms (i.e., information technology, finance, facilities, etc.) to create economies of scale. The front offices and legal practices of the two firms were to remain separate. The partners had told the board that the organizational cultures of the two firms differed widely, so the board wanted to know whether such differences would create problems for the merger. Partners from both firms were asked independently about their experiences with mergers. Those who had been involved in one or more mergers stated that cultural differences did matter and could cause serious culture clashes between professionals.

How Scientific Evidence Helped

A search of online scientific databases yielded a meta-analysis based on 46 studies with a combined sample size of 10,710 mergers and acquisitions. The meta-analysis confirmed the partners' judgment that a negative association existed between cultural differences and the effectiveness of postmerger integration. However, the study also indicated that this association was only the case when the intended level of integration was high. In mergers that required a low level of integration, cultural differences were found to be positively associated with integration benefits. In the case of the two law firms, the planned integration concerned only back office functions, making the likelihood of a positive outcome higher.

Organizational Evidence

A second source of evidence is the organization itself. Whether for a business, hospital, or governmental agency, organizational evidence comes in many forms. It can be financial data, such as cash flow or costs, or it can be business measures, such as return on investment or market share. It can come from customers or clients in the form of customer satisfaction, repeat business, or product returns statistics. It can also come from employees through information about retention rates or levels of job satisfaction. Organizational evidence can consist of "hard" numbers such as staff turnover rates, medical errors, or productivity levels, but it can also include "soft" elements such as perceptions of the organization's culture or attitudes toward senior management. Organizational evidence is essential to identifying problems that require managers' attention. It is also essential to determining likely causes of problems, plausible solutions, and what is needed to implement these solutions.

Case Example

Considering a Change in Structure

The board of a large insurance company had plans to change from a regionally focused structure to a product-based one. According to the board, the restructuring would improve the company's market presence and drive greater customer focus. The company's sales managers, however, strongly disagreed with the change. They argued that ditching the regional structure would hinder the building of good relationships with customers and therefore harm customer service.

How Organizational Evidence Helped
Analysis of organizational data revealed that the company's customer satisfaction was well above the industry average. Further data analysis revealed a strong negative correlation between account managers' monthly travel expenses and the satisfaction rates of their customers, suggesting that sales managers who lived close to their customers scored higher on customer satisfaction. This evidence convinced the board to retain the regional structure after all.

Experiential Evidence
A third source of evidence is the professional experience and judgment of managers, consultants, business leaders, and other practitioners. Different from intuition, opinion, or belief, professional experience is accumulated over time through reflection on the outcomes of similar actions taken in similar situations. This type of evidence is sometimes referred to as "tacit" knowledge.

Professional experience differs from intuition and personal opinion because it reflects the specialized knowledge acquired through repeated experience and the practice of specialized activities—whether playing the violin or making a cost estimate. Many practitioners take seriously the need to reflect critically on their experiences and distill the practical lessons. Their knowledge can be vital for determining whether a management issue really does require attention, if the available organizational data are trustworthy, whether research findings apply in a particular situation, or how likely a proposed solution is to work in a particular context.

Case Example

Personal Development Plans

A university hospital decided to ask its nurses to compile personal development plans, which were to include a statement of each nurse's aspirations and career priorities. The human resources (HR) director pointed out that, according to Abraham Maslow's hierarchy of needs (a well-known theory about motivations), basic levels of needs (e.g., health, safety) must be met before an individual can focus on higher-level needs (e.g., career and professional development). The nurses at the emergency department were increasingly exposed to serious safety hazards, including physical violence. The HR director therefore recommended that these nurses be excluded from the program until the safety hazards had been substantially reduced.

How Experiential Evidence Helped
Experienced managers and nurses were asked independently for their views on the HR director's recommendation. Most of them disagreed with the recommendation, and they indicated that their experience suggested that the opposite was often the case—that nurses who worked in difficult circumstances tended to be strongly interested in professional development and self-improvement. Additional evidence was harvested from online scientific databases, where a range of studies showed a lack of empirical evidence supporting Maslow's theory. The nurses' view therefore prevailed.

Stakeholder Evidence
A fourth source of evidence is stakeholder values and concerns. Stakeholders are any individuals or groups who may be affected by an organization's decisions. Internal stakeholders include employees, managers, and board members. Stakeholders outside the organization may include suppliers, customers, shareholders, the government, and the public at large. Stakeholder

values and concerns reflect what stakeholders believe to be important, which in turn affects how they tend to react to the possible consequences of the organization's decisions.

Certain stakeholders may place more or less importance on, for example, short-term gain versus long-term sustainability, employee well-being versus employee output, organizational reputation versus profitability, and participation in decision making versus top-down control. Organizations that serve or respond to different stakeholders can reach very different decisions on the basis of the same evidence (compare ExxonMobil and Greenpeace, for example). Gathering evidence from stakeholders is not just important for ethical reasons; it also provides a frame of reference from which to analyze evidence from other sources. It provides important information about the ways in which decisions will be received and about whether those decisions are likely to produce the desired outcomes.

Case Example

Employee Satisfaction Survey

To assess employees' satisfaction with their supervisors, a telecommunications company conducted a survey among its 12,500 employees. The survey contained some questions about demographics, such as postal code, date of birth, and job title, as well as five questions about employees' satisfaction with their immediate supervisor. The introductory letter by the CEO stated that all answers would remain anonymous. After the survey was sent out, only 582 employees responded—a response rate of less than 5 percent.

How Stakeholder Evidence Helped

To find out why so many people did not participate in the survey, the company held a focus group discussion with employees from different parts of the organization. The employees expressed concerns that the demographic data would make it possible to identify the individuals behind the answers. Given the sensitive nature of the survey's topic, they therefore decided not to participate. Based on this outcome, the survey was modified by dropping the postal code and replacing the date of birth with an age range. The modified survey yielded a response rate of 67 percent.

Why Do We Have to Critically Appraise Evidence?

Evidence is never perfect, and it can often be overstated or misleading. A seemingly strong claim might turn out to be based on a single and not particularly reliable piece of information. A colleague's confident opinion about the effectiveness of a practice might turn out to be based on little more than an anecdote. A long-standing way of doing things in an organization might never have been actually evaluated to make sure it works. All evidence should be critically appraised in a process that carefully and systematically assesses its trustworthiness and relevance.

The way a piece of evidence is evaluated may differ slightly depending on its source. However, critical appraisal always involves asking the same basic questions: Where and how is the evidence gathered? Is it the best available evidence? Is there enough evidence to reach a conclusion? Are there reasons that the evidence could be biased in a particular direction?

If we are critically appraising a colleague's experiences with a particular problem, we may wonder how many times she has experienced that issue and whether those situations were comparable. For example, if a colleague proposes a solution to high levels of staff absenteeism but his experience relates only to a single instance that involved migrant workers picking fruit, then that colleague's experience likely would not have much to teach you about dealing with absenteeism of orthopedic surgeons in a hospital.

Similar questions need to be asked about organizational evidence such as sales figures, error rates, and cash flow. How were these figures calculated? Are they accurate? Are they reliable? In the case of scientific evidence, we should ask about how the study was designed. How were the data collected? How was the outcome measured? To what extent are alternative explanations for the outcome possible? Evidence-based practice is about using the best available evidence, and critical appraisal plays an essential role in discerning and identifying such evidence.

Why Focus on the Best Available Evidence?

In almost any situation, we can gather different types of evidence from various sources, and sometimes in quite large quantities. But which evidence should we pay more attention to and why? A fundamental principle of evidence-based practice is that the quality of our decisions is likely to improve when we make use of trustworthy evidence—in other words, the best available evidence.

This principle is apparent in everyday decision making, whether we are buying someone a birthday present or wondering where to go for dinner. In most cases, we actively seek out information from multiple sources, such as our partner's opinion, the experiences of friends, or the comments of a local food critic. Sometimes this information is so weak that it is hardly convincing at all; other times, the information is so strong that no one doubts its correctness. We therefore must be able to determine, through critical appraisal, what evidence is the most trustworthy. For instance, the most trustworthy evidence about what part of Ireland has the least chance of rain in early August will obviously come from average monthly rainfall statistics, not from the personal experience of a colleague who visited the country once.

Exactly the same is true for management decisions. Imagine you are making a decision about whether to use a quality management method such as Six Sigma to reduce medical errors in a British university hospital. Information from a study of 150 European university hospitals in which medical errors were measured before and after the introduction of Six Sigma is more trustworthy than the professional experience of a colleague who works at a small private hospital in Sydney. However, such a study might never have been done. Instead, the best *available* evidence could be case studies from just one or two hospitals.

For some decisions, we might not have any scientific or organizational evidence at all; thus, we may have no option but to make a decision based on the professional experience of a colleague or to pilot test some different approaches and see for ourselves what might work best. Given the principles of evidence-based practice, even limited-quality evidence can lead to a better decision than we would reach by not using it, as long as we are aware of the limitations of the evidence when we act on it.

Some Common Misconceptions About Evidence-Based Practice

Misconceptions about evidence-based practice are a major barrier to its uptake and implementation. For this reason, we must ensure that such misconceptions are challenged and corrected. In most cases, the misconceptions reflect a narrow or limited understanding of the principles of evidence-based practice.

Misconception #1: Evidence-Based Practice Ignores the Practitioner's Professional Experience

This misconception directly contradicts the key point of evidence-based practice, which is that decisions should be made through the conscientious, explicit, and judicious use of evidence from four sources, including experience. Evidence-based practice does not establish that any one source of evidence is more valid than any other. Experiential evidence—the aggregated professional experience and judgment of practitioners—can be extremely important if it is appraised to be trustworthy and relevant. Experiential evidence is also essential in appropriately interpreting and using evidence from other sources.

If we are trying to identify effective ways of sharing information with colleagues, scientific and organizational evidence can be informative; however, we might rely on experiential evidence to determine what practices make good sense if we are working with professionally trained colleagues or lower-skilled workers. At the same time, scientific evidence can help us understand the extent to which our experiential evidence is trustworthy. Research indicates that many years of experience in a technical specialty can lead to considerable expertise and tacit knowledge. On the other hand, an individual holding a series of unrelated jobs over the same number of years may have far less trustworthy and reliable expertise. Evidence-based practice is hence about using evidence from multiple sources, rather than relying on only one.

Misconception #2: Evidence-Based Practice Is All About Numbers and Statistics

Evidence-based practice involves seeking out and using the best available evidence from multiple sources. It is not exclusively about numbers and quantitative data, and you do not need to become a statistician to undertake it. An understanding of basic statistical concepts is useful in critically evaluating some types of evidence, but the principles behind such concepts as sample size, statistical versus practical significance, confidence intervals, and effect sizes can be understood without any mathematics. Evidence-based practice is not about doing statistics, though statistical thinking is an important element.

Misconception #3: Managers Need to Make Decisions Quickly and Do Not Have Time for Evidence-Based Practice

Sometimes, evidence-based practice is about taking a moment to reflect about the degree to which the evidence you have can be trusted. More often, it is about preparing yourself (and your organization) to make key decisions well by identifying the best available evidence you need, preferably before you need it. Some management decisions do need to be made quickly, but even split-second decisions require trustworthy evidence. Making a good, fast decision about when to evacuate a leaking nuclear power plant or how to make an emergency landing requires up-to-date knowledge of emergency procedures and reliable instruments that provide trustworthy evidence about radiation levels or altitude. When important decisions need to be made quickly, an evidence-based practitioner anticipates the kinds of evidence that good decisions require.

The need to make an immediate decision is generally the exception rather than the rule. The vast majority of management decisions are made over much longer time periods—sometimes weeks or even months—and often require consideration of legal, financial, strategic, logistical, or other organizational issues. This time provides plenty of opportunities to collect and critically evaluate evidence about the nature of the problem and the decision most likely to produce the desired outcome. For evidence-based practice, time is not normally a deal breaker.

Misconception #4: Each Organization Is Unique, so the Usefulness of Scientific Evidence Is Limited

One reason that practitioners might resist using research evidence is the belief that their own organization is unique. And because their organization is different from the ones being studied, they feel that research findings simply would not apply to them. This belief, too, is a misconception. Although organizations do in fact differ, they also tend to face very similar issues, sometimes repeatedly, and they often respond to those issues in similar ways. Peter Drucker, a seminal management thinker, was perhaps the first to assert that most management issues are "repetitions of familiar problems cloaked in the guise of uniqueness" (Lowenstein 2006).

The truth of the matter is that organizations commonly have myths and stories about their own uniqueness, when, in reality, they tend to be neither unique nor exactly alike, but somewhere in between (Martin et al. 1983). Evidence-based practitioners need to be flexible enough to take any such similar-yet-different qualities into account. A thoughtful practitioner, for instance, might develop a system that uses individual financial incentives for independent salespeople but rewards knowledge workers with opportunities for development or personally interesting projects. Such an approach could stem from knowing that financial incentives tend to lower performance for knowledge workers while increasing the performance of less-skilled workers (Ariely et al. 2009; Joseph and Kalwani 1998).

Misconception #5: If You Do Not Have High-Quality Evidence, You Cannot Do Anything

Sometimes, very little or no high-quality evidence is available. Such evidence is often lacking in cases involving new management practices or the implementation of new technologies. In some areas, the organizational context changes rapidly, limiting the relevance and applicability of scientific and experiential evidence that derived from a context different than that of today. In such cases, the evidence-based practitioner has no other option but to work with the limited evidence at hand and supplement it through learning by doing. This approach involves pilot testing and treating any course of action as a prototype. The practitioner systematically assesses the outcomes of decisions through a process of constant experimentation, punctuated by critical reflection about which things work and which things do not (Pfeffer and Sutton 2010; Weick and Sutcliffe 2007).

Misconception #6: Good-Quality Evidence Gives You the Answer to the Problem

Evidence is not an answer. It does not speak for itself. To make sense of evidence, we need an understanding of the context and a critical mind-set. You might take a test and find out you scored 10 points, but if you don't know the average or total possible score, it's hard to determine whether you did well. You may also want to know what doing well on the test actually means. Does it indicate or predict anything important to you and in your context? And why? Your score in the test is meaningless without this additional information. At the same time, evidence is never conclusive. It does not prove things, which means that no piece of evidence can be viewed as a universal or timeless truth. In most cases, evidence comes with a large degree of uncertainty. Evidence-based practitioners therefore make decisions not based on conclusive, solid, up-to-date information but on probabilities, indications, and tentative conclusions. Evidence does not tell you what to decide, but it does help you to make a better-informed decision.

What Is the Evidence for Evidence-Based Practice?

Sometimes people ask whether we have evidence that an evidence-based practice approach is more effective than the other ways managers typically make decisions. This is, of course, a very important question. Assessing the effect of evidence-based practice would require an evaluation of a large number of situations and contexts where evidence-based practice was applied and the measurement of a wide range of outcomes, preferably by means of a double-blind, randomized, controlled study. Such a study might well be too difficult to carry out. However, plenty of scientific evidence suggests that taking an evidence-based approach to decisions is more likely to be effective.

We noted earlier in this chapter that the human mind is susceptible to systematic errors. We have cognitive limits and are prone to biases that impair the quality of the decisions we make. We must continuously ask ourselves, How can we make decisions without falling prey to our biases? Are there decision practices or processes that can improve decision quality? Fortunately, a large number of studies indicate the following:

- Forecasts or risk assessments that are based on the aggregated (averaged) professional experience of many people are more accurate than forecasts based on one person's personal experience, provided the forecasts are made independently before being combined (Armstrong 2001; Bauer et al. 2003; Servan-Schreiber et al. 2004; Silver 2012; Yaniv and Choshen-Hillel 2012).

- Professional judgments based on hard data or statistical models are more accurate than judgments based on individual experience (Ayres 2007; Grove 2005; Lewis 2003).

- Knowledge derived from scientific evidence is more accurate than the opinions of experts (Antman et al. 1992).

- A decision based on the combination of critically appraised experiential, organizational, and scientific evidence yields better outcomes than a decision based on a single source of evidence (McNees 1990; Tetlock 2006).

- Evaluating the outcome of a decision improves both organizational learning and performance, especially in novel and nonroutine situations (Anseel, Lievens, and Schollaert 2009; Ellis and Davidi 2005).

Summary

We started this chapter by explaining what evidence-based practice was about—that it involved decision making through the conscientious, explicit, and judicious use of the best available evidence from multiple sources. By using and critically appraising evidence from multiple sources, you increase the likelihood of an effective decision.

We also discussed why we need evidence-based practice. Most managers prefer to make decisions solely based on personal experience, but personal judgment alone is not a particularly reliable source of evidence. It is prone to cognitive biases and thinking errors. In addition, managers and consultants are often not aware of the current scientific evidence; in fact, large discrepancies seem to exist between what managers and consultants think is effective and what the current scientific research shows. As a result, billions of dollars are spent on management practices that are ineffective or even harmful to organizations.

We then discussed what counts as evidence. Evidence, simply, is information, whether from scientific research, the organization itself, or the professional experience of managers. Evidence regarding the values and concerns of stakeholders may also be important to take into account. We also noted that evidence is never perfect and that we must critically appraise the trustworthiness of evidence, regardless of whether it is drawn from scientific research or from experience. We can appraise evidence by asking how it was gathered, if it could be biased in a particular direction, and whether it is the best available evidence.

Sometimes the best available evidence is hardly convincing at all, but other times it is so compelling that no one doubts it. In other situations, little or no high-quality evidence is available. In those cases, we have no other option but to work with the limited evidence at hand and supplement it through learning by doing—that is, by pilot testing and systematically assessing the outcomes of the decisions we take. Evidence is not an answer, and in most cases it comes with a large degree of uncertainty. Evidence-based practitioners therefore make decisions not based on conclusive, solid, up-to-date information but on probabilities, indications, and tentative conclusions.

The most important learning point is that evidence-based practice starts with a critical mind-set. It means questioning assumptions, particularly where someone asserts some belief as a fact. So, from now on, always ask: What is the evidence for that, how trustworthy is it, and is this the best available evidence?

Notes

1. This example is partly adapted from Pfeffer and Sutton (2011).
2. More educated managers do, however, show somewhat greater knowledge of scientific findings.

References

Anseel, F., F. Lievens, and E. Schollaert. 2009. "Reflection as a Strategy to Enhance Task Performance After Feedback." *Organizational Behavior and Human Decision Processes* 110 (1) 23–35.

Antman, E. M., J. Lau, B. Kupelnick, F. Mosteller, and T. C. Chalmers. 1992. "A Comparison of Results of Meta-analyses of Randomized Control Trials and Recommendations of Clinical Experts." *Journal of the American Medical Association* 268 (2): 240–48.

Ariely, D., U. Gneezy, G. Loewenstein, and N. Mazar. 2009. "Large Stakes and Big Mistakes." *Review of Economic Studies* 76 (2): 451–69.

Armstrong, J. S. 2001. *Principles of Forecasting: A Handbook for Researchers and Practitioners.* New York: Kluwer Academic Publishers.

Ayres, I. 2007. *Super Crunchers.* New York: Bantam Books.

Barnett-Hart, A. K. 2009. "The Story of the CDO Market Meltdown: An Empirical Analysis." PhD diss., Harvard University.

Bauer, A., R. A. Eisenbeis, D. F. Waggoner, and T. Zha. 2003. "Forecast Evaluation with Cross Sectional Data: The Blue Chip Surveys." *Economic Review* 88 (2): 17–31.

Bazerman, M. H. 2009. *Judgment in Managerial Decision Making.* New York: Wiley.

Choudhry, N. K., R. H. Fletcher, and S. B. Soumerai. 2005. "Systematic Review: The Relationship Between Clinical Experience and Quality of Health Care." *Annals of Internal Medicine* 142 (4): 260–73.

Clements, M. P. 2002. "An Evaluation of the Survey of Professional Forecasters Probability Distribution of Expected Inflation and Output Growth." Published November 22. www2.warwick.ac.uk/fac/soc/economics/staff/academic/clements/wp/spf2comp.pdf.

Dawes, M., W. Summerskill, P. Glasziou, A. Cartabellotta, J. Martin, K. Hopayian, F. Porzsolt, A. Burls, and J. Osborne. 2005. "Sicily Statement on Evidence-Based Practice." *BMC Medical Education.* Published January 5. http://bmcmededuc.biomedcentral.com/articles/10.1186/1472-6920-5-1.

Ellis, S., and I. Davidi. 2005. "After-Event Reviews: Drawing Lessons from Successful and Failed Experience." *Journal of Applied Psychology* 90 (5): 857–71.

Grove, W. M. 2005. "Clinical Versus Statistical Prediction." *Journal of Clinical Psychology* 61 (10): 1233–43.

Joseph, K., and M. U. Kalwani. 1998. "The Role of Bonus Pay in Salesforce Compensation Plans." *Industrial Marketing Management* 27 (2): 147–59.

Kahneman, D. 2011. *Thinking, Fast and Slow.* London: Penguin Group.

Lewis, M. 2003. *Moneyball: The Art of Winning an Unfair Game.* New York: W. W. Norton & Company.

Loungani, P. 2000. "The Arcane Art of Predicting Recessions." *Financial Times* via International Monetary Fund. Accessed June 3, 2016. www.imf.org/external/np/vc/2000/121800.htm.

Lowenstein, R. 2006. "When Business Has Questions, Drucker Still Has Answers." *New York Times.* Published January 22. www.nytimes.com/2006/01/22/business/yourmoney/22shelf.html.

Martin, J., M. S. Feldman, M. J. Hatch, and S. B. Sitkin. 1983. "The Uniqueness Paradox in Organizational Stories." *Administrative Science Quarterly* 28 (3): 438–53.

McNees, S. K. 1990. "The Role of Judgment in Macroeconomic Forecasting Accuracy." *International Journal of Forecasting* 6 (3): 287–99.

Mintzberg, H. 1990. "The Manager's Job: Folklore and Fact." *Harvard Business Review* 53 (4): 49–61.

Pfeffer, J., and R. I. Sutton. 2011. "Trust the Evidence, Not Your Instincts." *New York Times.* Published September 3. www.nytimes.com/2011/09/04/jobs/04pre.html.

———. 2010. "Treat Your Organization as a Prototype: The Essence of Evidence-Based Management." *Design Management Review* 17 (3): 10–14.

Rynes, S. L., A. E. Colbert, and K. G. Brown. 2002. "HR Professionals' Beliefs About Effective Human Resource Practices: Correspondence Between Research and Practice." *Human Resource Management* 41 (2): 149–74.

Servan-Schreiber, E., J. Wolfers, D. M. Pennock, and B. Galebach. 2004. "Prediction Markets: Does Money Matter?" *Electronic Markets* 14 (3): 243–51.

Silver, N. 2012. *The Signal and the Noise: Why So Many Predictions Fail—but Some Don't.* London: Penguin.

Simon, H. A. 1997. *Models of Bounded Rationality.* Cambridge, MA: MIT Press.

Tetlock, P. E. 2006. *Expert Political Judgement.* Princeton, NJ: Princeton University Press.

Weick, K. E., and K. Sutcliffe. 2007. *Managing the Unexpected: Resilient Performance in an Age of Uncertainty.* New York: Wiley.

Yaniv, I., and S. Choshen-Hillel. 2012. "Exploiting the Wisdom of Others to Make Better Decisions: Suspending Judgment Reduces Egocentrism and Increases Accuracy." *Journal of Behavioral Decision Making* 25 (5): 427–34.

RAPID EVIDENCE ASSESSMENTS IN MANAGEMENT: AN EXAMPLE

by Eric Barends, Karen Plum, and Andrew Mawson

Evidence-based practice is about making decisions through the conscientious, explicit, and judicious use of the best available evidence from multiple sources. Much of this evidence may come from scientific research. However, data, facts, and figures from local organizations and even professional experience also constitute evidence. Over the past few decades, the volume of management research in healthcare has increased dramatically, with topics ranging from the impact of leadership training programs on physicians (Straus, Soobiah, and Levinson 2013) to strategies for improving patient safety culture (Morello et al. 2013). From the start of the evidence-based medicine movement in the early 1990s, however, it was clear that not every practitioner would be able to search in research databases and critically appraise the scientific evidence found (Daly 2005). After all, searching in research databases can be a laborious and time-consuming task, and critically appraising a study's trustworthiness requires specialized skills that not all practitioners possess. For this reason, the movement promoted the development of so-called preappraised evidence, presented in the form of evidence summaries that enable practitioners to quickly consult the best available scientific evidence on issues of concern. The summaries are regularly used to answer questions about the effectiveness of healthcare interventions and have now become a cornerstone of evidence-based practice.

Evidence Summaries

Preappraised evidence summaries come in many forms. One of the best-known types is the conventional literature review, which provides an overview of relevant scientific literature published on a topic. However, a conventional literature review's trustworthiness is often low: Clear criteria for inclusion are often lacking, studies are selected based on researchers' individual preferences, and the research results are generally not subjected to a critical appraisal (Antman 1992; Bushman and Wells 2001; Chalmers, Enkin, and Keirse 1993; Fink 1998). As a result, most conventional literature reviews are prone to severe bias and considered unsuitable for answering questions about the effectiveness of interventions. Many evidence-based disciplines therefore use so-called systematic reviews instead of conventional reviews.

The systematic review methodology aims to identify all the relevant studies on a specific topic as comprehensively as possible and to select appropriate studies based on explicit criteria. In addition, two researchers, independently of each other, assess the quality of the studies included on the basis of specific criteria, such as the presence of a pretest or a control group (Higgins and Green 2011; Petticrew and Roberts 2006). In contrast to a conventional literature review, a systematic review is transparent, verifiable, and reproducible. As a result, the likelihood of bias is considerably smaller. Most systematic reviews also include a meta-analysis, in which statistical analysis techniques are used to combine the results of individual studies to arrive at a more accurate estimate of the effect.

Although the systematic review methodology was originally developed in the field of medicine, it has also shown its added value in such disciplines as nursing, education, policing, criminology, public policy, and management (Petticrew 2001). In disciplines where evidence-based practice is well established, systematic reviews are provided by global communities such as the Cochrane and Campbell collaborative and by organizations such as the Evidence for Policy and Practice Information and Co-ordinating (EPPI) Centre. In healthcare management, however, the systematic review methodology is not yet widely adopted, and such reviews consequently are scarce.

Rapid evidence assessments (REAs) and critically appraised topics (CATs) are two other types of evidence summaries that are used to inform practice. Both REAs and CATs apply the same systematic approach to selecting the studies: The methodological quality and practical relevance of the studies are assessed on the basis of explicit criteria, and the summaries are therefore transparent, verifiable, and reproducible.

The main ways in which these three types of summaries vary involve the time and resources used to produce them and the length and the depth of the results produced. A CAT is the quickest to produce: It might take one skilled person a few days. An REA might take several people a few weeks. A systematic review or meta-analysis usually takes a team many months, because it aims to identify all relevant studies (both published and unpublished).

In general, a healthcare organization will not have the time or the financial means to assign a team of social researchers to conduct a systematic review on a managerial topic of interest. An organization might be able to use a CAT, on the other hand, to get a quick impression of available scientific evidence about the effect of a specific intervention—for instance, determining whether hourly ward rounds decrease the number of patient falls. However, a CAT might lack the rigor needed to address a larger question that has a major impact on the organization as a whole—for instance, "What strategies for improving patient safety culture in hospitals are most widely studied and what is known about their effect?" Because of these practical limitations, many organizations choose to conduct REAs instead.

Rapid Evidence Assessments

An REA provides a balanced assessment of what is known in scientific literature about an intervention or practical issue by using the systematic review method to search and critically appraise primary studies. However, in order to be *rapid*, an REA makes concessions in the breadth and depth of the search process. Aspects of the process that may be limited to reduce the timescale include the following:

- *The question.* Even more than a systematic review, an REA calls for the question to be focused and specified (in terms of population, intervention, comparison, outcome, and context).
- *Searching.* The assessment might consult only a limited number of databases, and unpublished research may be excluded. Sometimes, an REA is limited to only meta-analyses or systematic reviews.
- *Data extraction.* The assessment might extract only a limited amount of key data, such as year, population, sector, sample size, moderators/ mediators, main findings, and effect size.
- *Critical appraisal.* Quality appraisal may be limited to methodological appropriateness (e.g., "Does the study's research design match the research question?") and methodological flaws.

Because of these limitations, an REA may be more prone to selection bias than a systematic review. Therefore, to justify an REA, the need to obtain evidence rapidly and at relatively limited costs must be greater than the risk associated with lacking a completely comprehensive review of all the evidence.

To illustrate how an REA can be conducted and how the outcome can inform management practice, this chapter features a sample REA about knowledge worker performance. The REA was conducted by a group of eight large UK- and US-based companies, and it focused on academic research about the determinants of knowledge worker performance. Although none of the eight organizations was a healthcare organization, the topic is of great importance to the practice of healthcare management. In recent decades, the number of healthcare workers engaged in knowledge work has increased substantially. Most workers in healthcare organizations today—whether they are nurses, physicians, managers, or staff members—are highly dependent on information and communication technology, and their work involves a high level of cognitive activity. In fact, for most healthcare organizations, an important part of core business involves processing existing knowledge to create new knowledge that can be used to develop diagnostic tools and treatments. Healthcare managers clearly have a responsibility to optimize work processes and enhance performance, yet many struggle to empower knowledge workers. In fact, when healthcare managers are asked what factors contribute to improving knowledge worker performance, most of them remain silent (Davenport, Thomas, and Cantrell 2002). The REA presented in the rest of this chapter will provide an evidence-based answer.

A Rapid Evidence Assessment of Research Literature About Factors Influencing Knowledge Worker Performance

Background

In the summer of 2013, a group of eight companies wanted to know what academic research had discovered about the determinants of knowledge worker performance. For each company, the payoff for enhancing knowledge worker performance would be huge—not only in terms of finance but also in terms of innovation, which often is a key success factor for long-term profitability and growth. Although the organizations all used various measures and controls to address the issue, they lacked a basic understanding of what really drives knowledge worker performance. For this reason, the organizations commissioned the Center for Evidence-Based Management (CEBMa)[1] and Advanced Workplace Associates (AWA)[2] to answer the following questions:

1. What is "knowledge work"?
2. Which of the factors that have an impact on the performance of knowledge workers are most widely studied, and what is known of their effect?
3. How do these factors enhance the performance of knowledge workers, how can they be measured, and what are the implications for management practice?

Reviewers from CEBMa conducted an REA of the available scientific literature, and AWA used its knowledge and experience to translate the academic findings into practical guidelines. Consequently, the results of this work can be relied upon as the "best available evidence" about this subject at this time.

Search Strategy: How Was the Research Evidence Sought?

The following databases were used to identify studies: ABI/INFORM Global from ProQuest, Business Source Premier from EBSCO, and Psyc-INFO from Ovid. The following generic search filters were applied to all databases during the search:

- Scholarly journals, peer-reviewed
- Published in the period 1980 to 2013
- Articles in English

A search was conducted using combinations of search terms, such as *productivity*, *performance*, *knowledge work*, and *knowledge based business*. Five search queries yielded a total of 570 studies.

Selection: How Were the Studies Selected for Inclusion?

The following inclusion criteria were applied to the selection of studies:

- Only quantitative studies were included.
- The only studies included were those in which the effect of an independent variable on the productivity, performance, or innovation of individual employees, teams, or organizations was measured.

Study selection took place in two phases. First, the titles and abstracts of the 570 studies were screened for their relevance to the REA. In cases of doubt, lack of information, or disagreement, the study was included. Duplicate publications were removed. This first phase yielded 109 single studies and 52 meta-analyses. In the second phase, studies were selected for inclusion based on the full article text. This phase yielded 24 single studies and 35 meta-analyses. A meta-analysis is a study that uses statistical techniques to combine the results of a number of studies published on the same topic to obtain a pooled quantitative estimate of the overall effect of a particular variable on a specific outcome.

Critical Appraisal and Classification: How Was the Quality of the Evidence Judged?

From each study, the information relevant to the REA question was extracted and interpreted. Such information included sample size, population, research design, independent variable, outcome measures, effect size, and findings. The research design of the included studies was systematically assessed and categorized according to Campbell's and Petticrew's classification system (Petticrew and Roberts 2006; Shadish, Cook, and Campbell 2002); the system helped ensure a good understanding of the robustness of each study. When looking to identify cause and effect (e.g., "If I do A, will it result in B?"), a study that uses both a control group and random assignment is regarded as the "gold standard." Next most valuable are nonrandomized studies and before-after studies. Cross-sectional studies (surveys) are considered to have the greatest chance of bias in their outcomes and thus have lower rankings in terms of robustness. Meta-analyses in which statistical analysis techniques are used to pool the results of controlled studies are regarded as the highest-quality evidence.

Limitations of the Evidence Base

Most of the studies reviewed in the 35 meta-analyses employed cross-sectional studies and controlled studies. The overall quality of the evidence was therefore moderate to high. However, concessions were made in relation to the breadth and depth of the search process—for instance, unpublished research was excluded. As a result, this REA may be prone to selection bias and is not a completely comprehensive assessment of all the published and unpublished evidence on the topic.

Results: What Was Found?

Question 1: What Is Knowledge Work?

Peter Drucker (1959) coined the term *knowledge work* to describe work that occurs primarily because of mental processes rather than physical labor. In the past century, organizations have moved from manual production to more knowledge-driven production, and the percentage of the workforce engaged in knowledge work has increased dramatically. In 1920, an estimated 30 percent of workers engaged in knowledge work (Davenport, Thomas, and Cantrell 2002). That number increased to 50 percent by 1956 (Naisbitt 1982) and to 70 percent by 1980 (Thomas and Baron 1994).

Since Drucker coined the term, authors have put forward a variety of definitions of both *knowledge work* and *knowledge workers*. When examined closely, most definitions seem to incorporate the following elements:

• Distribution or application of knowledge

- Highly educated, autonomous professionals
- Use of information technology as an integral part of the work process
- A work process that is difficult to standardize
- Complex and intangible outcomes

Most studies acknowledge that the differences between manual work and knowledge work are best considered on a continuum. In addition, even the highest level of knowledge work includes mundane tasks such as storing information, returning telephone calls, and composing and responding to e-mails (Heerwagen et al. 2004). To assess the level of knowledge work, different aspects of the job should be examined (Ramirez 2006):

- Autonomy—the degree of worker control over how a task is done
- Structure—the degree to which established rules, policies, or procedures determine how a task is done
- Knowledge—the degree to which possessing knowledge and executing cognitive processes are part of a task
- Complexity—the degree to which a task presents difficulty in understanding or has confusing interrelated subtasks
- Routine and repetitiveness—the degree to which a task is part of a regular or established procedure characterized by habitual or mechanical performance of steps
- Physical effort—the degree to which a task requires body strength, coordination, and skill

Question 2: Which of the Factors That Have an Impact on the Performance of Knowledge Workers Are Most Widely Studied, and What Is Known of Their Effect?

A total of 76 factors were identified, accounting for more than 145 effect sizes. Based on the analysis of the 59 studies selected, we can determine that the following six factors with the highest association to knowledge worker performance were most widely studied: (1) social cohesion, (2) perceived supervisory support, (3) information sharing / transactive memory, (4) vision and goal clarity, (5) external communication, and (6) trust.

Information about these factors is presented in exhibit 2.1.

EXHIBIT 2.1
Six Factors
Influencing
Knowledge
Worker
Performance

Factor	Performance Measure	Number of Studies	Mean Correlation Weighted by Sample Size
1. Social cohesion	Team performance, hard outcome	40+	.49
	Team performance, behavioral		.70
2. Perceived supervisory support	Employee performance	50+	.53
3. Information sharing / transactive memory	Team performance	60+	.51
4. Vision and goal clarity	Team innovation	80+	.49
5. External communica-tion	Team performance, innovation	30+	.48
6. Trust	Team performance	200+	.32 to .62

Question 3: How Do These Factors Enhance the Performance of Knowledge Workers, How Can They Be Measured, and What Are the Implications for Management Practice?

Factor 1. Social Cohesion
Social cohesion refers to a shared liking of or attraction to the group, emotional bonds of friendship, caring and closeness among group members, and enjoyment of one another's company (Chiocchio 2009). Social cohesion is not a stable trait. It can—and most likely does—change over time in both its form and its intensity throughout the processes of group formation, group development, group maintenance, and group dissolution (Carron and Chelladurai 1981). However, even though social cohesion is dynamic, it is unlikely to change dramatically on a moment-to-moment basis.

How does social cohesion enhance performance?

A high level of social cohesion among team members creates a psychologically safe environment in which team members feel free to explore new ways of doing things (Hülsheger, Anderson, and Salgado 2009). A person is more willing to take risk in a situation in which she has a reliable bond with an important other. This notion has been confirmed in other areas of psychology, such as developmental psychology (e.g., child development theories suggests that children who are well bonded with their parents engage in more exploratory and learning behavior). Furthermore, knowledge workers who have strong feelings of belongingness and attachment to their colleagues are more likely to cooperate and interact with each other, and thus more likely to exchange ideas and share information (Hülsheger, Anderson, and Salgado 2009). For example, operating room nurses are more likely to share innovative ideas to improve patient safety with surgeons when there is a high level of social cohesion between these two professional groups.

How can social cohesion be measured?

The level of social cohesion can be measured through the use of five survey statements adapted from the Group Cohesion Questionnaire (GCQ) by Carless and De Paola (2000). These survey statements—and statements for measuring the other factors examined in this REA—are listed in exhibit 2.2 at the end of this chapter.

What are the implications for management practice?

- *Team familiarity.* Team-familiarity activities can help enhance social cohesion, which in turn enhances performance (Carron and Spinks 1995). One longitudinal study, for instance, demonstrated that surgical team familiarity contributes to reductions in operative time and improvement of clinical performance (Xu et al. 2013). Team familiarity can be achieved through a variety of socially based activities, such as sports, entertainment, charitable events, meals together, or drinks after work (Klein et al. 2009). Additional tools offer more formal and structured ways for team members to learn about one another.
- *A safe psychological environment.* A safe psychological environment enables knowledge workers to feel comfortable contributing freely and challenging where appropriate (Moore and

Mamiseishvili 2012). For instance, a manager who begins meetings by encouraging each team member to contribute (i.e., "checking in" with them individually) can help give quiet employees a better chance to speak. A safe psychological environment can also be reinforced by team members who consider the impact of one another's emotions. Such consideration encourages the team to take responsibility for the "tone" of their discussions, rather than leaving it solely to the manager.

- *Physical spaces to help knowledge workers to connect.* The physical workplace has an impact on the development of social cohesion. It provides the spaces where knowledge workers form and maintain a large part of their working relationships. The workplace should include social areas for networking and talking, and it should enable team members to see one another when traveling between facilities or meetings. Social cohesion becomes harder to achieve, for instance, when nurses feel uncomfortable going into a space that is perceived as the exclusive territory of physicians (and vice versa!).

Factor 2. Perceived Supervisory Support

When knowledge workers interact with and receive feedback from their manager, they form perceptions about how the manager supports them. Perceived supervisory support (PSS) reflects the workers' feelings about how the manager helps in times of need, praises individuals or the team for a task well done, or recognizes them for extra effort.

How does strong supervisory support enhance performance?

The PSS construct stems from the norm of reciprocity, which states that people treat others as they would like to be treated, repaying kindness with kindness and retaliating against those who inflict harm (Brunell et al. 2013; Gouldner 1960). Put differently, when a manager helps his employees well in times of need or recognizes them for extra effort, the employees will feel inclined to act in a way that is of value to the manager (e.g., meeting goals and objectives) and thus the organization as a whole (Edmondson and Boyer 2013; Eisenberger et al. 1986). Not surprisingly, physicians experiencing inadequate supervisory support tend to describe their commitment to the hospital and its patients in negative terms—suggesting a negative effect on performance (Tayfur and Arslan 2013).

How can perceived supervisory support be measured?
The level of perceived supervisory and organizational support can be measured with six survey statements adapted from the validated Survey of Perceived Organizational Support (SPOS) by Eisenberger and colleagues (1986). The statements are listed in exhibit 2.2.

What are the implications for management practice?

- *People management skills.* Research demonstrates that asking good questions, taking time to meet with workers, and caring about employees' lives and careers are important attributes of effective managers. Managers of knowledge workers should therefore be equipped with excellent people management skills and make regular one-to-one discussions part of routine management. Other ways that managers can contribute in this area include being available to the team, being proactive with problem solving so problems don't fester, setting the tone in which the team operates, and managing conflict.
- *Communication skills.* Good communication skills enable managers leading knowledge workers to enter into dialogue with the team members and helps them address difficult situations. Research suggests that good communication is about consistency and a regular flow of information. The worst scenario is that only bad news is communicated.

Factor 3. Information Sharing / Transactive Memory
Information sharing (IS) refers to the extent to which teams utilize the individual members' distinctive knowledge for the team's benefit. Especially if complex problems have to be addressed, IS is indispensable; it allows team members to share their knowledge and experiences, to exchange their thoughts, and to generate new ideas (Hülsheger, Anderson, and Salgado 2009).

The transactive memory system (TMS), an important concept related to IS, was originally observed through the study of dating couples. Researchers noticed that people in a close relationship treated their partners as an external memory device. Within a team, the TMS refers to a form of knowledge that is embedded in a team's collective memory. This collective memory works like an indexing system that tells members who has what knowledge.

How does information sharing enhance performance?
Researchers believe that the sharing of information leads to better group decisions and, as a result, better overall group performance (Hackman 1990). In addition, IS leads to increased awareness of who in the group possesses what knowledge. A well-developed TMS is thought to improve team performance because it gives members quick and coordinated access to one another's specialized expertise, enabling them to effectively combine knowledge to solve complex problems (Hsu et al. 2012).

How can information sharing and transactive memory be measured?
The level of IS and TMS can be measured via five survey statements adapted from questionnaires by Bock and colleagues (2005); Choi, Lee, and Yoo (2010); Lewis (2003); and Bunderson and Sutcliffe (2002). The statements are listed in exhibit 2.2.

What are the implications for management practice?

- *Identifying workers' areas of expertise.* Once the team recognizes the value in knowing more about one another's expertise, the challenge is to find ways to make that expertise *visible.* The most effective methods of achieving this goal are methods the team members choose for themselves; team members are more likely to perceive value in something they have cocreated and bought into. Examples include "show and tell" sessions or other informal gatherings where knowledge workers share their areas of expertise and become recognized among the group as experts. In addition, networking media such as internal directories, intranet pages, LinkedIn, social media, and blogs are all means of identifying skills, exchanging knowledge, and developing the vital TMS.

- *Supporting the development of a TMS.* A TMS is deeply rooted in social relationships, interactions, and the processes and procedures used to get work done. The development of a TMS can therefore be supported by bringing knowledge workers with different areas of expertise together for a specific task; engaging in social interaction to promote bonding; and generally deepening relationships upon which workers will depend in the future. One study, for instance, demonstrated that the TMS in geriatric teams increased when its members attended a greater number of interprofessional team meetings in which patient cases were discussed and specialized knowledge was shared with the whole team (Tan et al. 2014). Teams should also have mechanisms or processes that keep the knowledge about team members' expertise current; if the information becomes out of date, it ceases to be relevant and reliable.

Factor 4. Vision and Goal Clarity

The notion of vision refers to an idea of a valued outcome that represents a higher-order goal and motivating force at work (Kouzes and Pozner 1987; West 1990). Several studies have demonstrated that a clear vision at the team level tends to have a positive effect on team performance. In this sense, the notion of vision refers to the extent to which knowledge workers have a common understanding of objectives and display high commitment to team goals. For this reason, vision at the team level is closely related to the idea of goal clarity.

Why do a clear vision and goal clarity enhance performance?

Several researchers have pointed out that, for a team to be effective, team members need to be committed to team objectives and share a sense of purpose and responsibility (Hülsheger, Anderson, and Salgado 2009). Such commitment can help point a team of knowledge workers in the same direction, which enhances cooperative and goal-directed behavior. In addition, clear goals help knowledge workers see connections between their personal values and the values of the team, which increases the degree to which they find meaning in their work (Wright and Pandey 2011). A clear vision and commitment to long-term objectives play an important role in allowing "freedom to act" while at the same time ensuring that knowledge workers are responsible for producing results (Simon, Stachel, and Covin 2011).

How can vision and goal clarity be measured?

The level of vision and (perceived) goal clarity can be measured with five survey statements adapted from validated questionnaires by Lee and colleagues (1991); Locke and Latham (1984); Rainey (1983); and Simon, Stachel, and Covin (2011). The statements are listed in exhibit 2.2.

What are the implications for management practice?

- *Team vision.* Ensuring that members share the team vision is not a one-off occurrence. Even if team members have a common understanding of objectives, the members might not all buy into them! Once the overall vision is understood, teams should work together to set team goals. Doing so provides an important element of cocreation, which enables more buy-in and ownership, even if the goals are the same ones the manager would have set. This approach also enables greater alignment with personal goals, which is important in bringing meaning to the work carried out by each team member. Managers, therefore, must encourage open discussions to clarify how each person's work contributes to the team's long-term goals.

- *Achievable, specific, and challenging goals.* Research demonstrates that the highest performance results from goals that are both challenging and specific (Latham 2009). Knowledge workers perform at higher levels when asked to meet a specific goal (e.g., "a reduction in the hospital-acquired infection rate of 20 percent," as opposed to simply "do your best"). In addition, challenging goals facilitate pride in accomplishment. The degree of challenge, however, must be balanced with realism, because failure is potentially more damaging than setting a goal that is too easy.

- *Regular feedback.* Regular feedback about achievement of goals—particularly as part of an open, two-way discussion—tends to enhance team member motivation and performance (Locke and Latham 1990). In fact, without feedback, the positive effect of goal setting wears off quickly (Erez 1977). Given constructively, feedback increases self-esteem and improves the performance of a wide range of outcomes. One study, for instance, showed that combined goal setting and feedback improved the safe passing of sharp instruments among hospital operating room personnel from a rate of 31 percent to 70 percent. A follow-up study suggested that the positive effect remained five months after implementation (Cunningham and Austin 2007).

Factor 5. External Communication

External communication refers to the ability of teams to span boundaries (both between teams and between organizations) to seek information and resources from others. Research has demonstrated a link between innovation and the amount of external communication that knowledge workers have with colleagues outside their team or organization (Hülsheger, Anderson, and Salgado 2009). For example, a study of over 400 California hospitals over ten years found considerable support for the relationship between interorganizational links and innovation in hospital services and technology (Goes and Park 1997).

How does external communication enhance performance?
External communication enhances the likelihood of obtaining new knowledge and discloses new perspectives. These perspectives in turn spark the development of new ideas (creativity) or the adoption of new ways of doing things (innovation). Knowledge worker teams whose tasks require creativity and innovation tend to experience enhanced performance when they undertake external communication (Ancona and Caldwell 1992).

How can external communication be measured?
The level of external communication can be measured with three statements adapted from validated questionnaires by Teigland and Wasko (2003) and Ancona and Caldwell (1992). The statements are listed in exhibit 2.2.

What are the implications for management practice?
Knowledge workers who have the support of management are more willing to communicate with others outside their team or organization (Burton et al. 2012). Encouraging knowledge workers to build relationships with colleagues outside their team or organization and to participate in professional networks can be effective ways of building external connections from which to draw information, ideas, and experiences. Managers can facilitate the development of these professional networks by arranging events (e.g., face-to-face meetings, video conferences) or facilitating webinars on important topics. They can also encourage knowledge workers to regularly visit other organizations or participate in other teams. Research suggests that healthcare organizations that promote and support "boundary spanners" are more likely to become aware of and implement innovations quickly (Greenhalgh et al. 2004).

Factor 6. Trust
Trust is a feeling created by the expectation that the actions of another individual or group will be for your benefit, or at least not detrimental to your interests (Gambetta 1988). Knowledge workers generally have two groups of people within the organization to which they can direct the feeling of trust: their colleagues and management. Trust in colleagues

and teammates is called *horizontal trust*. In organizations with a high level of horizontal trust, knowledge workers expect their colleagues to take collective interests into account when making decisions; workers do not simply act out of self-interest. *Vertical trust* refers to the trust knowledge workers have in management.

How does trust enhance the level of performance?

Trust is particularly crucial for the performance of knowledge workers because it influences whether individual group members are willing to share and exchange information with one another (Robertson, Gockel, and Brauner 2012). As a result, the performance of knowledge workers is indirectly dependent on the level of horizontal trust. In addition, vertical trust helps in aligning the team goals with the goals of management. If the team lacks trust in management, it may also lack alignment between these goals.

What determines the level of trust in a group or team?

Positive exchange experiences are important antecedents of trust. When team members have experienced several positive exchanges, the sharing of knowledge and ideas is facilitated. In addition, trust is more likely to develop when teams are composed of individuals with similar characteristics. An important rule states that trust begets trust, while distrust begets distrust (March and Olsen 1975). When a manager trusts her employees, employees are more likely to reciprocate this feeling—and vice versa. Laschinger and colleagues (2000), for instance, found that empowered nurses reported higher levels of vertical trust. Similar findings hold for trust in colleagues.

     Another important factor that determines the level of trust is procedural justice—that is, the fairness of the procedures used to determine organizational outcomes (Connell, Ferres, and Travaglione 2003). For instance, the perception of the fairness of organizational systems and processes involving performance appraisal, professional development opportunities, and job security are important elements of trust toward management (Korsgaard, Schweiger, and Sapienza 1995).

How can trust be measured?

Both horizontal and vertical trust can be measured with seven statements adapted from the Copenhagen Psychological Questionnaire, or COPSOQ II (National Research Centre for the Working Environment 2014). The statements are listed in exhibit 2.2. The two types of trust must be measured separately because they are different constructs and might not be positively related.

What are the implications for management practice?
Colleagues can strengthen trust by (1) communicating often and openly, (2) telling the truth and keeping agreements, (3) using participative decision making, (4) showing genuine interest in and respect toward all coworkers, and (5) providing organizational support toward employees (Dirks and Ferrin 2002; Robertson, Gockel, and Brauner 2012). In addition, for issues related to performance appraisal, professional development, or job security, managers should strive for maximum procedural justice. In healthcare, for instance, performance appraisals of medical staff play a key role in clinical governance, which in turn is critical to containing costs and ensuring high-quality patient care. Research has demonstrated that the medical staff's perception of fairness plays a key role in the successful implementation of an appraisal system (Clarke, Harcourt, and Flynn 2013).

Finally, the practical implications discussed in the sections about social cohesion and supervisory support may also apply here, as they address the deepening of relationships and the building of trust.

EXHIBIT 2.2
Survey for Measuring the Six Factors

The six factors identified in this REA can be measured by having team members read the following statements and indicate their level of agreement. The levels can be scored as follows: Strongly agree = 5; somewhat agree = 4; neither agree nor disagree = 3; somewhat disagree = 2; strongly disagree = 1. A low aggregate team score (e.g., below 3.5) is an indication of low team performance.

Social Cohesion
1. Members of our team like to spend time together outside of work hours.
2. Members of our team get along with each other.
3. Members of our team would rather get together as a team than go out on their own.
4. Members of our team defend each other from criticism by outsiders.
5. Members of our team help each other on the job.

(continued)

EXHIBIT 2.2

Survey for
Measuring the
Six Factors
(Continued)

Perceived Supervisory Support

1. My supervisor is willing to extend himself or herself in order to help me perform my job to the best of my ability.
2. My supervisor takes pride in my accomplishments at work.
3. My supervisor tries to make my job as interesting as possible.
4. The organization values my contribution to its well-being.
5. The organization strongly considers my goals and values.
6. The organization really cares about my well-being.

Information Sharing / Transactive Memory

1. Our team members share their work reports and official documents with other team members.
2. Our team members share their experience or know-how with other team members.
3. Information to make key decisions is freely shared among the members of the team.
4. Our team members trust that other members' knowledge is credible.
5. Our team members are confident relying on the information that other team members bring to the discussion.

Vision and Goal Clarity

1. Our team has clearly defined goals.
2. Our team goals are clear to everyone who works here.
3. It is easy to explain the goals of this team to outsiders.
4. I have specific, clear goals to aim for in my job.
5. If I have more than one goal to accomplish, I know which ones are most important and which are least important.

External Communication

1. Our team members use information obtained from external teams every day.
2. Our team is contacted by outside teams for knowledge and information.
3. Our team scans the external environment for ideas and solutions.

Trust

Horizontal Trust

1. Our team members withhold information from each other.
2. Our team members withhold information from the management.
3. Our team members in general trust each other.

Vertical Trust

1. The management trusts the team to do their work well.
2. The team members can trust the information that comes from the management.
3. The management withholds important information from the team members.
4. The team members are able to express their views and feelings toward management.

Sources: Ancona and Caldwell (1992); Bock et al. (2005); Bunderson and Sutcliffe (2002); Carless and De Paola (2000); Eisenberger et al. (1986); Lee et al. (1991); Lewis (2003); Locke and Latham (1984); National Research Centre for the Working Environment (2014); Rainey (1983); Simon, Stachel, and Covin (2011); Teigland and Wasko (2003); Choi, Lee, and Yoo (2010).

EXHIBIT 2.2
Survey for
Measuring the
Six Factors
(Continued)

Some Final Thoughts About the Implications of This REA

The six factors outlined here were derived through a scientifically robust review of more than 500 research studies. The studies were undertaken in leading academic institutions across the world and were published in peer-reviewed journals. We believe the findings of this REA therefore represent the best available scientific evidence in relation to knowledge worker performance at this time.

The power of these findings became clear during our discussions with the companies that commissioned the REA. Imagine if a management team were to address the six factors across all aspects of the organization to create the conditions that gave knowledge workers their best chance of being effective? What if senior managers and leaders were brave enough to start again with a blank sheet of paper? What would it mean for leadership, communication, recruitment, and the ways objectives and goals are set?

However, the six factors are not simply for leaders prepared to take a "blank sheet" approach. They also provide guidance for managers who want to improve their teams' performance and for business leaders seeking to take a more evolutionary approach. Some of the managers and business leaders who participated in this REA pointed out that the findings provide an evidence-based framework relating to "what to do differently or stop doing in my job to enhance performance."

Some Final Thoughts About Implications Specific to Healthcare

All healthcare organizations use indicators to monitor and enhance performance. This REA, however, demonstrates that most of the indicators that healthcare organizations use—such as job satisfaction and employee engagement—correlate poorly with knowledge worker performance and are therefore of limited value (Bowling 2007). Thus, most healthcare organizations are doing a poor job at creating the conditions for their doctors and nurses to be effective.

We hope that this REA will contribute to a better understanding of the factors that affect knowledge worker performance. Furthermore, we hope it will serve as a convincing example of how REAs can prevent healthcare organizations from spending money on management practices that are ineffective or even harmful to members and patients.

Acknowledgments

The authors would like to thank everyone who contributed to this REA: AWA's team members; CEBMa, particularly Professor Rob Briner and Professor Denise Rousseau; and the managers and business leaders of AllSteel, Allied Bakeries, BDO, BP, Old Mutual Wealth, Telereal Trillium, and the Royal Bank of Scotland. Their feedback and inputs were highly valuable in guiding the research.

Notes

1. Center for Evidence-Based Management (CEBMa) is a nonprofit member organization dedicated to promoting evidence-based practice in the field of management.
2. Advanced Workplace Associates (AWA) is a UK-based workplace management consultancy.

References

Ancona, D. G., and D. F. Caldwell. 1992. "External Activity and Performance in Organizational Teams." *Administrative Science Quarterly* 37 (4): 634–65.

Antman, E. M. 1992. "A Comparison of Results of Meta-analyses of Randomized Controlled Trials and Recommendations of Clinical Experts." *Journal of the American Medical Association* 286 (2): 240–48.

Bock, G. W., R. W. Zmud, Y. G. Kim, and J. N. Lee. 2005. "Behavioral Intention Formation in Knowledge Sharing: Examining the Roles of Extrinsic Motivators, Social-Psychological Forces, and Organizational Climate." *MIS Quarterly* 29 (1): 87–111.

Bowling, N. A. 2007. "Is the Job Satisfaction–Job Performance Relationship Spurious? A Meta-analytic Examination." *Journal of Vocational Behavior* 71 (2): 167–85.

Brunell, A. B., M. S. Davis, D. R. Schley, A. L. Eng, M. H. M. van Dulmen, K. L. Wester, and D. J. Flannery. 2013. "A New Measure of Interpersonal Exploitativeness." *Frontiers in Psychology* 4 (May): article 299.

Bunderson, J. S., and K. M. Sutcliffe. 2002. "Comparing Alternative Conceptualizations of Functional Diversity in Management Teams: Process and Performance Effects." *Academy of Management Journal* 45 (5): 875–93.

Burton, P., A. Wu, V. R. Prybutok, and G. Harden. 2012. "Differential Effects of the Volume and Diversity of Communication Network Ties on Knowledge Workers' Performance." *IEEE Transactions on Professional Communication* 55 (3): 239–53.

Bushman, B., and G. Wells. 2001. "Narrative Impressions of Literature: The Availability Bias and Corrective Properties of Meta-analytic Approaches." *Personality and Social Psychology Bulletin* 27 (9): 1123–30.

Carless, S. A., and C. De Paola. 2000. "The Measurement of Cohesion in Work Teams." *Small Group Research* 31 (1): 71–88.

Carron, A. V., and P. Chelladurai. 1981. "The Dynamics of Group Cohesion in Sport." *Journal of Sport Psychology* 3 (2): 123–39.

Carron, A. V., and K. S. Spinks. 1995. "The Group Size–Cohesion Relationship in Minimal Groups." *Small Group Research* 26 (1): 86–105.

Chalmers, I., M. Enkin, and M. J. Keirse. 1993. "Preparing and Updating Systematic Reviews of Randomized Controlled Trials of Health Care." *Millbank Quarterly* 71 (3): 411–37.

Chiocchio, F. 2009. "Cohesion and Performance: A Meta-analytic Review of Disparities Between Project Teams, Production Teams, and Service Teams." *Small Group Research* 40 (4): 382–420.

Choi, S. Y., H. Lee, and Y. Yoo. 2010. "The Impact of Information Technology and Transactive Memory Systems on Knowledge Sharing, Application, and Team Performance: A Field Study." *MIS Quarterly* 34 (4): 855–70.

Clarke, C., M. Harcourt, and M. Flynn. 2013. "Clinical Governance, Performance Appraisal, and Interactional and Procedural Fairness at a New Zealand Public Hospital." *Journal of Business Ethics* 117 (3): 667–78.

Connell, J., N. Ferres, and T. Travaglione. 2003. "Engendering Trust in Manager–Subordinate Relationships: Predictors and Outcomes." *Personnel Review* 32 (5): 569–87.

Cunningham, T. R., and J. Austin. 2007. "Using Goal Setting, Task Clarification, and Feedback to Increase the Use of the Hands-Free Technique by Hospital Operating Room Staff." *Journal of Applied Behavior Analysis* 40 (4): 673–77.

Daly, J. 2005. *Evidence-Based Medicine and the Search for a Science of Clinical Care.* Berkeley, CA: University of California Press.

Davenport, T., R. Thomas, and S. Cantrell. 2002. "The Mysterious Art and Science of Knowledge-Worker Performance." *MIT Sloan Management Review.* Published October 15. http://sloanreview.mit.edu/article/the-mysterious -art-and-science-of-knowledgeworker-performance/.

Dirks, K. T., and D. L. Ferrin. 2002. "Trust in Leadership: Meta-analytic Findings and Implications for Research and Practice." *Journal of Applied Psychology* 87 (4): 611–28.

Drucker, P. 1959. *The Landmarks of Tomorrow.* New York: Harper & Row.

Edmondson, D. R., and S. L. Boyer. 2013. "The Moderating Effect of the Boundary Spanning Role on Perceived Supervisory Support: A Meta-analytic Review." *Journal of Business Research* 66 (11): 2186–92.

Eisenberger, R., R. Huntington, S. Hutchison, and D. Sowa. 1986. "Perceived Organizational Support." *Journal of Applied Psychology* 71 (3): 500–507.

Erez, M. 1977. "Feedback: A Necessary Condition for the Goal Setting–Performance Relationship." *Journal of Applied Psychology* 62 (5): 624–27.

Fink, A. 1998. *Conducting Research Literature Reviews: From Paper to the Internet.* London: Sage Publications.

Gambetta, D. G. 1988. "Can We Trust Trust?" In *Trust: Making and Breaking Cooperative Relations,* edited by D. G. Gambetta, 213–17. New York: Basil Blackwell.

Goes, J. B., and S. H. Park. 1997. "Interorganizational Links and Innovation: The Case of Hospital Services." *Academy of Management Journal* 40 (3): 673–96.

Gouldner, A. W. 1960. "The Norm of Reciprocity: A Preliminary Statement." *American Sociological Review* 25 (2): 161–78.

Greenhalgh, T., G. Robert, F. Macfarlane, P. Bate, and O. Kyriakidou. 2004. "Diffusion of Innovations in Service Organizations: Systematic Review and Recommendations." *Milbank Quarterly* 82 (4): 581–629.

Hackman, J. R. (ed.). 1990. *Groups That Work (and Those That Don't): Creating Conditions for Effective Teamwork.* San Francisco: Jossey-Bass.

Heerwagen, J., K. Kampschroer, K. Powell, and V. Loftness. 2004. "Collaborative Knowledge Work Environments." *Building Research & Information* 32 (6): 510–28.

Higgins, J., and S. Green (eds.). 2011. *Cochrane Handbook for Systematic Reviews of Interventions: Version 5.1.0.* Updated March. http://handbook .cochrane.org/.

Hsu, J. S.-C., S.-P. Shih, J. C. Chiang, and J. Y.-C. Liu. 2012. "The Impact of Transactive Memory Systems on IS Development Teams' Coordination, Communication, and Performance." *International Journal of Project Management* 30 (3): 329–40.

Hülsheger, U. R., N. Anderson, and J. F. Salgado. 2009. "Team-Level Predictors of Innovation at Work: A Comprehensive Meta-analysis Spanning Three Decades of Research." *Journal of Applied Psychology* 94 (5): 1128–45.

Klein, C., D. DiazGranados, E. Salas, L. Huy, C. S. Burke, R. Lyons, and G. F. Goodwin. 2009. "Does Team Building Work?" *Small Group Research* 40 (2): 181–222.

Korsgaard, A. M., D. M. Schweiger, and H. J. Sapienza. 1995. "Building Commitment, Attachment, and Trust in Strategic Decision-Making Teams: The Role of Procedural Justice." *Academy of Management Journal* 38 (1): 60–84.

Kouzes, J. M., and B. Z. Pozner. 1987. *The Leadership Challenge.* San Francisco: Jossey-Bass.

Laschinger, H. K., R. N. Spence, J. Finegan, J. Shamian, and S. Casier. 2000. "Organizational Trust and Empowerment in Restructured Healthcare Settings: Effects on Staff Nurse Commitment." *Journal of Nursing Administration* 30 (9): 413–25.

Latham, G. 2009. "Motivate Employee Performance Through Goal Setting." In *Handbook of Principles of Organizational Behavior,* edited by E. A. Locke, 161–79. Chichester, UK: Wiley.

Lee, C., P. Bobko, C. Early, and E. A. Locke. 1991. "An Empirical Analysis of a Goal Setting Questionnaire." *Journal of Organizational Behavior* (12) 6: 467–82.

Lewis, K. 2003. "Measuring Transactive Memory Systems in the Field: Scale Development and Validation." *Journal of Applied Psychology* 88 (4): 587–604.

Locke, E. A., and G. P. Latham. 1990. *A Theory of Goal-Setting and Task Performance.* Englewood Cliffs, NJ: Prentice Hall.

———. 1984. *Goal Setting: A Motivational Technique That Works.* Englewood Cliffs, NJ: Prentice Hall.

March, J. G., and J. Olsen. 1975. "The Uncertainty of the Past: Organizational Learning Under Ambiguity." *European Journal of Political Research* 3 (2): 149–71.

Moore, A., and K. Mamiseishvili. 2012. "Examining the Relationship Between Emotional Intelligence and Group Cohesion." *Journal of Education for Business* 87 (5): 296–302.

Morello, R. T., J. A. Lowthian, A. L. Barker, R. McGinnes, D. Dunt, and C. Brand. 2013. "Strategies for Improving Patient Safety Culture in Hospitals: A Systematic Review." *BMJ Quality and Safety* 22 (8): 11–18.

Naisbitt, J. 1982. *Megatrends*. New York: Warner Books.

National Research Centre for the Working Environment. 2014. "Copenhagen Psychological Questionnaire—COPSOQ II." Updated February 4. www .arbejdsmiljoforskning.dk/~/media/Spoergeskemaer/copsoq/uk/copsoq-ii -medium-size-questionnaire-english.pdf#.

Petticrew, M. 2001. "Systematic Reviews from Astronomy to Zoology: Myths and Misconceptions." *British Medical Journal* 322 (7278): 98–101.

Petticrew, M., and H. Roberts. 2006. *Systematic Reviews in the Social Sciences: A Practical Guide*. Oxford, UK: Blackwell Publishing.

Rainey, H. G. 1983. "Private Agencies and Private Firms: Incentive Structures, Goals, and Individual Roles." *Administration and Society* 15 (2): 207–42.

Ramirez, Y. W. 2006. "Defining Measures for the Intensity of Knowledge Work in Tasks and Workers." PhD diss., Department of Industrial Engineering, University of Wisconsin–Madison.

Robertson, R., C. Gockel, and E. Brauner. 2012. "Trust Your Teammates or Bosses? Differential Effects of Trust on Transactive Memory, Job Satisfaction, and Performance." *Employee Relations* 35 (2): 222–42.

Shadish, W. R., T. D. Cook, and D. T. Campbell. 2002. *Experimental and Quasi-Experimental Designs for Generalized Causal Inference*. Boston: Houghton Mifflin Company.

Simon, M., C. Stachel, and J. G. Covin. 2011. "The Effects of Entrepreneurial Orientation and Commitment to Objectives on Performance." *New England Journal of Entrepreneurship* 14 (2): article 3.

Straus, S. E., C. Soobiah, and W. Levinson. 2013. "The Impact of Leadership Training Programs on Physicians in Academic Medical Centers: A Systematic Review." *Academic Medicine* 88 (5): 710–23.

Tan, K. T., F. Adzhahar, I. Lim, M. Chan, and W. S. Lim. 2014. "Transactive Memory System as a Measure of Collaborative Practice in a Geriatrics Team: Implications for Continuing Interprofessional Education." *Journal of Interprofessional Care* 28 (3): 239–45.

Tayfur, O., and M. Arslan. 2013. "The Role of Lack of Reciprocity, Supervisory Support, Workload and Work–Family Conflict on Exhaustion: Evidence from Physicians." *Psychology, Health & Medicine* 18 (5): 564–75.

Teigland, R., and M. M. Wasko. 2003. "Integrating Knowledge Through Information Trading: Examining the Relationship Between Boundary Spanning Communication and Individual Performance." *Decision Sciences* 34 (2): 261–86.

Thomas, B. E., and J. P. Baron. 1994. "Evaluating Knowledge Worker Productivity: Literature Review." *USACERL Interim Report FF-94/27*: 1–27.

West, M. A. 1990. "The Social Psychology of Innovation in Groups." In *Innovation and Creativity at Work: Psychological and Organizational Strategies*, edited by J. L. Farr, 309–33. Chichester, UK: Wiley.

Wright, B. E., and S. K. Pandey. 2011. "Public Organizations and Mission Valence: When Does Mission Matter?" *Administration & Society* 43 (1): 22–44.

Xu, R., M. J. Carty, D. P. Orgill, S. R. Lipsitz, and A. Duclos. 2013. "The Teaming Curve: A Longitudinal Study of the Influence of Surgical Team Familiarity on Operative Time." *Annals of Surgery* 258 (6): 953–57.

3

THE BALDRIGE: WHAT WE'VE LEARNED FROM THE MOST RIGOROUS EVIDENCE-BASED MANAGEMENT IN HEALTHCARE ORGANIZATIONS

by John R. Griffith

This chapter reviews the processes involved in winning the Malcolm Baldrige National Quality Award, and it argues that the process and the publicly available winners' applications represent the current epitome of evidence-based management—a set of comprehensive processes for managing any healthcare provider organization. The applications show that the processes have been carefully structured to produce effective outcomes, repeatedly studied and improved, successfully implemented in a variety of settings, and audited. The management system the Baldrige winners have collectively created constitutes a model that can be effectively installed in most US healthcare organizations. If universally implemented, the model would raise performance medians to the current top quartiles.

The Baldrige Process and Its Results as Evidence-Based Management

Several hundred healthcare provider organizations (HCOs) are pursuing the "Baldrige journey." They begin at the state level and reapply annually, improving as they implement suggestions from the previous year. Each year, several are recognized at the state level, and one or two are selected as national winners. The 19 winners through 2016 represent a diverse array, including every kind of care, from intake clinics to palliative care and hospices, in a broad spectrum of American communities.

Evidence-based management is the "conscientious, explicit, and judicious use of the best available evidence from multiple sources" (Barends, Rousseau, and Briner 2014). The process followed by the Baldrige is entirely consistent. Organizations on the journey file 50-page, single-spaced applications that describe work processes according to a rigorous outline in the Baldrige Excellence Framework (formerly the Baldrige Criteria) (Baldrige

Performance Excellence Program 2015). The applications are reviewed in painstaking depth by at least a dozen trained examiners, who evaluate each process against specific criteria, score it, and suggest *opportunities for improvement* (OFIs) to justify their scoring. Applicants receive a detailed summary of OFIs. They are encouraged to seek *best practice,* including successful processes from previous winners' applications. As they implement solutions and reapply, their applications receive higher scores and win reviews by more senior examiners. The top few each year receive a site visit by a team of seven experienced reviewers, who spend five full days on site, verifying the accuracy of the application. The applications of the winners are publicly available, though the winners' scores and OFIs are kept confidential (Baldrige Performance Excellence Program 2016). All other applicant information is totally confidential. Organizations that receive state-level awards can allow their names to be recognized.

Application scoring is heavily (45 percent) weighted to results, which include outcomes and process measures of quality of care, patient satisfaction, market support, worker and physician satisfaction, cost, and financial performance. The winners are top quartile in most measures, and often top decile (Foster and Chenoweth 2011; Griffith 2015; Schulingkamp and Latham 2015). The remaining score is divided across six major categories of organizational work processes: Leadership, Strategy, Customers, Measurement Analysis and Knowledge Management, Workforce, and Operations (Baldrige Performance Excellence Program 2015).

The systematic pursuit of excellence—with careful process descriptions, multiple reviews, and field audits—makes Baldrige winners the epitome of evidence-based management. They demonstrate validated, measured performance across a well-tested framework of systematically acquired, repeatedly tested work processes, addressing both clinical care and the maintenance of critical resources—customers, workers, logistics, and finance. Many HCOs pursue evidence-based management without seeking the Baldrige, documenting substantial excellence (Institute of Medicine 2013). The Baldrige process is unequalled in rigorous structure, external review, field audit, and published results.

The Ethical Framework of the Baldrige Is Consistent with Medical Professionalism

Evidence-based management and evidence-based medicine are both founded on empiricism and the scientific method, philosophies that led to extraordinary twentieth-century achievements (Montori and Guyatt 2008). They also have another philosophical foundation that is often left implicit: healthcare as a *mitzvah*, or duty to fellow humans. Most physicians, nurses, and other care-givers have personal commitments to help the sick, to refrain from exploiting their information asymmetry, and to provide full value for their compensation. These precepts are built into the Hippocratic Oath, the criteria of the Accreditation Council for Graduate Medical Education (2014), the *Code of Ethics* of the American College of Healthcare Executives (2011), and many other value statements. They depart substantially from the "caveat emptor" ethics of the marketplace. The Baldrige Framework is explicitly founded on similar values (Baldrige Performance Excellence Program 2015, 39):

- Systems perspective
- Visionary leadership
- Patient-focused excellence
- Valuing people
- Organizational learning and agility
- Focus on success
- Managing for innovation
- Management by fact
- Societal responsibility and community health
- Ethics and transparency
- Delivering value and results

The scoring emphasis on quality of care, beginning with care outcomes, is clear evidence that the commitment to "Patient-focused excellence," "Societal responsibility and community health," "Ethics and transparency," and "Delivering value and results" is not in any sense superficial or secondary. Plainly stated, this is evidence-based management for patient care, not for profit.

The Winners Represent All of Healthcare and Much of America

The HCOs that won the Baldrige Award between the years of 2002 and 2015 are listed below (Baldrige Performance Excellence Program 2016):

2015: Charleston Area Medical Center Health System, Charleston, WV

2014: Hill Country Memorial, Fredericksburg, TX
St. David's HealthCare, Austin, TX

2013: Sutter Davis Hospital, Davis, CA

2012:   North Mississippi Health Services, Tupelo, MS

2011:   Henry Ford Health System, Detroit, MI
        Schneck Medical Center, Seymour, IN
        Southcentral Foundation, Anchorage, AK

2010:   Advocate Good Samaritan Hospital, Downers Grove, IL

2009:   AtlantiCare, Atlantic City, NJ
        Heartland Health, St. Joseph, MO

2008:   Poudre Valley Health System (now part of University of Colorado Health), Fort Collins, CO

2007:   Mercy Health System (now part of MercyRockford Health System), Janesville, WI
        Sharp HealthCare, San Diego, CA

2006:   North Mississippi Medical Center, Tupelo, MS

2005:   Bronson Methodist Hospital, Kalamazoo, MI

2004:   Robert Wood Johnson University Hospital, Hamilton, NJ

2003:   Baptist Hospital, Inc., Pensacola, FL
        Saint Luke's Health System, Kansas City, MO

2002:   SSM Health Care, St. Louis, MO

These organizations collectively provide comprehensive healthcare, from initial patient contact through acute, rehabilitation, continuing, and palliative care. Several of them operate health insurance plans. They provide many medical fellowships and substantial nursing education. Several are also Magnet hospitals. Geographically, the range is impressive. It includes rural and urban communities, every US region, several places with economic challenges (e.g., Atlantic City, Detroit, Janesville, Charleston), and one organization with an exceptional geographic challenge (the Southcentral Foundation serves a Native American population across the Aleutian Islands).

The Baldrige Model, a Comprehensive System for Managing HCOs

The Baldrige emphasis on finding and copying best practice has led to the Baldrige Model, a documented, audited system that can produce excellent results on a balanced scorecard of strategic measures, across the spectra of clinical requirements and operating environments.

The model emphasizes eight critical practices:

1. *An explicit consensus committing to mission and values.* The winners summarize their missions as either "healthy community" or "excellent care" (White and Griffith 2016). They achieve stakeholder consensus through widespread review and discussion and sustain it both by regular use and by requiring new associates to review and accept both the mission and the values. The fact that all associates of the organization are committed to a common mission provides a foundation for discussion and decision making that supports the other practices.

2. *A culture of empowerment that encourages associates to raise any work-related concern.* Empowerment is supported by "servant leadership," whereby management is expected to respond constructively to concerns expressed by any associate, patient, guest, or vendor (Studer 2008). The concepts of empowerment and servant leadership implement "service excellence," a management philosophy stating that meeting worker needs supports worker satisfaction, retention, commitment, and effectiveness in meeting patient needs (White and Griffith 2016).

3. *A system of multidimensional performance measures and external benchmarks, with scorecards reported regularly for every permanent work unit.* The measures are rigorously defined to focus on elements within the work group's control. Each unit scorecard provides regular reports of performance and easy identification of goal achievement or unanticipated difficulty. The strategic scorecard reports organization-wide aggregates for about 30 outcomes-oriented measures of quality, patient satisfaction, associate satisfaction, and cost. It is aggregated from unit scorecards and reported to the governing board at each meeting.

4. *A top-down/bottom-up negotiation process where strategic goals are established by the governing board from benchmarks and an environmental review, and where unit goals are identified from local OFIs.* "Benchmark" is the best known performance; there is proof that the benchmark has been, and can be, achieved. The strategic and unit perspectives on goals are reconciled in a three- to five-month negotiation process, leading to improvement commitments for the coming year. The final goals are realistic progress toward benchmark. They are almost universally achieved at both the unit and strategic level.

5. *"Continuous improvement," the systematic pursuit of OFIs.* Multidisciplined performance improvement teams (PITs) use

analytic processes such as Lean and Six Sigma to seek and correct "root causes." Any measure less than benchmark is an OFI; even Baldrige winners have several hundred or thousand OFIs at any given time. The OFIs must be prioritized, and the PITs staffed and managed. PIT recommendations are tested and implemented in improvement goals.

6. *Evidence-based medicine, with clinical protocols to guide the care of common conditions and to standardize tasks from hand washing to neurosurgery.* The protocols are detailed descriptions of clinical work processes. Patient management protocols are often adapted from publicly available guidelines (Agency for Healthcare Research and Quality 2016; Mutter, Rosko, and Wong 2008). Task protocols are adapted from published documentation and managed by the clinical specialty most often involved. Protocols facilitate the training of associates and the supervised delegation of tasks to lower cost providers. They promote safety, prompt essential actions, discourage unnecessary care, prevent delays, reduce rework, and improve efficiency.

7. *Expanded training.* Baldrige winners typically provide ten days of training per full-time equivalent (FTE) per year, several times the traditional level. The training includes applying protocols and other work processes, learning servant leadership, understanding performance measures and statistical interpretation, serving on and leading performance improvement teams, and negotiating improvement goals. It is supplemented with individual development plans and support for formal education.

8. *Extensive use of rewards for achievement and for exceptional effort.* Baldrige winners strongly emphasize rewards, ranging from personal thanks and encouragement to public recognition and celebration to cash prizes and annual bonuses. Most winners pay substantial bonuses to units that achieve their goals, to managers whose units are successful, and to senior executives who contribute to strategic goal achievement. The amounts are not publicly released but are believed to be in the range of 5 to 10 percent—equivalent to several weeks' pay. Many Baldrige winners also give small gifts to patients and families who have experienced service failures, such as excessive delays or lost personal property. These gifts are part of the "service recovery" system to address failures in customer relations.

Although we know little about "typical" processes in these areas, Baldrige processes clearly represent major changes in activities, attitudes, and behaviors. The activity changes are fairly obvious:

- The consensus is maintained by near constant repetition and extensive dialogue. Bronson Methodist Hospital, for example, lists 35 different mechanisms for communicating ideas (Bronson Methodist Hospital 2005). Most of these mechanisms are two-way, creating participation and commitment and improving learning. They complement the standard promotional communications.

- Performance measures are multidimensional, precisely defined, and highly reliable. If they are not, the organization will fail. Even a few examples of misleading or erroneous data will destroy confidence. Larger HCOs, like Sharp and Henry Ford, must deliver thousands of values each month. Benchmarks are used wherever possible.

- Robust problem-solving systems such as Lean require trained support—not just on a few projects, but on enough to respond effectively to important OFIs. PITs are closely monitored; extra resources are used to keep them productive and on schedule.

- Evidence-based medicine requires a reasonably effective electronic health record (EHR). The protocol, the individualized plan of care, provision for orders and notes, and reports must be convenient to support effective dialogue in caregiving teams.

- Training is carefully developed, readily available, and rigorous. It includes assessment of learning and application.

- The reward systems are designed to pay out. The negotiated goals are almost always met; 90-day plans come into play whenever achievement is in danger.

- The use of rewards increases several kinds of fraud risks, so it requires a sophisticated audit system, covering not only financial data but also work processes and performance data. Incentive payment systems are notoriously fragile. When workers do not believe the system is fair, the consensus cannot be maintained.

Basically, these changes mean that all the HCO's support systems must work effectively, and they must be perceived as effective by all associates. Everything the clinical teams need—patients, supplies, information, equipment—must be there, on time and in good order.

Even more demanding is what might be called the "soft side" of the transition, the change in attitude and behavior of the entire leadership. Servant leadership is not the tradition of American organizations, but it must be sustained and universal. Representatives from three winners—Hill Country Memorial, Schneck, and Sutter Davis—expanded on these challenges in the *Frontiers of Health Services Management* issue from the fall of 2015. Their thoughts, presented in the sections that follow, confirm that the change constitutes a profound mental redirection.

Hill Country Memorial

Pope, Padula, and Wallace-Dooley (2015) share observations from Hill Country Memorial's Baldrige journey:

> [Success] requires a significant level of commitment, perseverance, and willingness to learn from mistakes, as well as the ability to motivate a team toward a vision (Pope, Padula, and Wallace-Dooley 2015, 4).

> We also implemented a "just culture," one in which people are not judged by the outcome of their behavior but by the quality of their decisions. Our goal was to encourage the team to share their mistakes and the lessons learned so we could all improve together. We developed a council structure across the entire organization, empowering frontline employees, volunteers, and physicians with tools to find, develop, and implement best practices. (Pope, Padula, and Wallace-Dooley 2015, 8–9)

> Maintaining good relationships with [physician] stakeholders is essential to our long-term sustainability. . . . [W]e found that we did not really have systematic processes for two-way communication. Of course, we had physician engagement surveys, a physician liaison, and informal meetings in the hallways, but no systematic mechanisms for senior leaders to engage in ongoing two-way communication with providers. . . . So we started going to them—not to speak, just to listen and make ourselves available. Doing so led to more opportunities for connecting with providers, which we made a requirement for leadership. (Pope, Padula, and Wallace-Dooley 2015, 9)

> Every quarter, team members' behaviors are rated for alignment with our values, and we develop action plans for improvement as necessary. Physicians and volunteers are evaluated similarly. We integrated our values into reward and recognition programs . . . that offer peer-to-peer or patient recognition, quarterly awards for exemplary demonstration of values, and annual True North Values Awards for employees, volunteers, and providers. (Pope, Padula, and Wallace-Dooley 2015, 10)

> Few days go by when the question "How does this align with our values?" does not come up in conversation. This steadfast and systematic focus on "doing the right thing" is the foundation of our culture of Remarkable Always. (Pope, Padula, and Wallace-Dooley 2015, 10)

> [The] goals are then shared with the team and patients via the departmental alignment boards, which are posted publicly in every department. The boards display . . . how well the department is currently performing on a specific goal. The department leader then repeats this process with employees, helping them set measurable personal goals that are aligned with the department and organizational goals. These quarterly coaching conversations help to maintain our alignment across the entire organization. (Pope, Padula, and Wallace-Dooley 2015, 13)

[W]e found that people often forgot what they learned because they were not applying the knowledge daily. To overcome this challenge, we developed simple process management and improvement tools that guide team members through the process, similar to the way a facilitator might. . . . This hands-on approach to learning process management has been far more educational and effective for our team than have classroom courses, and it has engaged people at all levels in process leadership. (Pope, Padula, and Wallace-Dooley 2015, 15)

Schneck Medical Center

Describing Schneck Medical Center's Baldrige journey, Forgey and Dye (2015) report substantial changes in employee attitudes about leadership, the mission, and dealing with burnout. They detail innovative solutions for cardiac catheterizations, readmissions, and chronic disease management, and they candidly admit that their thinking changed radically as they progressed:

Building engagement and alignment among key stakeholders is a critical step on the performance excellence journey. It is not something that happens by chance; it involves a great deal of effort and thought. (Forgey and Dye 2015, 18)

Employees at all levels must understand that the Baldrige journey is not about adding to people's daily work; instead, it is about making daily work easier and providing better care to patients. It is about actively incorporating performance excellence into people's work instead of just talking about it. Schneck uses dashboards at the department, service line, and organizational levels to link employees, results, plans, and processes so people can see the results and the impact of their efforts. (Forgey and Dye 2015, 19–20)

Do not misunderstand: Receiving the Baldrige Award is wonderful, but our drive did not come from chasing it. Instead, it came from improving the value we provide to our patients, their families, and our workforce. (Forgey and Dye 2015, 20)

When we first sat down as a leadership team to complete our organization profile, we saw very quickly how mistaken we had been. We stated that we wanted to be an organization of excellence, yet when our senior executives discussed this topic, we each had our own definition of what we perceived excellence to be. (Forgey and Dye 2015, 24–25)

Baldrige is not a quick fix; it is a systematic process that involves changing the organizational culture. Situations may arise where you need to slow down, wait, or let something go and move on. Doing what is right for the organization at the wrong time will fail just as not doing what is right will. Confusion and discomfort are normal and to be expected. (Forgey and Dye 2015, 27)

Sutter Davis

Wagner (2015) shares insights from Sutter Davis's transformation:

> I am frequently asked, "How do you sustain the journey, year after year?" The answer lies in leadership and the strength of the commitment to be the best and to earn the recognition. (Wagner 2015, 41)
>
> Just as the Baldrige Award is earned, so too is the trust of the workforce. Credible leadership is built on trust, consistency, fairness, and equitability, and it is demonstrated through role modeling. (Wagner 2015, 41)
>
> I believe the journey develops the team better than any other framework, operating system, or leadership model. . . . During the journey, the leadership team becomes proficient at accepting feedback on how they are managing and leading the business, and they actively seek out the best performers, develop the desire to benchmark, . . . and look for ways to improve performance. . . . This process is transformational. (Wagner 2015, 42–43)
>
> Mature teams are willing to confront the brutal facts, learn to benchmark against the best, and realize that the results are about improving performance on the basis of quantifiable outcomes. (Wagner 2015, 44)
>
> Many operating systems can take an organization only so far, and many, if not most, focus on the return on investment. The Baldrige Criteria offer a much more balanced framework for leadership. . . . [O]ne of my key takeaways from the Baldrige journey was how important it is to simply stop and take the time to define words. At Sutter Davis, we defined our systems and processes, which led to speaking and understanding more clearly about how our processes were integrated and how we contributed to the results. (Wagner 2015, 44)

What these people are saying is that the transition involves hearts and minds as much as processes and systems.

The Consensus Directly Improves Patient Care and Reduces Cost

Several elements in the Baldrige Model are expensive. Exact details are not available, but maintaining the information system and EHR, providing ten days training per FTE, and paying the bonus could easily add more than 10 percent to operating costs. PITs take people from their primary jobs, and Lean fact-finding can get expensive. Emphasizing mission and servant leadership pulls the focus of budgeting away from inputs and cost-cutting, and toward improving outputs. Nevertheless, all winners, even those in economically challenging environments, report at least satisfactory financial operations. What offset the costs?

The answer is not completely clear. (Winners are allowed to conceal competitive details.) However, their data show that length of stay and readmissions are reduced and market share is increased. The Baldrige Model systematically eliminates errors, delays, and rework in patient care as well as in support activities. The traditional hierarchy of individual caregivers—doctor, nurse, aide, clerk—becomes a team collectively following evidence-based best practice. The team members like their work and stay with the organization, leading to turnover of less than 10 percent per year. They benefit from the training and are comfortable with learning and change. Because they believe in the mission, know more, relate better to each other, and have fewer logistic problems, they share and implement a commitment to excellence. In simplistic terms, the winners balance the books not by cutting the nursing staff but by helping the staff treat people more efficiently and more effectively. Cost per case drops as outcomes improve. Patient satisfaction and physician satisfaction improve as well. Many of the winners have converted their improvement to increased market share.

Several Factors Impair the Spread of the Consensus

If a physician knew that a specific protocol moved survival, readmission, patient satisfaction, and cost from the median to the top quartile, she would follow that protocol and insist that the HCO support it. Evidence-based medicine and medical ethics require her to insist. The Baldrige Model is a specific protocol that is documented not for a single patient or disease but for overall HCO operations. Yet data from sources such as www.WhyNotThe Best.org show that it is not widely practiced. The spread of evidence-based management has been agonizingly slow (Institute of Medicine 2013). The slowness can be attributed to several factors:

- The Baldrige Model is complex, and it requires major changes in attitude and practice for all associates.
- It is not clear how many professional HCO managers understand the opportunity.
- Before the shift in focus from "volume" to "value" in payment systems, organizations had little financial incentive to make the changes.
- Governing boards have a serious information asymmetry. "Public" members generally know only what they have been told. Insiders, including the senior management and medical leadership, have control of all of the information needed for the strategic scorecard.

Despite these obstacles, the Baldrige Model can be spread. Several of the winners have acquired HCOs and incorporated them successfully.

Winners are attractive to both hospitals and physician practices seeking stronger partners. Once the deal is signed, the winners implement the model in new organizations, without the Baldrige process. (Winners cannot reenter the process for five years.)

How the Spread of the Model Can Be Encouraged

Spread of the Baldrige Model requires transition organizations capable of installing the model in tens or hundreds of HCOs. The Baldrige process is highly labor intensive and not easily scaled. Transition organizations should take the place of the Baldrige process: They should be evidence-based groups that can effectively support any given HCO, enabling it to implement the cultural and procedural changes that the model requires.

A successful transition organization must do the following:

- Acquire the knowledge and skill to provide client HCOs with guidance and encouragement, similar to that the winners received on their journeys.
- Implement the empowerment and servant leadership concepts in operations, building the associate loyalty and commitment that represent a central component of success.
- Be able to identify promising OFIs, support PITs, and set realistic interim improvement goals. The transition organization can provide guidance from a growing knowledge base of best practice. It should be able to draw upon experts in the various processes, including hands-on care, logistic and financial systems, and strategic planning. A model site with training, examples, and consultant experts would be helpful, possibly through affiliation with Baldrige winners.
- Be prepared for a multiple-year "journey" at each site. Evidence from the winners shows that, though the model requires substantial investments, it generates savings as it goes. Transition does not require a large financial reserve, but the winners have required several years of repetition to deploy the concepts and incorporate them firmly into the organization culture.
- Invest in marketing and promotion to build interest. The empowerment concept requires that local governing boards, physicians, and employees be convinced, not coerced.

The transition organizations' most critical challenge may be the marketing. The proposition is that the Baldrige Model meets all stakeholders' needs better. The stakeholders need to be persuaded. Associate stakeholders need to know that their colleagues working under the Baldrige Model are more satisfied than they are and that success can be achieved under the full range of caregiver affiliations, from employment to privileging for fee-for-service. The winners' applications provide striking documentation; the challenge is to disseminate it.

Community stakeholders are a bigger challenge. Transition organizations need to stimulate a broader understanding of realistic improvement possibilities. Efforts to brand the "learning organization" image could reach public members directly. Demonstration sites, with committed trustees, physicians, nurses, and other workers, would be a valuable marketing tool.

Transition organizations should negotiate long-term management contracts with existing provider corporations. The offer must begin, "Your patients and your caregivers will be delighted with our model, and as citizens and employers, you will like it because it improves health, increases caregiver satisfaction, and minimizes cost." The contract needs to include realistic performance guarantees and continued employment assurances. The company must deliver on those commitments to sustain sales.

A transition management organization could potentially take several forms:

- A contract management company (The percentage of hospitals managed by contract companies has been stable for many years. Offering and promoting "guaranteed excellence" could support a new entrant or the expansion of existing firms.)
- A subsidiary or affiliate of a Baldrige winner
- A healthcare consulting company (An established consulting company could affiliate with a winner, or winners.)
- A subsidiary or affiliate of an insurance company, such as UnitedHealth Group or the not-for-profit Blue Cross plan, Health Care Service Corporation
- A subsidiary founded by an existing healthcare system, such as Kaiser Permanente, Trinity Health, or Ascension Health
- A consortium, like the Health Care Transformation Task Force (www.hcttf.org), establishing the transition organization as a vehicle to achieve its goals
- A venture by large employers, such as the Healthcare Marketplace Collaborative (McDonald, Mecklenburg, and Martin 2015) or an expansion of the Leapfrog Group (www.leapfroggroup.org /about)

Limitations

The proposition is that the Baldrige Model constitutes evidence-based managerial practice that (1) produces results that are substantially superior to those of other practices across all important dimensions and (2) is transportable and should be transported to most HCO sites in the United States. The documentation for the first part of the proposition speaks for itself. The second part of the proposition has more serious limitations.

The set of Baldrige winners does not represent an experimental design and does not prove that the model can be universalized. However, it does prove that the results are not a fluke. The healthcare markets in San Diego, Tupelo, Chicago, Kansas City, Detroit, Sacramento, and Atlantic City, plus dozens of smaller ones, are sufficiently diverse to suggest that the model can be spread more broadly.

We need a better understanding of how and why the Baldrige Model works. We need a clearer grasp of the ways in which the model supports superior clinical practice, both in patient results and practitioner satisfaction. We need a better understanding of corporate incentives, to uncover why a given HCO's governance would support the model and what would make them continue pursuing excellence. We need documentation of risk factors—which HCOs quit the journey, and why? We need to know how to apply the model in safety-net HCOs and academic medical centers—two important HCO types that have not yet had Baldrige winners. These important frontiers would expand on the existing evidence that aggressive pursuit of the Baldrige Model can produce substantially superior HCO performance.

References

Accreditation Council for Graduate Medical Education. 2014. "ACGME Common Program Requirements." Updated September. www.acgme.org/What-We-Do/Accreditation/Common-Program-Requirements.

Agency for Healthcare Quality and Research. 2016. "National Guideline Clearinghouse." Accessed June 10. www.guideline.gov.

American College of Healthcare Executives. 2011. *Code of Ethics*. Amended November 14. www.ache.org/abt_ache/code.cfm.

Baldrige Performance Excellence Program. 2016. "Baldrige Award Recipient Information." Accessed June 9. http://patapsco.nist.gov/Award_Recipients/index.cfm.

———. 2015. *2015–2016 Baldrige Excellence Framework (Health Care): A Systems Approach to Improving Your Organization's Performance*. Gaithersburg, MD: US Department of Commerce, National Issue of Standards and Technology.

Barends, E., D. M. Rousseau, and R. B. Briner. 2014. *Evidence-Based Management: The Basic Principles*. Center For Evidence-Based Management. Accessed June 9, 2016. www.cebma.org/wp-content/uploads/Evidence-Based-Practice-The-Basic-Principles.pdf.

Bronson Methodist Hospital. 2005. *2005 Malcolm Baldrige National Quality Award Application Summary*. Accessed June 10, 2016. http://patapsco.nist.gov/Award_Recipients/PDF_Files/Bronson_Methodist_Hospital_Application_Summary.pdf.

Forgey, W. L., and T. Dye. 2015. "Small-Town Touch, Big-City Innovation, World-Class Aspirations." *Frontiers of Health Services Management* 32 (1): 17–29.

Foster, D. A., and J. Chenoweth. 2011. "Comparison of Baldrige Award Applicants and Recipients with Peer Hospitals on a National Balanced Scorecard." Thomson Reuters. Published October. www.nist.gov/baldrige/upload/baldrige-hospital-research-paper.pdf.

Griffith, J. R. 2015. "Understanding High-Reliability Organizations: Are Baldrige Recipients Models?" *Journal of Healthcare Management* 60 (1): 44–61.

Institute of Medicine. 2013. *Best Care at Lower Cost: The Path to Continuously Learning Health Care in America*. Washington, DC: National Academies Press.

McDonald, P. A., R. S. Mecklenburg, and L. A. Martin. 2015. "The Employer-Led Health Care Revolution." *Harvard Business Review* 93 (7/8): 38–50.

Montori, V. M., and G. H. Guyatt. 2008. "Progress in Evidence-Based Medicine." *Journal of the American Medical Association* 300 (15): 1814–16.

Mutter, R. L., M. D. Rosko, and H. S. Wong. 2008. "Measuring Hospital Inefficiency: The Effects of Controlling for Quality and Patient Burden of Illness." *Health Services Research* 43 (6): 1992–2013.

Pope, J. E., E. Padula, and D. Wallace-Dooley. 2015. "Improving Ourselves for the Sake of Others: Our Baldrige Journey." *Frontiers of Health Services Management* 32 (1): 3–16.

Schulingkamp, R. C., and J. R. Latham. 2015. "Healthcare Performance Excellence: A Comparison of Baldrige Award Recipients and Competitors." *Quality Management Journal* 22 (3): 6–22.

Studer, Q. 2008. *Results That Last: Hardwiring Behaviors That Will Take Your Company to the Top*. Hoboken, NJ: Wiley.

Wagner, J. 2015. "Sharing Leadership Insights on Our Baldrige Journey to Excellence." *Frontiers of Health Services Management* 32 (1): 40–44.

White, K. R., and J. R. Griffith. 2016. *The Well-Managed Healthcare Organization*, 8th ed. Chicago: Health Administration Press.

SCIENTIFIC EVIDENCE— DOING THE WORK

RESEARCH OPPORTUNITIES AND EXAMPLES

by Thomas Rundall and Terese Otte-Trojel

Introduction

Evidence-based management involves a rigorous process for making management decisions through the conscientious, explicit, and judicious use of four types of information (Briner, Denyer, and Rousseau 2009; Rousseau 2012a):

1. The best available scientific evidence pertaining to the management decision: studies with research designs that are strong with respect to measurement reliability and internal validity (and, in rare cases, external validity) and that enable assessments of causal relationships or associations between independent and dependent variables while controlling for confounding factors
2. The best available organizational evidence: organizational data, facts, figures, and business analytics that describe community healthcare needs, organizational capabilities, performance on quality and financial indicators, and other factors that might influence decisions
3. The best available experiential evidence: professional insight, understanding, skill, and expertise that are accumulated by practitioners over time
4. Organizational values and stakeholder concerns: the strongly held beliefs and ethical values that permeate an organization's culture and the concerns of internal and external stakeholders that may influence decisions

This chapter will identify research opportunities associated with each of these four categories of information. It will also provide opportunities to study and learn from the efforts of health organization managers to use evidence-based management in making important decisions.

The Healthcare Management Research Context

A great deal of management research in the healthcare field has focused on programs, policies, and practices that directly affect what is commonly known as the "Triple Aim." The three goals of the Triple Aim are as follows (Berwick, Nolan, and Whittington 2008):

- Improving the patient experience of care, including quality and satisfaction
- Improving the health of populations
- Reducing the cost of healthcare per capita

The Triple Aim has become widely accepted among policymakers and thought leaders in the organizations that provide and pay for healthcare services. Pursuit of the aim is difficult for healthcare organizations, given the complexity of their structures and operations and the fragmented service delivery and payment systems in which they function. The goals identify high-value management challenges that influence the performance of specific organizations and to some extent the performance of the healthcare system as a whole; as a result, they represent major opportunities for healthcare management researchers.

A number of other management issues are only indirectly related to the Triple Aim but are crucial to a healthcare organization's viability. Such issues include

- human resource management, including hiring, training, assessing, retaining, and compensating employees;
- efforts to establish a preferred brand in the community being served;
- supply chain management;
- the strengthening of hospital–physician relationships;
- revenue cycle management;
- the outsourcing of services;
- organizational mergers, joint ventures, and partnerships;
- investment of the organization's financial reserves;
- development of a culture supportive of innovation;
- placement and design of new facilities; and
- compliance with legal and regulatory requirements.

These and other important issues suggest research needs and opportunities that could contribute to evidence-based decision making beyond the areas directly related to the Triple Aim. They remind us that the four types of evidence described at the start of this chapter can lead to improvements across virtually the entire range of an organization's operational and strategic decisions.

Research Opportunities Across the Four Types of Evidence

In the sections that follow, we identify research opportunities within each of the four evidence types: scientific evidence, organizational evidence, experiential evidence, and evidence from organizational values and stakeholder concerns. We also discuss opportunities to study evidence-based management in action and see how the four types of evidence are explicitly or implicitly used in decision making. Finally, we present some ideas about where and how to secure funding for management research.

We use the widely accepted goals of the Triple Aim to provide focus to our suggested research opportunities. However, we also suggest research topics that are of fundamental importance to healthcare organizations but only indirectly related to the Triple Aim. In addition, we provide examples of published management research related to the opportunities identified. All the examples we include deal specifically with management issues in healthcare organizations; for a discussion of general management research literature, we recommend the writings by Rousseau (2012a, 2012b) and Madhavan and Mahoney (2012) in *The Oxford Handbook of Evidence-Based Management.*

The healthcare management examples presented in this chapter were identified through a search of published healthcare management literature. We searched using Google Scholar, PubMed, and ABI/INFORM Global, and we reviewed tables of contents from the past five years in journals such as the *Journal of Healthcare Management, Health Services Management Research, Medical Care Research and Review,* the *International Journal of Healthcare Management,* and *Health Care Management Review.* The selected research examples are representative of the types of evidence and the reported research on managerial issues as described above. The examples were drawn from research conducted in the United States and numerous other countries, illustrating the global nature of healthcare management research.

When considering the various research opportunities and examples, note that the four categories of evidence are not mutually exclusive. Scientific evidence is generated by studies with experimental or quasi-experimental designs that attempt to identify causal relationships or significant associations among independent and dependent variables. However, the data for a scientific study can come from any number of sources within or outside an organization, depending on the management action being studied, the possible effects of the decision, and the variables that the researcher believes may mediate or moderate an action's effects.

For example, a scientific study examining the relationship between performance appraisal practices and employee satisfaction, commitment, and on-the-job behavior at several hospitals would likely involve the collection and analysis of organizational evidence (e.g., employee participation, satisfaction, commitment, on-the-job behavior) while controlling for the confounding effects of differing organizational values across the study hospitals. This single study would likely involve at least three of the four types of evidence. Hence, the scientific evidence category is cross-cutting in the sense that organizational, experiential, and values-related data could be included as independent, control, or dependent variables in a given study, depending on the management issue or decision being addressed.

Scientific Evidence

The key strength of scientific evidence is its ability to provide information about causal effects of policies, practices, and programs on organizational outcomes of interest (generated, for instance, when randomized controlled experiments are performed) and information about the strength of relationships among variables (generated when statistical methods are applied to control for the simultaneous effects of confounding factors). The healthcare field features two broad types of scientific evidence: (1) findings regarding the effects of managerial decisions or estimates of causal relationships or associations among various independent and dependent variables derived from a single primary study and (2) findings regarding effects and relationships among variables synthesized from a systematic review of multiple studies of the same (or very similar) managerial policy or program. Systematic reviews are exceptionally important for understanding the effects of managerial decisions—just as they are for medical decisions as well. They combine findings from numerous studies of different health organizations and contexts to help us understand the overall strength of an observed policy or program effect and how that effect may be moderated by organizational and contextual factors.

Research Opportunities

Scientific evidence is especially important in (1) assessing whether management policies, practices, and programs that have already been implemented have achieved their intended effects and (2) assessing the likelihood that a new policy, practice, or program is sufficiently likely to achieve desired effects that are worth the monetary and other costs of going forward with implementation. In the section that follows, we briefly describe a primary study and a systematic review that have generated scientific evidence for healthcare management. We also identify several other examples to show the range of topics that these types of scientific research may address.

Examples of Primary Studies

Using a randomized controlled trial design, Dodge and colleagues (2014) assessed the impact of a brief postnatal home-visiting intervention on the use of emergency healthcare services and family outcomes. The intervention, which was implemented between July 2009 and December 2010 in Durham, North Carolina, consisted of five to seven postnatal home visits. A total of 4,777 births within that period were assigned to either an intervention group or a control group. Eighty percent of the families participated in the intervention, and adherence was 84 percent. The impact of the intervention was evaluated through blinded interviews with a random subset of 549 families, as well as through review of hospital records. Compared to families in the control group, families in the intervention group reported fewer infant emergency care visits, lower rates of anxiety, and more community connections, positive parenting behaviors, and participation in higher-quality childcare. Blinded home-care visits confirmed higher-quality home environments in intervention families. Further, hospital records showed that infants in the intervention group had 59 percent fewer emergency medical care episodes than control infants. In conclusion, the study demonstrated that a brief home-visiting program can lower emergency medical care and improve family outcomes.

Other examples of research in this category of scientific evidence include studies dealing with physical work conditions and nurse turnover (Vardaman et al. 2014); cost-efficiency reporting and physician behavior (Goodman 2012); factors that can reduce hospital readmissions (Carey and Lin 2014); the effect of physician panel size on health outcomes (Stefos et al. 2011); costs and quality of care in multispecialty medical groups (Weeks et al. 2010); and financial performance of hospitals that belong to health networks and systems (Bazzoli et al. 2000).

Examples of Systematic Reviews

McMillan and colleagues (2013) conducted a systematic review to assess the nature and efficacy of patient-centered care interventions for chronic disease patients. The aim of the review was to synthesize all randomized controlled trials that had been conducted on this topic to identify the types of interventions, the ways the concept of patient-centeredness had been operationalized, and the outcomes the interventions had produced. The review included 30 studies. The studies revealed that most interventions focused on promoting patient empowerment and aimed to educate patients and encourage them to participate in their own care. In addition, several interventions focused on providers—particularly on training providers to deliver empowering care. The authors pointed to some promising findings linking patient-centered care approaches with patient satisfaction and perceived quality of care. Findings regarding other outcomes (such as health, clinical, functional, personal, and system outcomes) were more complex and mixed.

Other examples of systematic reviews include reviews of studies on dissemination of performance information and continuous improvement (Lemire, Demers-Payette, and Jefferson-Falardeau 2013), the effect of community-based pharmacy interventions on patient outcomes (Blalock et al. 2013), and organizational transformation in healthcare and other industries (Lee et al. 2013).

Organizational Evidence

The key strength of organizational evidence is the ability to monitor organizational performance on key indicators and track changes over time. Organizational data from clinical and administrative databases are essential to assessing patient acuity, adequacy of nurse staffing, and, more generally, employee workload, performance, and satisfaction; assessing patient care service use, process quality, patient safety, outcomes, cost of care, and other organizational characteristics with quantitative and qualitative data; and assessing the organization's operating and nonoperating financial performance.

Research Opportunities

The following sections describe five examples of important research opportunities that can be addressed with organizational evidence: (1) use of clinical and administrative databases to assess patient risk; (2) use of medical record data about patient conditions and service provision to design, implement, and monitor new programs; (3) use of an organization's financial and administrative data to estimate the cost of care and measures of efficiency; (4) use of data on an organization's safety culture and data from medical records about serious error events to improve safety; and (5) use of internal employee survey data and other human resources data to assess employee work life and job satisfaction.

Example: Use of Clinical and Administrative Databases to Assess Patient Risk

Rana and colleagues (2014) used routine hospital data captured within a large regional health service in Australia to establish a framework for predicting risk of unplanned readmission for acute myocardial infarction (AMI) patients. The study, which included 1,660 consecutive AMI patients, followed two steps. In the first step, a predictive model was established based on randomly selected records of two-thirds (1,107) of the patients. In the second step, the model was tested on the last one-third (553) of patient records. At the time of the study, the best existing predictive models for AMI readmission were the seven-factor HOSPITAL score and the Elixhauser comorbidity score, both of which build on evidence from known biomarkers. Rana and colleagues aimed to test the newly generated hospital data model against the two existing models in terms of the ability to predict 30-day ischemic heart disease readmission and all-cause readmission after 12 months of initial AMI hospitalization. The study concluded that the hospital data model had significantly higher predictive qualities than the two other models, for both the 30-day and the 12-month readmissions. The model showed that important factors associated with readmission included emergency department attendances, cardiac diagnoses and procedures, renal impairment, and electrolyte disturbances.

Another example of research on this topic within the category of organizational evidence is a study on predictive modeling and team care for high-need patients at HealthCare Partners (Feder 2011).

Example: Use of Medical Record Data on Patient Conditions and Service Provision to Design, Implement, and Monitor New Programs

David and colleagues (2015) set out to assess the degree to which adoption of the patient-centered medical home (PCMH) model reduces utilization of emergency department services. The study examined data from 460,000 Independence Blue Cross patients enrolled in 280 primary care practices that adopted the PCMH model between 2008 and 2012. The results of the analysis showed that adoption of the PCMH model was associated with lower emergency department utilization for patients with chronic diseases but not for those without. Among patients with chronic diseases, transition to the PCMH model was associated with reductions in emergency department utilization of 5 to 8 percent; however, the effectiveness of the model varied by chronic condition. The largest reductions in emergency department utilization were found among chronic patients with diabetes and hypertension. The study concluded that these observed reductions likely stem from better management of chronic illness.

Other examples of research on this topic within the category of organizational evidence include studies on improving patient satisfaction in hospital care settings (Otani, Herrmann, and Kurz 2011); assessing accountable care organizations' efforts to engage patients and their families (Shortell et al. 2015); and a team-based, quality-focused compensation model for primary care providers (Greene, Hibbard, and Overton 2014).

Example: Use of an Organization's Financial and Administrative Data to Estimate the Cost of Care and Measures of Efficiency

Relying on claims data and hospital administrative data sets, McCarthy and colleagues (2015) sought to quantify the potential cost savings of providing palliative care consults in five hospitals in a Texas region. In addition, the research team aimed to identify relationships between cost savings and team structure, patient diagnosis, and timing of the consults. The study included hospital administrative records on all inpatient stays at the five hospitals from the start of 2009 through mid-2012. Data were restricted to patients over the age of 18 years with inpatient stays of between 7 and 30 days. In the analysis, patients who received palliative care were matched with patients who did not receive such care, and they were compared across several observable characteristics including age, gender, diagnosis, and hospital. The analysis showed significant cost savings of $3,426 per patient for those who received a palliative care consult in the hospital compared to those who did not. This effect was only significant for patients dying at the hospital and especially for patients who received the consult within 15 days of admission. Interdisciplinary care team structures were associated with higher cost savings. Contrary to what existing literature suggested, no significant cost savings were found for patients who were discharged alive, with the exceptions of patients with a pulmonary or infection diagnosis and those receiving a palliative care consult after ten days in the hospital.

Other examples of research on this topic within the category of organizational evidence include studies estimating the cost of diabetes mellitus-related events from inpatient admissions in Sweden (Gerdtham et al. 2009) and those examining the association between hospital costs and quality of care (Jha et al. 2009).

Example: Use of Data on an Organization's Safety Culture and Data from Medical Records on Serious Error Events to Improve Safety

Rathert, Fleig-Palmer, and David (2006) used survey data to assess health service providers' perceptions of patient safety and attributors to medical errors that compromise patient safety. Specifically, the authors examined data collected in a larger study of patient safety in three hospitals in the eastern United States that were part of the same health system. The study reported on responses to two open-ended questions from a survey filled in by 1,089 frontline healthcare providers. The first question asked about conditions that could increase the chances for medical errors, and the second question asked about conditions that could decrease the chances for errors. Coding of the answers led to the identification of 18 categories including "staffing," "hiring," "policies and procedures," and "technology." The results showed that staffing was seen as the top concern across all three hospitals and that policies and procedures ranked second among the perceived attributors to medical errors. Paradoxically, at the same time, focusing on policies and procedures was considered to be the most important approach to decreasing medical errors across all the hospitals. The remaining categories were consistent across all three hospitals, although their relative importance differed.

Another example of research on this topic within the category of organizational evidence is a study on safety subcultures in healthcare organizations and the management of medical error (Sirriyeh et al. 2012).

Example: Use of Internal Employee Survey Data and Other Human Resources Data to Assess Employee Work Life and Job Satisfaction

Mosadeghrad, Ferlie, and Rosenberg (2011) conducted a study within a hospital network in Iran with the intent to delineate the relationships among employee job stress, quality of working life, and turnover intention. Using a cross-sectional design, the authors collected data from hospital employees through a validated questionnaire. An analysis of the collected data showed that about one fourth of the respondents rated their job stress as high, largely due to inadequate pay, inequality at work, work overload, staff shortage, lack of recognition and promotion prospects, time pressure, lack of job security, and lack of management support. Further, the analysis pointed to an inverse relationship between job stress and employees' quality of working life. Though quality of working life reduced the probability of turnover intentions, job stress was positively related to employees' turnover intention.

Other examples of research on this topic within the category of organizational evidence include studies on high performance work practices in the healthcare sector (Boselie 2010) and innovative human resource practices in US hospitals (Platonova and Hernandez 2013).

Experiential Evidence

The strengths of experiential evidence are the tacit knowledge, insight, understanding, skill, and expertise that experienced managers, and managers from differing backgrounds, can bring to important decisions. This type of evidence helps managers understand problems and devise solutions in the form of policies, programs, and practices that are appropriate for the particular organization in which a managerial issue is identified and acceptable to the stakeholders involved. Experiential evidence can also contribute to an understanding of the implications of scientific and organizational evidence for the specific circumstances that pertain in a given organization.

Research Opportunities

The following two research topics are examples of important research opportunities that can examine and refine the way that experiential evidence is used by managers: (1) use of qualitative, experience-based information for decision making and (2) interviews with managers of healthcare-related organizations to gain a detailed understanding of how decisions are made in various contexts.

Example: Use of Qualitative, Experience-Based Information for Decision Making

Using survey methods, Baghbanian, Hughes, and Khavarpour (2011) investigated the basis on which Australian healthcare administrators make decisions concerning allocation of resources. Specifically, the investigation aimed to assess the extent to which economic evaluations played a role in decision making. Ninety-one nationally representative healthcare administrators completed the survey. The results showed that more than three out of five administrators believed that formal economic considerations should play a larger role in decision making. However, more than four out of five believed that such information should have only a marginal influence on resource allocation decisions. The survey respondents identified several barriers that may limit the use of evidence from economic evaluations in resource allocation decisions. Such barriers included ethical considerations, policy guidelines, time and money constraints, methodological issues, the inflexibility of healthcare budgets, and the dominance of historical budgeting, as well as issues involving the nature and relevance of available evidence. The survey responses suggested that economic evaluations do not sufficiently take into account the broader organizational contexts in which decisions are made. Thus, the authors concluded that, until evidence from economic evaluations can be placed into broader sociopolitical and volatile contexts, the evidence will likely not influence resource allocation decisions to a large extent.

Other examples of research on this topic within the category of experiential evidence include studies on implementing high-performance work practices in healthcare organizations (McAlearney et al. 2013) and on perspectives on the enablers of e-health (electronic health) adoption (Moxham et al. 2012).

Example: Using Interviews with Managers of Healthcare-Related Organizations to Gain a Detailed Understanding of How Decisions Are Made in Various Contexts

Stephen O'Connor interviewed Dr. Kenneth R. White, associate dean for strategic partnerships and innovation at the University of Virginia Medical Center and professor of nursing at the University of Virginia School of Nursing, to gain his perspectives on several topics related to healthcare management (White 2014). When asked about strategies essential to ensuring delivery of high-value healthcare, White emphasized the importance of changing an organization's culture and shifting from a transactional management perspective to a transformational leadership focus. Underlying this shift must be a constant focus on achieving—and financially rewarding—outcomes that matter to patients. As such, White is a proponent of the thinking of

Michael Porter, including the idea of integrated practice units. Such thinking will, according to White, stimulate promotion of interprofessional teamwork and the breaking down of system silos. White believes these aspects to be critical for reducing fragmentation of care and separation of health professions; thus, they encourage safer and more patient-centered care.

Other relevant interviews with healthcare-related managers and decision makers include interviews with David Bernd, CEO of Sentara Healthcare (Bernd 2003); Daniel J. Wolterman, president and CEO of Memorial Hermann Health Care System (Wolterman 2010); and Anthony Armada, president of Advocate Lutheran General Hospital and Advocate Lutheran General Children's Hospital (Armada 2011).

Organizational Values and Stakeholder Concerns

Evidence regarding organizational values and stakeholder concerns provide contextual information about preferences, values, and ethical beliefs that helps managers understand the attitudes and behaviors of patients, employees, physicians, and others in the healthcare system. This type of evidence is important in helping managers define the nature of a performance problem and the types of interventions that are likely to be supported by key stakeholders over the long term, hence enhancing the chances of success.

Research Opportunities

The following two research topics provide opportunities to examine organizational values and stakeholder concerns as they are expressed through an organization's culture: (1) assessing the effects of organizational culture on performance and (2) assessing efforts to change the culture of healthcare organizations.

Example: Assessing the Effects of Organizational Culture on Performance

Shortell and colleagues (1995) assessed the relationships among organizational culture, quality improvement processes, and selected outcomes for a broad sample of hospitals in the West and Midwest of the United States. The research team collected primary data on measures related to quality improvement programs, organizational culture, implementation approaches, and degree of quality improvement implementation. Subsequently, the team merged these data with data on perceived impact and objective measures of clinical efficiency for six clinical conditions. An analysis showed that a participative, flexible, and risk-taking organizational culture was significantly related to implementation of quality improvement programs. Further, implementation of quality improvement programs was positively correlated with perceived patient outcomes and human resource development. Hospital size appeared to have an effect on the ability of hospitals to implement quality improvement programs; the more bureaucratic and hierarchical culture found in larger-size hospitals was believed to pose a barrier to implementation.

Other examples of research on this topic within the category of organizational values and stakeholder concerns include studies about the relationship between hospital-based emergency department culture and work satisfaction and intent to leave (Lin et al. 2012) and the impact of organizational culture and caregiver training on patient safety (Johnson 2004).

Example: Assessing Efforts to Change the Culture of Healthcare Organizations
Through a case study of the Oklahoma State University Center for Health Sciences, Bacigalupo, Hess, and Fernandes (2009) described efforts to change an existing top-down and internally oriented organizational culture toward a "change-ready" culture better able to adapt and respond to the external environment. Over several years, the executive leadership of the center worked with consultants to achieve this change. A key effort involved redistributing power within the organization by hiring new department leaders who were suitable and open to bringing about a more decentralized form of decision making. Yet this decentralized decision-making culture was not readily accepted. A main issue during the initial 12-month transition period was that the new leaders did not feel comfortable or equipped to make important decisions. During this time, in a process facilitated by the consultants, senior management worked closely with the department leaders to train and support them in their decision making. Following the transition period, the department leaders became increasingly swift and confident as decision makers, and they began focusing on making decisions that supported organization-wide objectives, rather than just departmental ones. According to Bacigalupo, Hess, and Fernandes, the changes to facilitate strategic and action-oriented decisions led to better quantitative performance; for example, the center went from being barely profitable to highly profitable.

Other examples of research on this topic within the category of organizational values and stakeholder concerns include a study on how to change the culture in medical education to teach patient safety (Kirch and Boysen 2010).

Evidence-Based Management in Action: Case Studies of Practice

Case studies can help inform the field of how evidence-based management is practiced and under what circumstances this approach to decision making has and has not been successful.

Research Opportunities

We currently know little about how managers systematically implement evidence-based management, the types of decisions that are made most frequently using evidence-based management, and the strategies that have been most successful at institutionalizing evidence-based management in healthcare organizations. Case studies involving the actual use of evidence-based management—incorporating interviews with managers and various qualitative and quantitative data from the process and outcomes of decisions—therefore represent an important research opportunity.

Examples of Cases

Several relevant and informative cases were presented in the first edition of *Evidence-Based Management in Healthcare*. In this section, we briefly summarize one of those cases, while also pointing the reader to the other relevant cases.

Grazier (2009) describes a case concerning the development, implementation, and evaluation of a chronic care management model of depression treatment. The model, which was put in place within several primary care group practices belonging to an academic medical center in the United States, built on an evidence-based management approach that followed five steps:

1. *Formulating the research question.* The guiding question for the study was: "How can we integrate the best approach to depression treatment within primary care?"
2. *Acquiring the evidence.* In this second step, the research team gathered evidence deriving from clinical research on treatment effects as well as from delivery system management research on primary and specialty mental health models.
3. *Assessing the validity, quality, and applicability of the evidence.* In an effort to test the feasibility and sustainability of a model combining depression treatment and primary care, the research team used a quasi-experimental design to implement an intervention. The intervention entailed a bundle of processes, which was given to patients assigned to the intervention group. The effect of the intervention was measured in terms of clinical outcomes and economic implications.
4. *Presenting the evidence.* The research team was able to demonstrate improved clinical depression scores in the intervention group. However, the intervention's impact on cost-savings was less clear.
5. *Applying the evidence in decision making.* To the degree employers and other decision makers were persuaded by the evidence on improved clinical outcomes and (potential) cost savings, this evidence might have weighed in on their decisions to integrate depression treatment into the overall health benefits package.

Other examples of relevant cases involve improving pain management in long-term care (Webb and Flaherty 2009), using evidence-based management to improve operating room scheduling (Wolfman 2009), and improving the health status of underserved children in Houston's East End (Bray 2009)—all of which appeared in the first edition of this book. The current edition of this book contains additional examples of evidence-based management in action.

Funding Opportunities

Although funding opportunities for healthcare management research are not nearly as numerous as for clinical and health policy research, they exist within individual health-related organizations, private foundations, and governmental agencies. In addition, depending on the nature of a given clinical or health policy study, opportunities may exist to build in management research components that address questions relevant to the larger clinical or policy issue.

A great deal of management research occurs within organizations as part of management's routine monitoring, problem identification, intervention development, implementation, and evaluation activities, and also as part of formative or summative evaluations of new managerial innovations. The funding for such research is typically included in the operating budget of the respective organizational unit. Some organizational research projects may be outsourced to researchers from universities or consulting organizations. But, increasingly, large provider organizations are developing in-house analytic capabilities and research centers to perform applied research using their clinical and managerial databases.

Health maintenance organizations and other healthcare delivery organizations that accept significant financial risk for the care they provide have been at the forefront of developing analytic capabilities in what has come to be called *delivery science*. The research is funded by a combination of internal health system funds and external funding, often via grants from government agencies. The research centers for many of these organizations—including those for several Kaiser Permanente regions, Baylor Scott and White Health, Geisinger Health System, the Marshfield Clinic, Harvard Pilgrim Health Care, Meyers Primary Care Institute, Group Health Cooperative, Henry Ford Health System, and the Palo Alto Medical Foundation—belong to the HMO Research Network that facilitates collaboration on research to improve healthcare delivery. As health systems continue to consolidate, integrate hospital services with physician organizations, and accept service delivery contracts from payers that place them at financial risk, these types of in-house research centers and collaborative networks, including partnerships with academic researchers, will proliferate.

In the United States, private, not-for-profit foundations provide funding for external research programs that help the foundations achieve their priorities. Such foundations may have a local, regional, state, or national orientation with respect to funding research projects. Much of their research portfolios tend to be oriented toward analyses of policies that affect access to affordable healthcare for disadvantaged populations and the development of community resources and structures to promote health and well-being. However, some foundations have also prioritized research on management policies and practices, particularly management strategies related to the way public policies, such as reimbursement for Medicaid services, affect healthcare organizations and the people they serve. The Robert Wood Johnson Foundation, the Commonwealth Fund, and the California Healthcare Foundation are examples of such funding sources.

In most developed countries, national government agencies provide funding for health services research and specifically for building the knowledge base for improving managerial decision making in healthcare. For example, the Institute of Health Services and Policy Research within the Canadian Institutes of Health Research (2015) is dedicated to "supporting innovative research, capacity-building, and knowledge translation initiatives designed to improve the way healthcare services are organized, regulated, managed, financed, paid for, used, and delivered" (see www.cihr-irsc.gc.ca/e/13733 .html). Similarly, the Centre for Health Service Development (2013) within the Australian Health Services Research Institute was established to undertake a program of research into methods to improve the management and provision of health services, with an emphasis on research supporting evidence-based management (see http://ahsri.uow.edu.au/chsd/index .html). In the United Kingdom, the Health Services and Delivery Research Programme within the National Institute for Health Research (2016) funds commissioned and researcher-initiated projects designed to produce evidence and evidence syntheses that will help managers and policymakers improve the organization and delivery of healthcare services (see www.nets.nihr .ac.uk/programmes/hsdr).

But perhaps the largest and most complex network of governmental agencies funding health services and management research is in the United States. Prominent federal funders of health services and management research include the Agency for Healthcare Research and Quality (see www.ahrq .gov/funding/index.html), the Health Services Research and Development Service of the US Department of Veterans Affairs (see www.hsrd.research .va.gov), the Health Resources and Services Administration (see www.hrsa .gov/grants/index.html), the Centers for Medicare & Medicaid Services (see www.cms.gov/cciio/resources/Funding-Opportunities/index.html), and the National Science Foundation (see www.nsf.gov/funding/). The

National Science Foundation's Industry/University Cooperative Research Center (I/U CRC) Program has been a particularly important source of seed funding for networks of health system managers and university-based researchers to collaborate on research projects. One notable I/U CRC is the Center for Health Organization Transformation at Texas A&M University (see www.chotnsf.org).

To help researchers locate funding opportunities, the US National Library of Medicine's National Information Center on Health Services Research and Health Care Technology provides a website called Health Services Research Information Central that consolidates information on federal grant opportunities from multiple federal agencies (see www.nlm.nih.gov/hsrinfo/grantsites.html).

Conclusion

In this chapter, we have identified numerous research opportunities that will contribute to each of the four categories of evidence used by managers. These research opportunities address important management issues that arise in healthcare organizations' efforts to achieve the Triple Aim, as well as other operational and strategic objectives. We have also identified examples of management research within each of the categories.

Our list of research opportunities is necessarily selective. Surely, one could identify other research opportunities by using a different framework for identifying management issues and related topics. Indeed, identification of research topics that will contribute to the evidence base for managerial decision making in healthcare is constrained only by the attention we give to the challenges faced by healthcare organizations, the concepts and theories we use to understand those challenges, and the imagination we bring to our research. We hope this chapter stimulates thinking about the challenges healthcare organizations face and the research that will help managers understand and respond to those challenges constructively.

References

Armada, A. A. 2011. "Interview with Anthony A. Armada, FACHE, President, Advocate Lutheran General Hospital and Advocate Lutheran General Children's Hospital." By S. J. O'Connor. *Journal of Healthcare Management* 56 (2): 85–88.

Bacigalupo, A., J. Hess, and J. Fernandes. 2009. "Meeting the Challenges of Culture and Agency Change in an Academic Health Center." *Leadership & Organization Development Journal* 30 (5): 408–20.

Baghbanian, A., I. Hughes, and F. A. Khavarpour. 2011. "Resource Allocation and Economic Evaluation in Australia's Healthcare System." *Australian Health Review* 35 (3): 278–83.

Bazzoli, G. J., B. Chan, S. M. Shortell, and T. D'Aunno. 2000. "The Financial Performance of Hospitals Belonging to Health Networks and Systems." *Inquiry* 37 (3): 234–52.

Bernd, D. L. 2003. "Interview with David L. Bernd, FACHE, CEO, Sentara Healthcare, Norfolk, Virginia." By K. L. Grazier. *Journal of Healthcare Management* 48 (3): 142–46.

Berwick, D. M., T. W. Nolan, and J. Whittington. 2008. "The Triple Aim: Care, Health, and Cost." *Health Affairs* 27 (3): 759–69.

Blalock, S. J., A. W. Roberts, J. C. Lauffenburger, T. Thompson, and S. K. O'Connor. 2013. "The Effect of Community Pharmacy-Based Interventions on Patient Health Outcomes: A Systematic Review." *Medical Care Research and Review* 70 (3): 235–66.

Boselie, P. 2010. "High Performance Work Practices in the Health Care Sector: A Dutch Case Study." *International Journal of Manpower* 31 (1): 42–58.

Bray, P. G. 2009. "Improving the Health Status of Underserved Children in Houston's East End." In *Evidence-Based Management in Healthcare,* edited by A. R. Kovner, D. J. Fine, and R. D'Aquila, 233–45. Chicago: Health Administration Press.

Briner, R. B., D. Denyer, and D. M. Rousseau. 2009. "Evidence-Based Management: Concept Cleanup Time?" *Academy of Management Perspective* 23 (4): 19–32.

Canadian Institutes of Health Research. 2015. "Institute of Health Services and Policy Research." Revised May 11. www.cihr-irsc.gc.ca/e/13733.html.

Carey, K., and M.-Y. Lin. 2014. "Hospital Length of Stay and Readmission: An Early Investigation." *Medical Care Research and Review* 71 (1): 99–111.

Centre for Health Service Development. 2013. "Primary Purpose and History." Reviewed May 16. http://ahsri.uow.edu.au/chsd/index.html.

David, G., C. Gunnarsson, P. A. Saynisch, R. Chawla, and N. Somesh. 2015. "Do Patient-Centered Medical Homes Reduce Emergency Department Visits?" *Health Services Research* 50 (2): 418–39.

Dodge, K. A., W. B. Goodman, R. A. Murphy, K. O'Donnell, J. Sato, and S. Guptill. 2014. "Implementation and Randomized Controlled Trial Evaluation of Universal Postnatal Nurse Home Visiting." *American Journal of Public Health* 104 (Suppl 1): 136–43.

Feder, J. L. 2011. "Predictive Modeling and Team Care for High-Need Patients at HealthCare Partners." *Health Affairs* 30 (3): 416–18.

Gerdtham, U. G., P. Clarke, A. Hayes, and S. Gudbjornsdottir. 2009. "Estimating the Cost of Diabetes Mellitus–Related Events from Inpatient Admissions in Sweden Using Administrative Hospitalization Data." *Pharmacoeconomics* 27 (1): 81–90.

Goodman, R. M. 2012. "Effect of Cost Efficiency Reporting on Utilization by Physician Specialists: A Difference-in-Difference Study." *Health Service Management Research* 25 (4): 173–89.

Grazier, K. L. 2009. "Using Evidence in Integrated Chronic Care Management." In *Evidence-Based Management in Healthcare,* edited by A. R. Kovner, D. J. Fine, and R. D'Aquila, 181–187. Chicago: Health Administration Press.

Greene, J., J. H. Hibbard, and V. Overton. 2014. "A Case Study of a Team-Based, Quality-Focused Compensation Model for Primary Care Providers." *Medical Care Research and Review* 71 (3): 207–23.

Jha, A. K., E. J. Orav, A. Dobson, R. A. Book, and A. M. Epstein. 2009. "Measuring Efficiency: The Association of Hospital Costs and Quality of Care." *Health Affairs* 28 (3): 897–906.

Johnson, K. 2004. "Keeping Patients Safe: An Analysis of Organizational Culture and Caregiver Training." *Journal of Healthcare Management* 49 (3): 171–78.

Kirch, D. G., and P. G. Boysen. 2010. "Changing the Culture in Medical Education to Teach Patient Safety." *Health Affairs* 29 (9): 1600–1604.

Lee, S. Y., B. J. Weiner, M. I. Harrison, and C. M. Belden. 2013. "Organizational Transformation: A Systematic Review of Empirical Research in Health Care and Other Industries." *Medical Care Research and Review* 70 (2): 115–42.

Lemire, M., O. Demers-Payette, and J. Jefferson-Falardeau. 2013. "Dissemination of Performance Information and Continuous Improvement: A Narrative Systematic Review." *Journal of Health Organization and Management* 27 (4): 449–78.

Lin, B. Y., T. T. Wan, C. P. Hsu, F. R. Hung, C. W. Juan, and C. C. Lin. 2012. "Relationships of Hospital-Based Emergency Department Culture to Work Satisfaction and Intent to Leave of Emergency Physicians and Nurses." *Health Services Management Research* 25 (2): 68–77.

Madhavan, R., and J. T. Mahoney. 2012. "Evidence-Based Management in 'Macro' Areas: The Case of Strategic Management." In *The Oxford Handbook of Evidence-Based Management,* edited by D. M. Rousseau, 79–91. New York: Oxford University Press.

McAlearney, A. S., J. Robbins, A. N. Garman, and P. H. Song. 2013. "Implementing High-Performance Work Practices in Healthcare Organizations: Qualitative and Conceptual Evidence." *Journal of Healthcare Management* 58 (6): 446–62.

McCarthy, I. M., C. Robinson, S. Hug, M. Philastre, and R. L. Fine. 2015. "Cost Savings from Palliative Care Teams and Guidance for a Financially Viable Palliative Care Program." *Health Services Research* 50 (1): 217–36.

McMillan, S. S., E. Kendall, A. Sav, M. A. King, J. A. Whitty, F. Kelly, and A. J. Wheeler. 2013. "Patient-Centered Approaches to Health Care: A Systematic Review of Randomized Controlled Trials." *Medical Care Research and Review* 70 (6): 567–96.

Mosadeghrad, A. M., E. Ferlie, and D. Rosenberg. 2011. "A Study of Relationship Between Job Stress, Quality of Working Life, and Turnover Intention Among Hospital Employees." *Health Services Management Research* 24 (4): 170–81.

Moxham, C., N. Chambers, J. Girling, S. Garg, E. Jelfs, and J. Bremner. 2012. "Perspectives on the Enablers of E-Health Adoption: An International Interview Study of Leading Practitioners." *Health Services Management Research* 25 (3): 129–37.

National Institute for Health Research. 2016. "Health Services and Delivery Research Programme." Accessed June 20. www.nets.nihr.ac.uk/programmes/hsdr.

Otani, K., P. A. Herrmann, and R. S. Kurz. 2011. "Improving Patient Satisfaction in Hospital Care Settings." *Health Services Management Research* 24 (4): 163–69.

Platonova, E. A., and S. R. Hernandez. 2013. "Innovative Human Resource Practices in US Hospitals: An Empirical Study." *Journal of Healthcare Management* 58 (4): 290–301.

Rana, S., T. Tran, W. Lou, D. Phung, R. L. Kennedy, and S. Venkatesh. 2014. "Predicting Unplanned Readmission After Myocardial Infarction from Routinely Collected Administrative Hospital Data." *Australian Health Review* 38 (4): 377–82.

Rathert, C., M. Fleig-Palmer, and K. David. 2006. "Minimizing Medical Errors: A Qualitative Analysis of Health Care Providers' Views on Improving Patient Safety." *Journal of Applied Management and Entrepreneurship* 11 (4): 5–17.

Rousseau, D. M. 2012a. "Envisioning Evidence-Based Management." In *The Oxford Handbook of Evidence-Based Management,* edited by D. M. Rousseau, 3–24. New York: Oxford University Press.

———. 2012b. "Organizational Behavior's Contributions to Evidence-Based Management." In *The Oxford Handbook of Evidence-Based Management,* edited by D. M. Rousseau, 61–78. New York: Oxford University Press.

Shortell, S. M., J. L. O'Brien, J. M. Carman, R. W. Foster, E. F. Hughes, H. Boerstler, and E. J. O'Connor. 1995. "Assessing the Impact of Continuous Quality Improvement/Total Quality Management: Concept Versus Implementation." *Health Services Research* 30 (2): 377–401.

Shortell, S. M., N. J. Sehgal, S. Bibi, P. P. Ramsay, L. Neuhauser, C. H. Colla, and V. A. Lewis. 2015. "An Early Assessment of Accountable Care Organizations' Efforts to Engage Patients and Their Families." *Medical Care Research and Review* 72 (5): 580–604.

Sirriyeh, R., R. Lawton, G. Armitage, P. Gardner, and S. Ferguson. 2012. "Safety Subcultures in Health-Care Organizations and Managing Medical Error." *Health Services Management Research* 25 (1): 16–23.

Stefos, T., J. F. Burgess Jr., M. F. Mayo-Smith, K. L. Frisbee, H. B. Harvey, L. Lehner, S. Lo, and E. Moran. 2011. "The Effect of Physician Panel Size on Health Care Outcomes." *Health Services Management Research* 24 (2): 96–105.

Vardaman, J. M., P. T. Cornell, D. G. Allen, M. B. Gondo, I. S. Muslin, R. N. Mobley, M. E. Brock, and T. L. Sigmon. 2014. "Part of the Job: The Role of Physical Work Conditions in the Nurse Turnover Process." *Health Care Management Review* 39 (2): 164–73.

Webb, A., and E. Flaherty. 2009. "Improving Pain Management in Long-Term Care." In *Evidence-Based Management in Healthcare,* edited by A. R. Kovner, D. J. Fine, and R. D'Aquila, 161–69. Chicago: Health Administration Press.

Weeks, W. B., D. J. Gottlieb, D. E. Nyweide, J. M. Sutherland, J. Bynum, L. P. Casalino, R. R. Gilles, S. M. Shortell, and E. S. Fisher. 2010. "Higher Health Care Quality and Bigger Savings Found at Large Multispecialty Medical Groups." *Health Affairs* 29 (5): 991–97.

White, K. R. 2014. "Interview with Kenneth R. White, PhD, FACHE, Associate Dean for Strategic Partnerships and Innovation and the University of Virginia Medical Center Professor of Nursing, University of Virginia School of Nursing." By S. J. O'Connor. *Journal of Healthcare Management* 59 (1): 3–8.

Wolfman, M. 2009. "Using Evidence-Based Management to Improve Operating Room Scheduling." In *Evidence-Based Management in Healthcare,* edited by A. R. Kovner, D. J. Fine, and R. D'Aquila, 207–17. Chicago: Health Administration Press.

Wolterman, D. J. 2010. "Interview with Daniel J. Wolterman, FACHE, President and Chief Executive Officer, Memorial Hermann Healthcare System." By S. J. O'Connor. *Journal of Healthcare Management* 55 (2): 73–76.

5

ACQUIRING EVIDENCE

by Susan Kaplan Jacobs

> *"Absence of evidence is not evidence of absence."*
>
> —Carl Sagan

This chapter aims to help you achieve the following objectives:

1. Recognize that engagement with the information ecosystem calls for "metaliteracy," an overarching set of core ideas that ground a way of thinking and practicing. Such ideas are considered "threshold concepts."

2. Be familiar with the steps of evidence-based management—*asking, acquiring, appraising, aggregating, applying,* and *assessing*—and recognize that the systematic search for, and retrieval of, evidence is nonlinear and iterative.

3. Understand that an initial information-seeking inquiry, or "scoping search," may begin with secondary background sources in print materials, electronic books and evidence summaries, review articles, and other specialized syntheses that aggregate and preappraise research evidence.

4. Use results of the scoping search to ask a research question that identifies a *problem* (or *population,* or *participants* of interest) and a proposed *intervention.* These elements provide a framework for locating evidence via specialized sources.

5. Exploit the architecture of the scholarly journal literature by understanding how it is produced, indexed, organized, disseminated, and accessed via specialized article databases. Use specialized article databases and their filtering functionalities to acquire evidence from the scientific literature.

6. Be familiar with specialized critiquing tools available to appraise applicability and actionability of evidence.

Note: This chapter references the research question in the evidence-based management demonstration provided by Bryce Clark in chapter 18. Please consult that chapter for additional background.

7. Understand the legal, ethical, and social issues surrounding the use of information and the need to cite source material in a standard format.

8. Develop a standard process and framework for a team collaboration to integrate evidence with management expertise and local "organizational" concerns. Aggregate, apply, and assess evidence.

Introduction

The information landscape presents an array of choices and has an often overwhelming presence in our daily existence. Ever-changing tools, apps, platforms, and resources in multiple formats can mask the important differences that distinguish materials that are rigorously peer-reviewed, formally published, and scholarly from those that are not, and that distinguish content that is freely available from that licensed by institutions. The increasingly collaborative and socially connected environment further blurs the distinctions among resources and their credibility. Naive searchers may not discern that there are vast distinctions among "everything that appears in a browser window" (Townsend, Brunetti, and Hofer 2011). A quest to locate the "best available evidence" exists in an environment of "one-stop" search portals (e.g., web-scale tools, general search engines) that promise comprehensiveness but often return an unmanageable number of results. Defining what exactly is meant by "evidence-based management" is critical and fundamental. Following from Straus and colleagues (2011) and Dawes and colleagues (2005), Barends, Rousseau, and Briner, in chapter 1 of this book, say that evidence-based practice is about making decisions through the "conscientious, explicit, and judicious use of the best available evidence" by taking the following steps to increase the likelihood of a favorable outcome:

1. Asking (translating a practical issue or problem into an answerable question)
2. Acquiring (systematically searching for and retrieving the evidence)
3. Appraising (critically judging the trustworthiness and relevance of the evidence)
4. Aggregating (weighing and pulling together the evidence)
5. Applying (incorporating the evidence into the decision-making process)
6. Assessing (evaluating the outcome of the decision taken)

Evidence-based healthcare practice is iterative; at any step, it may require redefining or modifying the question asked and returning to earlier steps. Step 1—the effort to formulate a focused question—determines how and where the search for evidence will begin. This task is fundamental, and for most questions it needs revisiting and revision. A dissonance exists between the ubiquitous perception that information is simply keystrokes away (e.g., by conducting a search through Google or Google Scholar and cherry-picking a few articles) and the execution of a systematic, informed, reproducible literature search that results in confidence that one has conscientiously and comprehensively *acquired* the best evidence.

In chapter 1, Barends, Rousseau, and Briner also describe four sources of evidence: scientific evidence, organizational evidence (internal data), experiential evidence (expertise and judgment of the practitioner), and the values and concerns of stakeholders (who may be affected by a decision to apply evidence). This chapter will focus on the first source—the findings from empirical studies published in academic journals. It will explore the larger context surrounding the first two steps of evidence-based process practice—asking and acquiring—and it will introduce a set of recommended knowledge practices for gaining the core ideas known as "metaliteracy" (ACRL 2015). The chapter also offers practical advice about conducting the search for healthcare management evidence, locating appraisal tools, and aggregating, applying, and assessing evidence for healthcare management research.

Prerequisites to Step 1

Formulation of the research question itself requires a process of inquiry. A prerequisite to "asking" is a preliminary investigation of background information, the "state of the science," the larger scope of the topic in context, and previously published evidence. Parallel prerequisites to the process of inquiry are experience, practice, and proficiency with technological tools and the information ecosystem, all of which contribute to metaliteracy (ACRL 2015).

Metaliteracy
A search of the literature to aid decision making for a healthcare management question differs from a search to answer a clinical question. It is less specifically about a patient and more about a population or group of participants. The participants might be healthcare providers, administrators, nonprofessional caregivers, researchers, or a patient group (Jaana, Vartak, and Ward 2014). Yet the information needs of clinicians and managers are similar in that they require information literacy skills. *Information literacy* can be defined as follows:

> The set of integrated abilities encompassing the reflective discovery of informa-
> tion, the understanding of how information is produced and valued, and the use of
> information in creating new knowledge and participating ethically in communities
> of learning (ACRL 2015).

Understanding how information is arranged is a central component of metaliteracy, and it is critical to the discovery of evidence and the evaluation of
its context and value. Capably navigating among sources of evidence is recognized as one of the "threshold concepts" for information literacy—a set of
competencies that are not as intuitive as they may appear. Other than through
direct instruction, understanding of threshold concepts is developed as one
experiences, often by trial and error, the organizing principles and contexts
associated with a discipline (Townsend, Brunetti, and Hofer 2011). Both
clinicians and managers also share the additional challenge of having limited
time to conduct an evidence search.

Research as Inquiry: The Scoping Search

Translating a practical issue into an answerable question requires a preliminary scoping search of the literature—a reconnaissance mission to survey
existing studies and the state of the science. At this point in the process,
even naive search strategies and serendipitous browsing can be useful. Scoping is a process of immersion and strategic exploration, during which one
notices the features and structure of the literature (e.g., vocabulary, filters)
and browses background information about a disease, condition, or policy or
management issue. Hence, the process of developing an answerable research
question—illustrated in exhibit 5.1—is *iterative*. Preliminary results may war-
rant broadening or narrowing the scope of the question. The scoping search
may identify some focal articles—perhaps some that are highly cited in the
literature—that lead to a set of searchable terms and synonyms, illuminating
the underlying infrastructure and complexity of the information landscape.

For example, an initial broad overview question might ask, "What is
the best evidence supporting effective preoperative patient education programs?" An initial exploration would seek evidence for the broad topic of
patient education programs or perhaps uncover a set of narrower topics—for
instance, preoperative patient education programs for a certain age group or
type of procedure, video-delivered patient education, printed materials for
patient education, nurse-delivered patient education, patient educator–delivered education, online tutorials for patients, disease-specific patient education, and so on.

A first recommended knowledge practice is to discover evidence that
has already been aggregated in some form of an evidence synthesis or a
summary.

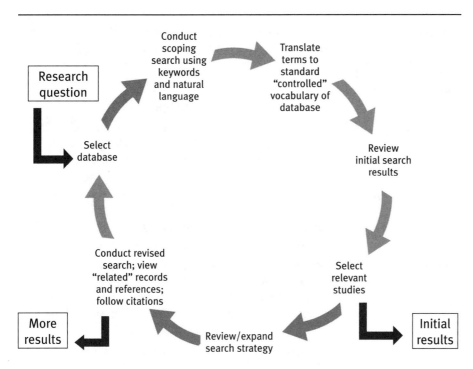

EXHIBIT 5.1
The Iterative
Nature of
Asking a
Question and
Acquiring
Evidence

Evidence Syntheses: Locating Background Information and Overviews

Evidence syntheses, summaries, review articles, critiqued abstracts, and other aggregated (often *secondary*) sources can often provide the first valuable discoveries in a search for the best evidence. Searchers are encouraged to consult books, evidence summaries, narrative reviews, and systematic review articles, such as the examples shown in exhibit 5.2. One source of systematic reviews, the Cochrane Library (www.cochranelibrary.com), offers free online searching of abstracts and serves as a good starting point for both the clinical and nonclinical aspects of a healthcare question. A rigorously conducted review will provide a summary, a critique of evidence, a synthesis, and a conclusion. In addition, a good systematic review will often include a reproducible search strategy for acquiring future evidence. A source's abstract and index terms—the descriptive *metadata*—go a long way toward defining or refining the research question, because they can point out the scope of relevant research.

In one of the sources listed in exhibit 5.2, McDonald and colleagues (2014) assemble, synthesize, and analyze 18 trials of participants undergoing a joint replacement following an educational intervention. The outcomes measured include "pain, function, health-related quality of life, anxiety, length of hospital stay, and the incidence of adverse events (e.g., deep vein

EXHIBIT 5.2
Selected
Examples
of Evidence
Syntheses for
a Research
Question

Research question: Does preadmission patient education reduce the length of stay for elective surgical patients?	
Evidence Synthesis or Background Source Type	Example
Print book	Hill, S., and Cochrane Collaboration (eds.). 2011. *The Knowledgeable Patient: Communication and Participation in Health; A Cochrane Handbook*. Chichester, UK: Wiley-Blackwell.
Electronic book collection	Source from Ebrary: MacKenzie, C. R., C. N. Cornell, and S. G. Memtsoudis (eds.). 2014. *Perioperative Care of the Orthopedic Patient*. New York: Springer. Available via http://proquest.libguides.com/ebrary.
Systematic review	McDonald, S., M. J. Page, K. Beringer, J. Wasiak, and A. Sprowson. 2014. "Preoperative Education for Hip or Knee Replacement." *Cochrane Database of Systematic Reviews*. Published May 13. http://doi.org/10.1002/14651858.CD003526.pub3.
Evidence summary of recommended practices	Slade, S. 2013. *Hip or Knee Replacement: Pre-Operative Education*. Joanna Briggs EBP Database. Available through www.ovid.com/site/catalog/databases/11299.jsp.

thrombosis)." The conclusion of the structured abstract summarizes the 88-page review and points to a more specific research question, assessing one particular outcome of interest.

Findings from the background overview for a research question can lead to a more specific search for individual studies, discussed in the next section. Additional metasearch tools and sources for evidence syntheses are suggested in exhibit 5.3.

Step 1: Asking—Translating a Practical Issue or Problem into an Answerable Question

Once some initial scoping for a broad topic has been conducted and some available syntheses have been identified, the research question can be more precisely framed to *ask* an answerable question. Background and overview questions inform narrower, more specific "foreground" questions (Straus et al. 2011). Based on the initial inquiry, a narrower research question might investigate one outcome measure—for example, "Does preadmission patient education reduce the length of stay for elective surgical patients?"

EXHIBIT 5.3
Metasearch
Tools and
Evidence
Syntheses

Health Services Research PubMed Queries
www.nlm.nih.gov/nichsr/hedges/search.html
A search interface for finding PubMed citations relating to healthcare quality
or healthcare costs; topics may include, for instance, appropriateness, process
assessment, outcomes assessment, costs, economics, qualitative research, and
quality improvement (PubMed is the interface for the US National Library of
Medicine's MEDLINE database)

TRIP
www.tripdatabase.com
A search engine for acquiring high-quality research evidence for both clinical and
nonclinical healthcare topics

McMaster Health Forum Health Systems Evidence
www.healthsystemsevidence.org
A free access point for evidence to support policymakers, stakeholders, and
researchers aiming to strengthen or reform health systems and deliver cost-
effective programs, services, and drugs to people who need them

PDQ-Evidence
www.pdq-evidence.org/en
A metasearch tool that facilitates rapid access to the best available evidence
for decisions about health systems and population health, offering systematic
reviews, overviews of reviews (including evidence-based policy briefs), primary
studies, and structured summaries of evidence (developed and maintained by
systematic searches on PubMed and other databases)

**Center for Evidence-Based Management (CEBMa) Database of Evidence
Summaries**
cebma-library.org
A continuously updated repository of syntheses of research evidence about governance, financial, and delivery arrangements within health systems, and about
implementation strategies that can support change in health systems

**Agency for Healthcare Research and Quality Evidence-Based Practice Center
(EPC) Reports**
www.ahrq.gov/research/findings/evidence-based-reports/index.html
Comprehensive information about medical conditions and healthcare technologies and strategies, generated by EPCs that review all relevant scientific literature on a wide spectrum of clinical and health services topics; EPCs also produce
technical reports on methodological topics and other types of reports

Cochrane EPOC Group
http://epoc.cochrane.org
A resource dedicated to systematic reviews of educational, behavioral, financial,
regulatory, and organizational interventions aiming to improve health professional practice and the organization of healthcare services

The PICO framework provides a structure for framing a searchable question (Straus et al. 2011). The letters *PICO* stand for

- population (or participants, patient, or problem);
- intervention;
- comparison group or standard practice; and
- outcomes.

When embarking on a literature search, focus on identifying the first two elements—*P* and *I*—which will ensure broad initial results. Including *C* and *O* terms at this point may initially limit the results retrieved and eliminate relevant citations; the limits can be added later and are discussed in the section about filtering.

The narrower question in our example—"Does preadmission patient education reduce the length of stay for elective surgical patients?"—identifies the problem (P) of "length of stay" for elective surgical patients and the intervention (I) of "preadmission patient education." In this example, the outcome (O) of interest has been specified (reduction of length of stay), and the population has been narrowed to "elective surgical patients." The comparison (C) is not specified but is understood to be an alternative intervention (e.g., education that is not delivered preoperatively or preadmission, a placebo, or no educational intervention at all).

Variations on the PICO model—with acronyms such as PICOC and PICOT—suggest additional limits to the research question for time period (T), context or circumstances (C), and other elements. Applying limits may improve the depth but decrease the breadth of initial search results (CEBMa 2015).

Step 2: Acquiring—Systematically Searching for and Retrieving the Evidence

The multidisciplinary nature of healthcare management research requires searchers to consider the wide dispersion of studies among myriad sources. Exhibit 5.4 lists selected article and web sources for discovery of the scientific literature for healthcare management. PubMed (the interface for the US National Library of Medicine's MEDLINE database) and the Science Citation Index (part of Web of Science) provide the best overall coverage of the most highly cited core journals for healthcare management; they can be supplemented by the Social Sciences Citation Index and Business Source Complete (Taylor, Gebremichael, and Wagner 2007). Health services research studies are widely dispersed and actually "constitute a tiny fraction of the MEDLINE database" (Wilczynski et al. 2004, 1179). Therefore, a searcher should consider multiple sources and have a carefully constructed search strategy that exploits the indexing language of the selected databases. The Cumulative Index to Nursing and Allied Health Literature (CINAHL) database indexes the major journals of interest to a nursing audience. PsycINFO and ABI/INFORM are interdisciplinary article databases that may be useful depending on the question asked.

Evidence-based practice sets out a clear set of steps and a variety of critiquing tools to ensure that appropriate research methodologies are employed. Nonetheless, searchers of scholarly literature often defeat these efforts at the onset and unwittingly bias their search results by neglecting to use specialized indexing sources such as those in exhibit 5.4. A general search engine such as Google or Google Scholar might be useful as a scoping tool, to help approach a new discipline or topic, to locate a known item by an author, or to discover some focal articles. But serendipitous browsing and the casual cherry-picking of results from a general web search are not only random and inefficient; they also cannot be documented and replicated. We must be cautious about the biases that such tendencies introduce.

Discovery Through Subject Terms: Translating a Focused Question to a Search Strategy

Returning to our research question—"Does preadmission patient education reduce the length of stay for elective surgical patients?"—an initial PubMed search strategy uses the problem (P) of "length of stay" and the intervention (I) of "patient education," and it links the terms with the Boolean connector *AND*. Using the *OR* connector, a searcher can broaden a search with synonyms or alternate terms (e.g., "length of stay" OR LOS). This strategy

---

EXHIBIT 5.4
Selected Resources for Locating Primary Studies and Reports About Healthcare Management Topics

PubMed (MEDLINE)
www.ncbi.nlm.nih.gov/pubmed (free public access to citations and abstracts; citations may include links to full text content in PubMed Central or open-access journals on publisher sites)
The premier source for bibliographic coverage of biomedical topics, including health administration

ProQuest Central
www.proquest.com/libraries/academic/databases/ProQuest_Central.html (requires institutional subscription)
Large multidisciplinary database that includes scholarly sources as well as newspapers and popular periodicals; includes ABI/INFORM Complete

(continued)

EXHIBIT 5.4
Selected
Resources
for Locating
Primary
Studies and
Reports About
Healthcare
Management
Topics
(Continued)

Science Citation Index and Social Science Citation Index (Web of Science)
http://ipscience.thomsonreuters.com/product/web-of-science (requires institutional subscription)
Multidisciplinary research platform with linked content citation metrics from multiple sources

Cumulative Index to Nursing and Allied Health Literature (CINAHL)
https://health.ebsco.com/products/the-cinahl-database (requires institutional subscription)
An index of nursing and allied health literature, including nursing journals and publications from the National League for Nursing and the American Nurses Association; covers a wide range of topics including nursing, biomedicine, health sciences librarianship, alternative/complementary medicine, and consumer health

Embase
www.elsevier.com/solutions/embase-biomedical-research (requires institutional subscription)
Biomedical database with journals from more than 90 countries, including many journals unique to Embase

PsycINFO
www.apa.org/pubs/databases/psycinfo (requires institutional subscription)
A collection of bibliographic records, ranging from 1806 to the present, centered on psychology and related disciplines, including medicine, psychiatry, nursing, sociology, pharmacology, physiology, and linguistics

Public Affairs Information Service (PAIS)
www.proquest.com/products-services/pais-set-c.html (requires institutional subscription)
Citations for journal articles, books, government documents, statistical directories, research reports, international agency publications, microfiche, Internet material, and more from countries throughout the world on topics related to public affairs and public administration

EBSCO Business Source Complete
www.ebscohost.com/academic/business-source-complete (requires institutional subscription)
Database covering management, economics, finance, accounting, and international business topics from 1886 to the present

Gray Literature
http://hlwiki.slais.ubc.ca/index.php/Grey_literature (information from HLWIKI International)
Materials not published commercially or indexed by major databases

is sometimes described as the "building blocks" method (Goodman, Gary, and Wood 2014). PubMed, as an initial database used, assists the search by mapping entered terms to a controlled vocabulary thesaurus—called MeSH (Medical Subject Headings)—in an attempt to disambiguate. Most specialized bibliographic databases (e.g., CINAHL, PsycINFO, Embase) have similar functionality. A search ("length of stay" OR LOS) AND "patient education" is translated, or mapped, to the standard MeSH terms "length of stay" AND "patient education as topic" (see www.ncbi.nlm.nih.gov /mesh/68010353). A sample PubMed result, with MeSH terms, publication type (PT), and abstract, is shown in exhibit 5.5 to illustrate the structure of a bibliographic database.

Complementary to the building blocks method is the "snowball method" of database searching (Goodman, Gary, and Wood 2014). From a focal article, a searcher can follow the reference list "backward" to other sources. A searcher can also use *cited reference searching* to search "forward," seeking articles that cite a seminal article or an article of particular interest (New York University Libraries 2016a). Database features that link a focal article to "similar articles" or "related articles" use metadata to "snowball" to articles that are similarly indexed. Article metrics, such as links by social media platforms, may be available.

In addition to the subject terms that describe an article, the added attributes of a citation, such as publication date, age group, and publication type (or methodology), can be instructive for the next step in search retrieval: filtering.

Advanced Searching: Filtering with Limits

One threshold concept for searchers points to knowledge of the "interrelatedness of something" (Meyer and Land 2003). An overly broad set of search results may present "too much"—a situation sometimes referred to as the "Goldilocks" dilemma. Fortunately, specialized health and business databases provide categorical filters—often presented as "limits"—that can be introduced into the iterative search process. For example, an article search can be limited to "peer-reviewed" or "research" articles in the CINAHL database. PubMed offers many more "publication type" limits, such as "multicenter study" or "clinical trial." Limits are also available for types of review articles (e.g., "systematic review," or "meta-analysis").

A published research study can be evaluated initially by noting the research methodology indicated in the citation or in the design section of the full article. Situating a primary study within the evidence hierarchy and noticing the publication type for a search result can make the structure of the literature more transparent to the searcher.

EXHIBIT 5.5

Sample PubMed
Citation

PMID- 19427164

DP - 2010 Jun

TI - Patient education before hip or knee arthroplasty lowers length of stay.

PG - 547-51

LID - 10.1016/j.arth.2009.03.012 [doi]

AB - From April 2006 to May 2007, 261 patients undergoing primary unilateral total hip arthroplasty or total knee arthroplasty were offered voluntary participation in a one-on-one preoperative educational program. Length of stay (LOS) and inpatient data were monitored and recorded, prospectively. Education participants enjoyed a significantly shorter LOS than nonparticipants for both total hip arthroplasty (3.1 +/- 0.8 days vs 3.9 +/- 1.4 days; P = .0001) and total knee arthroplasty (3.1 +/- 0.9 days vs 4.1 +/- 1.9 days; P = .001).
CI - Copyright 2010 Elsevier Inc. All rights reserved.
FAU - Yoon, Richard S
AU - Yoon RS
AD - Department of Orthopedic Surgery, Center for Hip and Knee Replacement (CHKR), New York-Presbyterian at Columbia University Medical Center, New York, NY 10032, USA.
FAU - Nellans, Kate W
AU - Nellans KW
FAU - Geller, Jeffrey A
AU - Geller JA
FAU - Kim, Abraham D
AU - Kim AD
FAU - Jacobs, Maiken R
AU - Jacobs MR
FAU - Macaulay, William
AU - Macaulay W
LA - eng
PT - Clinical Trial
PT - Journal Article
DEP – 20090508
PL - United States
TA - J Arthroplasty
JT - The Journal of arthroplasty
JID – 8703515
SB - IM
MH - Aged
MH - *Arthroplasty, Replacement, Hip
MH - *Arthroplasty, Replacement, Knee
MH - Female
MH - Humans

EXHIBIT 5.5
Sample PubMed
Citation
(Continued)

MH - *Length of Stay
MH - Male
MH - Middle Aged
MH - Osteoarthritis, Hip/*surgery
MH - Osteoarthritis, Knee/*surgery
MH - *Patient Education as Topic
MH - Preoperative Care
MH - United States
SO - J Arthroplasty. 2010 Jun;25(4):547-51. doi: 10.1016/j.arth.2009.03.012. Epub 2009May 8.

This sample PubMed citation, with selected MeSH terms highlighted, cites a journal article titled "Patient Education Before Hip or Knee Arthroplasty Lowers Length of Stay" by Yoon and colleagues (2010).
Source: National Center for Biotechnology Information, US National Library of Medicine, PubMed (2015).

Understanding the hierarchical nature of published studies is a threshold concept (Meyer and Land 2003). It is acquired as a searcher begins to contextualize evidence and realize that all evidence is not equally valid. Goodman, Gary, and Wood (2014, 324) write:

> Effective retrieval of relevant information about related concepts requires an iterative process of interrogation and refinement of queries, culminating in a unified final search statement. Along the way, evaluations are made about the relevance of records retrieved and whether and how to continue searching. Skilled searchers review retrieved records for relevant key words and use those terms and synonyms to refine their queries.

An initial search strategy should capture both the subject terms and the methodological aspects (often indicated by "publication type") of studies when gathering relevant records (Higgins and Green 2011).

Preformulated Searches and Summaries

Preformulated searches, also known as "hedges," are another tool for evidence retrieval. One of the tools listed in exhibit 5.3 is the Health Services Research (HSR) PubMed Queries site, which allows searchers to conduct a topic search followed by the application of filtering for broad categories of appropriateness, process assessment, outcomes assessment, cost, economics, qualitative research, and quality improvement. Furthermore, the searcher can select a "broad, sensitive" approach or a "narrow, specific" approach (National Information Center on Health Services Research and Health Care Technology 2013).

A number of online tutorials and learning resources are available for constructing strategies, using Boolean connectors, applying limits, using hedges, and seeking assistance in conducting a rigorous and thorough literature search. The list of references at the end of this chapter includes resources from the American Psychological Association (2016); EBSCO (2016); the National Center for Biotechnology Information, US National Library of Medicine, PubMed (2016); and the National Information Center on Health Services Research and Health Care Technology (2016).

Consulting with a health sciences librarian or a business librarian is always recommended. Librarians acting as intermediaries form "an essential part of the health care team by allowing knowledge consumers to focus on the wise interpretation and use of knowledge for critical decision making, rather than spending unproductive time on its access and retrieval" (Homan 2010, 51). The *Cochrane Handbook for Systematic Reviews of Interventions* points out the complexity of searching the literature and "highly recommends enlisting the help of a healthcare librarian when searching for evidence" (Higgins and Green 2011, section 6.3.1). Finally, there is no substitute for hands-on practice.

Steps 3 Through 6: Appraise, Aggregate, Apply, Assess

Barends's steps 3 through 6—appraise, aggregate, apply, and assess—complete the cycle of evidence-based healthcare practice. Appraisal of an article, a report, a protocol, or a printed recommendation involves the evaluation of the methodology and the source of the research. From the abstract and text of a research article, we can make an initial determination about the relevance of the subject to the research question and the level of evidence associated with the research design. We can then move on to appraise the methodology and appropriateness of the research methods. Appraisal tools should be matched to the methodology of the study. For the example in exhibit 5.5, for instance, the selection of an appraisal tool would be influenced by the publication type (PT) field that indicates "Clinical Trial." Exhibit 5.6 lists some resources for the appraisal and evaluation of evidence, including specialized tools to appraise nonrandomized controlled trials (Centers for Disease Control and Prevention 2016).

The range of healthcare evidence is often depicted hierarchically, with evidence pyramids that situate the randomized controlled trial as the gold standard for clinical medicine. However, public health, health management, and policy interventions involve groups of participants, are more complex, and do not lend themselves to that design. Studying the impact of an intervention on a community or group is complicated because groups are not as easily comparable as individuals; context becomes more important for the effectiveness of an intervention on one group or another (Kemm 2006). Thus, applying a filter for "randomized controlled trials" for a health management topic can inadvertently exclude the highest level of evidence for that topic. The best evidence may rely on a variety of research designs. Kemm (2006) points out that evidence "enlightens" health policy making rather than providing "the answer" to a problem. A focus on "methodological appropriateness" can be more helpful in assessing research involving such outcomes as "safety," "satisfaction," "cost," and other measures relevant to groups (Petticrew and Roberts 2003).

For our research question on preoperative education, outcomes such as "length of stay" and "adverse events" are measurable indicators to evaluate the preadmission intervention; however, more qualitative outcomes such as pain, postoperative anxiety, and quality of life are subjective, influenced by reporting bias, and more suited to other types of assessment. A specialized assessment tool—the Patient Education Materials Assessment Tool (PEMAT), for instance—might therefore be appropriate for evaluating the impact of patient education (Agency for Healthcare Research and Quality 2016). Specialized assessment tools range across the spectrum and should be matched to the methodology of a study.

An Overview of Knowledge Practices

As described earlier in the chapter, the iterative process of acquiring evidence involves navigation among multiple platforms, and it requires the searcher to engage in a variety of knowledge practices. The following is a list of key practices and guidelines:

- *Conduct a preliminary scoping search based on the key terms of the research question; consider preaggregated, preappraised sources, such as those suggested in exhibit 5.3.* From the reconnaissance, a searcher can begin to evaluate the breadth and depth of the evidence.
- *Frame a research question in PICO format.* Once a scoping search has established the existent evidence for an intervention, a broader or narrower research question can be identified.
- *Select an initial article database.* The major article databases for health services research journals and associated topics include PubMed (MEDLINE), Web of Science, CINAHL, EBSCO Business Source, PsycINFO, and ProQuest.
- *Develop proficiency with Boolean connectors to associate the "building blocks."* Narrow results with the Boolean *AND* and categorical

EXHIBIT 5.6

Critical
Appraisal Tools
and Resources

National Collaborating Centre for Methods and Tools
www.nccmt.ca/index-eng.html
A searchable online collection of evidence-informed methods (processes) and
tools (instruments) for knowledge translation in public health

Transparent Reporting of Evaluations with Nonrandomized Designs (TREND)
www.cdc.gov/trendstatement
A 22-item checklist specifically developed to guide standardized reporting of
nonrandomized controlled trials; complements the widely adopted CONsolidated
Standards of Reporting Trials (CONSORT) statement for randomized controlled
trials

Users' Guide to the Medical Literature
www.ncbi.nlm.nih.gov/pubmed/21098772
A resource by Fan and colleagues (2010) to guide the use of an article about
quality improvement

Critical Appraisal Skills Programme (CASP) tools
www.casp-uk.net
A collection of freely downloadable critical appraisal tools designed to be used
when reading and critiquing research; includes tools for systematic reviews, randomized controlled trials, cohort studies, case control studies, economic evaluations, diagnostic studies, qualitative studies, and clinical prediction rules

**Center for Evidence-Based Management Critical Appraisal Tools and
Questionnaires**
www.cebma.org/frequently-asked-questions/what-is-critical-appraisal
An overview of critical appraisal with links to a variety of tools and
questionnaires

limits. Use the Boolean *OR* connector to broaden a search term
with synonyms. Use available limits such as publication date, age of
participants (if relevant), methodology, and so on. Both ProQuest
and CINAHL have a "peer-reviewed" limit. CINAHL has a limit for
"research." Available search filters can go a long way toward improving
relevant article retrieval.

- *Consult database thesauri.* These resources can help you identify
  controlled vocabulary (index) terms and synonyms.
- *Exploit metadata.* Scan titles and abstracts of the initial search results.
  Notice the descriptive metadata (e.g., index terms, publication type,
  date of publication, journal type) for the most relevant results.
- *Make use of the "snowball method."* The method is complementary to
  the building blocks method, and it helps you move on from initial

search results by following the bibliography and/or cited references connected to a focal article (Goodman, Gary, and Wood 2014). Look for links to "related articles" or "similar articles," which can yield valuable related evidence.

- *Avoid cherry-picking!* Cherry-picking is random, inefficient, prone to bias, and not reproducible.

- *Start by seeking high sensitivity.* The *Cochrane Handbook for Systematic Reviews of Interventions*, which presents guidelines for comprehensive searches, states, "Searches should seek high sensitivity, which may result in relatively low precision" (Higgins and Green 2011, section 6.1).

- *Evaluate initial results for relevance, and then refine a search strategy to increase precision.* Refinements might add a search term, such as a comparative term (C), outcome measure (O), time period (T), or context/circumstances (C) following the PICO model and its variations.

- *Develop a refined and reproducible search strategy.* Keep a paper trail of the search strategy to include in a research paper appendix.

- *Locate appropriate critical appraisal tools.* Appraisal of an article, a report, a protocol, a printed recommendation, or another item begins with evaluation of the methodology and source of the research.

- *Attribute sources and cite evidence in a standard format* (e.g., APA, Vancouver). Use a citation management tool (e.g., EndNote, RefWorks, Zotero, Mendeley) to build a personal database of search results, to ease the burden of citing while writing, and to avoid inadvertent plagiarism.

- *Subscribe to alerting services for journals, publishers, and saved search strategies* (New York University Libraries 2016b).

- *Consult with a health sciences or business librarian.* Revisit the research question, review the search process, and ensure that a comprehensive and broad strategy has been used.

- *Remember that searching the literature takes work!* There is no easy way to conduct a thorough and comprehensive search for evidence. Choices are critical, beginning with keywords and question formulation, and continuing through database selection and later steps in the process.

These knowledge practices contribute to the concept of metaliteracy, and they require "ongoing adaptation to emerging technologies and an understanding of the critical thinking and reflection required to engage in these spaces as producers, collaborators, and distributors" (ACRL 2015). When they are not followed, search results can become skewed and the evidence distorted by careless decisions about search term selection, as well as by the "FUTON bias" that results from using and citing the literature that is most readily available in "full text on the net" (Wentz 2002). Practiced behavior and experience serve to avoid search bias and other problems. By applying and employing the knowledge practices outlined in this section, a more specific and precise research question can be developed and the most relevant evidence can be discovered.

Teamwork for Evidence-Based Healthcare Management

As the previous discussion points out, the framing of the research question, the discovery of evidence, assessment, appraisal, and integration into practice demand a variety of skills and knowledge practices. Like any "construction project," the process requires team collaboration. Differing levels of technological expertise and time constraints may point to the idea of identifying one team member to lead the evidence search, serve as a liaison with a healthcare librarian, and keep track of search strategies in various databases. Another team member might be charged with organizing the evidence into a shared citation management database. Critical appraisal of selected literature might be conducted by a subgroup of the team, applying inclusion or exclusion criteria to the evidence gathered. A team member with expertise as a facilitator might be designated to liaise with a client, a professor, or another consultant regarding the progress of the project, the assessment of evidence, or the need to modify the original research question or objective if necessary. The written report that synthesizes and carefully cites the published literature might be coordinated by yet another team member or group.

Efforts to embed information literacy competencies and evidence-based practice into academic curricula lend credence to the complex nature of evidence-based healthcare management. Managers can be empowered by the knowledge and expertise to navigate the hierarchy of evidence to support decision making and practice changes in the workplace. They can also gain a foundation for lifelong professional competence in the use of health services management research (Jacobs, Gano, and Kovner 2009).

Conclusion: Challenges for Locating Evidence

Searchers will encounter search portals and discovery tools that have less filtering functionality but greater recall or breadth—in other words, they lack precision, but they deliver more results. "Web-scale" tools have become increasingly available on web portals, and they deliver broader and more interdisciplinary search results, essentially promising "one-stop shopping."

However, such tools are generally inappropriate for the searchers of both healthcare and healthcare management literature. Searchers learn through the successful retrieval of evidence but also through the pitfalls they encounter; receiving false and irrelevant "hits" and revising the process can lead to a deeper understanding, the "aha!" moments, and the mastery of threshold concepts. This chapter has provided a framework to help teams engage, organize, and continually update their efforts to inform healthcare management with the best evidence available. Within this framework, essential knowledge practices are best strengthened through hands-on practice, continual engagement, collaboration, and a willingness to seek support from others.

References

Agency for Healthcare Research and Quality. 2016. "The Patient Education Materials Assessment Tool (PEMAT) and User's Guide." Updated May. www.ahrq .gov/professionals/prevention-chronic-care/improve/self-mgmt/pemat /index.html.

American Psychological Association. 2016. "Tutorials on APA Databases." Accessed March 30. www.apa.org/pubs/databases/training/tutorials.aspx.

Association of College & Research Libraries (ACRL). 2015. "Framework for Information Literacy for Higher Education." Accessed July 6. www.ala.org/acrl /standards/ilframework.

Center for Evidence-Based Management (CEBMa). 2015. "What is a PICOC?" Accessed October 26. www.cebma.org/frequently-asked-questions/what-is-a -picoc.

Centers for Disease Control and Prevention. 2016. "The TREND Statement." Updated April 15. www.cdc.gov/trendstatement.

Dawes, M., W. Summerskill, P. Glasziou, A. Cartabellotta, J. Martin, K. Hopayian, F. Porzsolt, A. Burls, and J. Osborne. 2005. "Sicily Statement on Evidence-Based Practice." *BMC Medical Education* 5 (1): 1–10.

EBSCO. 2016. "CINAHL Support Center." Accessed March 30. http://support .epnet.com/cinahl/training.php.

Fan, E., A. Laupacis, P. J. Pronovost, G. H. Guyatt, and D. M. Needham. 2010. "How to Use an Article About Quality Improvement." *Journal of the American Medical Association* 304 (20): 2279–87.

Goodman, J. S., M. S. Gary, and R. E. Wood. 2014. "Bibliographic Search Training for Evidence-Based Management Education: A Review of Relevant Literatures." *Academy of Management Learning & Education* 13 (3): 322–53.

Higgins, J. P., and S. Green (eds.). 2011. *Cochrane Handbook for Systematic Reviews of Interventions*. Updated March. http://handbook.cochrane.org.

Homan, J. M. 2010. "Eyes on the Prize: Reflections on the Impact of the Evolving Digital Ecology on the Librarian as Expert Intermediary and Knowledge Coach, 1969–2009." *Journal of the Medical Library Association* 98 (1): 49–56.

Jaana, M., S. Vartak, and M. M. Ward. 2014. "Evidence-Based Health Care Management: What Is the Research Evidence Available for Health Care Managers?" *Evaluation & the Health Professions* 37 (3): 314–34.

Jacobs, S. K., G. Gano, and A. R. Kovner. 2009. "Evidence-Based Health Services Management for Nurse Leaders: An Intracampus Partnership and Curriculum." In *Proceedings of the 10th International Congress on Medical Librarianship (ICML) 2009*. Published August/September. http://espace.library.uq.edu.au/view/UQ:179758.

Kemm, J. 2006. "The Limitations of 'Evidence-Based' Public Health." *Journal of Evaluation in Clinical Practice* 12 (3): 319–24.

McDonald, S., M. J. Page, K. Beringer, J. Wasiak, and A. Sprowson. 2014. "Preoperative Education for Hip or Knee Replacement." *Cochrane Database of Systematic Reviews*. Published May 13. http://doi.org/10.1002/14651858.CD003526.pub3.

Meyer, J., and R. Land. 2003. *Threshold Concepts and Troublesome Knowledge: Linkages to Ways of Thinking and Practising Within the Disciplines*. Enhancing Teaching–Learning Environments in Undergraduate Courses Project, University of Edinburgh. Published May. www.colorado.edu/UCB/Academic Affairs/ftep/documents/ETLreport4-1.pdf.

National Center for Biotechnology Information, US National Library of Medicine, PubMed. 2016. "PubMed Online Training." Updated March 1. www.nlm.nih.gov/bsd/disted/pubmed.html.

———. 2015. PubMed ID: 19427164. Accessed October 22. www.ncbi.nlm.nih.gov/pubmed/?term=19427164.

National Information Center on Health Services Research and Health Care Technology (NICHSR). 2016. "Outreach and Training Activities in NICHSR." Updated February 11. www.nlm.nih.gov/nichsr/outreach.html.

———. 2013. "Health Services Research (HSR) PubMed Queries." Updated September 19. www.nlm.nih.gov/nichsr/hedges/search.html.

New York University Libraries. 2016a. "Health (Nursing, Medicine, Allied Health): Cited Reference Searching." Research Guides at New York University. Accessed March 30. http://guides.nyu.edu/citedreferencesearching.

———. 2016b. "Research Guides: Alerting Services." Accessed March 30. http://guides.nyu.edu/alertingservices.

Petticrew, M., and H. Roberts. 2003. "Evidence, Hierarchies, and Typologies: Horses for Courses." *Journal of Epidemiology and Community Health* 57 (7): 527–29.

Straus, S. E., P. Glasziou, W. S. Richardson, and R. B. Haynes. 2011. *Evidence-Based Medicine: How to Practice and Teach It*, 4th ed. Edinburgh, UK: Churchill Livingstone.

Taylor, M. K., M. D. Gebremichael, and C. E. Wagner. 2007. "Mapping the Literature of Health Care Management." *Journal of the Medical Library Association* 95 (2): e58–65.

Townsend, L., K. Brunetti, and A. R. Hofer. 2011. "Threshold Concepts and Information Literacy." *Portal: Libraries and the Academy* 11 (3): 853–69.

Wentz, R. 2002. "Visibility of Research: FUTON Bias." *Lancet* 360 (9341): 1256.

Wilczynski, N. L., R. B. Haynes, J. N. Lavis, R. Ramkissoonsingh, A. E. Arnold-Oatley, and HSR Hedges Team. 2004. "Optimal Search Strategies for Detecting Health Services Research Studies in MEDLINE." *CMAJ: Canadian Medical Association Journal / Journal de l'Association Médicale Canadienne* 171 (10): 1179–85.

Yoon, R. S., K. W. Nellans, J. A. Geller, A. D. Kim, M. R. Jacobs, and W. Macaulay. 2010. "Patient Education Before Hip or Knee Arthroplasty Lowers Length of Stay." *Journal of Arthroplasty* 25 (4): 547–51.

BARRIERS TO THE USE OF EVIDENCE-BASED MANAGEMENT IN HEALTHCARE . . . AND HOW TO OVERCOME THEM

by Thomas D'Aunno

This chapter aims to advance managers' ability to overcome common barriers to the use of evidence-based decision making in healthcare organizations. In many instances, sufficient empirical evidence is available to guide managerial decision making. Some instances have less evidence available than one might like, but cases with little or no evidence for managers to draw on are rare. At a minimum, managers can, and should, take guidance from even limited available evidence. Perhaps most importantly, in the absence of evidence, managers should launch projects to create needed evidence. Still, in spite of mounting evidence to guide managerial behavior, organizational performance does not seem to be improving fast enough. In fact, the gap between what we know to work well in management and what managers actually do may be increasing (Pfeffer and Sutton 2006). What are the key barriers to the uptake of evidence-based management, and more importantly, how can these obstacles be overcome?

I divide this chapter into three parts. First, I discuss barriers to the use of evidence-based management in healthcare organizations. I argue that understanding key barriers can promote efforts to limit or overcome them—in other words, one should have a good diagnosis of the causes of a problem before one tries to solve it. Second, I discuss practices that managers can engage in to promote the use of evidence-based decision making in their work. This discussion draws heavily on recent studies about ways to improve managerial and organizational performance in the healthcare field through organizational learning (Nembhard and Tucker 2016; Selker et al. 2011). The chapter concludes by outlining initial steps to take in promoting the use of evidence-based management.

Barriers to the Practice of Evidence-Based Management

To begin, this chapter follows the definition of *evidence-based management* used by Barends (2016) and his colleagues at the Center for Evidence-Based

Management, which states that management decisions should be based on a combination of critical thinking and the best available evidence. By "evidence," Barends means information, facts, or data supporting (or contradicting) a claim, assumption, or hypothesis. Evidence may come from scientific research, internal organizational information, or even professional experience.

Drawing on a medical model of practice as an analogy, I argue that an important first step in advancing the use of evidence-based management is for managers to diagnose the factors that limit the use of evidence in decision making. Armed with an understanding of the particular barriers they face, individuals can then develop a "treatment" plan to take steps to improve behavior. Research from a variety of disciplines shows a long list of factors that limit evidence-based management and decision making (Crossan and Apaydin 2010; Damschroder et al. 2009; Meyers, Durlak, and Wandersman 2012; Rye and Kimberly 2007). For practical reasons, this section focuses only on a few of the more common and powerful factors.

Policy Contexts

Regulations and incentives put in place by federal, state, and local policies can—and often do—limit the use of evidence-based management among individual managers and organizations. Though health and health-related policies may seem distant to many managers, their effects, both direct and indirect, often are substantial. Fee-for-service payment systems, for instance, can inhibit the use of both evidence-based management and evidence-based clinical practices by encouraging the overuse of services and focusing narrowly on illness, rather than using health promotion programs (Chan et al. 2013; Powell et al. 2013). Of course, Medicare and other payers are trying to move away from payment systems that reward healthcare providers simply for the volume of services they produce; however, this reform is a work in progress.

In another important example, states that have made policy decisions not to expand their Medicaid program place financial stress on individuals who need health services, as well as on managers and clinicians who face the burden of providing uncompensated care. In turn, stress is a well-documented cause of poor decision making that, in this example, affects all involved.

In many instances, policymakers with good intentions aim to promote the use of evidence-based practices but, unfortunately, do not provide adequate support for implementation. D'Aunno and colleagues (2014), for example, show that state policies aiming to make HIV testing more routine in substance abuse treatment clinics had mixed results. On the one hand, clinics had higher rates of testing in states that followed Centers for Disease Control guidelines to streamline testing practices (e.g., by dropping pretest counseling). On the other hand, most states do not provide resources to support the costs of testing (e.g., training or hiring specialized staff members). On the whole, testing rates have declined in the past several years.

These examples highlight a general problem: The use of evidence-based management practices requires supportive policy contexts. In other words, they need policymakers and policies that take into account the resources and incentives that healthcare providers and managers need to perform effectively. To the extent that policies are not aligned with organizational capacity, managers have incentives to take shortcuts that might promote short-term efficiency at the expense of long-term performance—an objective of many evidence-based management practices.

A final point may seem obvious, but it is worth reinforcing: Healthcare organizations and their managers should not be passive recipients of policies that limit evidence-based management and clinical practice. Advocacy is needed at all levels to support evidence-based policies that can increase the effectiveness and efficiency of healthcare services.

Community and Market Environments

Community and local market environments play a significant role in inhibiting the use of evidence-based management. One important factor is the extent to which communities are characterized by social and organizational networks that have closed, as opposed to open, structures (Burt 1992). In closed networks, strong social and professional ties draw individuals to one another but limit their external focus. For instance, a closed structure might limit individuals' travel to professional conferences or participation in training and educational programs. In contrast, loose or open networks are characterized by ties among individuals that are not as strong locally. Individuals in these networks are more cosmopolitan: They travel, seek information from diverse sources, and are in contact with a more diverse set of people. Research shows that individuals and groups in open networks are more innovative and more likely to adopt evidence-based practices.

In short, strong social ties that act as "glue" in a community certainly have benefits. For instance, once individuals in a closed network decide to adopt new practices, they implement those practices more quickly and thoroughly than individuals in an open network. However, closed networks often come at the cost of the adoption and use of newer, evidence-based managerial practices.

A second feature of community and market environments that might limit the use of evidence-based practices is the extent to which the environments are competitive. Competition for scarce resources (e.g., patients with generous private insurance coverage) creates uncertainty and, often, anxiety for managers. In turn, these forces accentuate the importance of power and politics in decision making within organizations and their communities. For example, conditions in the current environment seem to have prompted an increase in hospital mergers and acquisitions. Managers have incentives to make their healthcare provider systems larger so they can use their market power to bargain with insurers for higher payment rates. However, a wealth of evidence shows that mergers among hospitals do not result in improved efficiency or quality of care (Burns et al. 2015).

Organizational Factors

Organizational culture, structure (including rules and incentives), and resources—both individually and collectively—can limit the practice of evidence-based management (Walshe and Rundall 2001). Such considerations may include managerial background, professional culture, training, and decision-making limitations. I focus below on a few particularly important factors.

Researchers have developed useful tools to measure and manage "patient safety culture"—that is, the extent to which individual members of a healthcare organization or unit share awareness of, and take responsibility for, practices (e.g., hand washing) that promote quality of care (Vogus and Sutcliffe 2007). One key element in these assessments is the extent to which individuals feel free to speak up when they sense that something is amiss that might affect patient care (e.g., when a surgeon is about to make a wrong-side incision). Edmondson (1999) labeled this element "psychological safety."

I argue that the same kind of culture is necessary for management decisions. Organizational cultures that lack psychological safety create conditions in which individual managers do not feel free to challenge one another's decision making, even when decisions are made blatantly in the absence of evidence or run counter to evidence. Cultures that stifle open discussion and the expression of differing views have produced disastrous management decisions—consider, for example, the Challenger space shuttle (Vaughan 1990) or the Bay of Pigs invasion (Janis 1982). Lack of psychological safety likely contributes to poor management decisions on a daily basis in healthcare organizations.

Organizational structure plays a similarly strong role in inhibiting evidence-based management. Structures, and related incentives, can create silos that prevent managers from seeing the effects of their decisions on organizations as a whole and, indeed, on the patients their organizations or units serve. In some ways, organizations in the modern world thrive on specialization and the structures (i.e., the division of roles and responsibilities) that support specialized work. These arrangements not only increase efficiency; they also promote the autonomy of specialized professional managers (e.g., accountants, financial analysts, marketing personnel). However, organizational designs in typical healthcare organizations also create barriers to effective communication and to the coordination of managerial work. Perhaps most perniciously, they can create divisions based on power and politics as individuals jockey for resources for themselves and their units.

Unfortunately, organizational politics are common in the healthcare field not only because of organizational designs and incentives, but also because organizational goals are often difficult to measure. Such conditions can prevent managers from receiving and providing meaningful and timely feedback on organizational performance, making learning difficult. Further, healthcare organizations typically have many stakeholders (e.g., patients and their families, professional groups, payers) whose interests do not always align.

In short, complex structures in many of today's healthcare organizations encourage competition among managers and their units, with deleterious effects on decision making. Engaging in evidence-based management in these circumstances is risky: It takes time and resources that other managers might be using to "get ahead." Why should the manager of a marketing department, for example, examine evidence for the effectiveness of an advertising campaign when she could instead be advocating for a larger share of the hospital budget for her unit?

Managers seeking to introduce evidence-based decision making and practices often face challenges that are common to individuals who seek organizational change and improvement. In particular, managers may not be rewarded if a new evidence-based practice replaces an established practice that enjoyed support from powerful groups or individuals. Indeed, in organizations with poor cultures, managers seeking change may be personally penalized if a new evidence-based practice they champion fails for some reason—even if they were not responsible for the failure.

Likewise, incentive systems for managers—including promotions, pay raises, and bonuses—often focus on individual performance rather than on individuals' contributions to team or organizational performance. Moreover, incentive systems often encourage short-term thinking and short-term efficiency at the expense of longer-term planning and effectiveness. In short, poorly designed organizational incentive systems, whether formal or informal, hamper managers' efforts to engage in evidence-based decision making in the same way that poorly designed policies limit managerial and organizational effectiveness.

Individual Managerial Factors

When we consider the increasingly well-documented, "hard-wired" limits of human decision making (Kahneman 2011), the picture darkens even more for the prospects of evidence-based management. The list of biases and decision traps that characterize human decision making and cognition seems to grow daily. For example, much research shows that individuals often engage in *confirmation bias*, or *confirmatory bias*—the tendency to search for, interpret, favor, and recall information in a way that confirms one's beliefs or hypotheses while giving disproportionately less consideration to alternative possibilities.

Fittingly, the field of *behavioral economics*, which focuses heavily on how to engineer decision making to overcome individuals' limitations, is one of the fast-growing fields in academia. Malcolm Gladwell's (2005) best seller *Blink* provides an extremely useful review of research on the limits of human decision making. He aims to show how individuals can use the limits of their decision making to their advantage, but most critics agree that this is a fool's errand.

Summary

A variety of forces—many of them complex—can stand in the way of the use of evidence-based decision making and management, both among individuals and among organizations. Proponents of evidence-based management might wonder, "Who can be against data-driven decision making?" The answer is that, sadly, no one needs to be consciously against evidence-based management to inhibit its practice. Individuals often simply engage in "business as usual" to continue suboptimal management. Fortunately, newer streams of research suggest some promising ways forward. I now turn to these approaches.

How to Increase the Use of Evidence-Based Management in Healthcare Organizations

This section draws heavily on recent studies about improving managerial and organizational performance in healthcare through organizational learning (Nembhard and Tucker 2016; Selker et al. 2011), as well as on prior work that focused on overcoming barriers to the use of evidence-based management (Pfeffer and Sutton 2006; Walshe and Rundall 2001).

My main argument is that practicing evidence-based management is a form of organizational learning (Pfeffer and Sutton 2006). Managers who generate and use evidence to make decisions are engaging in learning: They attempt to improve performance using the codified experience of others or by problem solving on the basis of data analyses they conduct themselves. By drawing on research about how to create learning organizations, we can inform our work to promote the practice of evidence-based management.

Lessons from Organizational Learning

Organizational learning is the process of creating, retaining, and transferring knowledge within an organization (Fiol and Lyles 1985; Levitt and March 1988). When learning occurs, an organization improves. Organizational improvement on any dimension, such as cost or quality of care, can occur over time because of accumulated experience. In contrast, improvement can also come from *deliberate* learning, which results from intentionally engaging in processes that aim to produce better outcomes.

Engaging in learning and evidence-based decision making is challenging for many organizations. Indeed, most organizations, especially those in rapidly changing fields, do not learn, adapt, or thrive (Argote 2012). Part of the problem stems from the difficulty that many managers have in admitting that their performance is suboptimal. Aware of the difficulty and importance of learning for organizations, management researchers have devoted significant attention to understanding drivers of successful organizational learning (Lapré and Nembhard 2010). By extension, this work also suggests several steps to increase the use of evidence-based management. We can ask: How can organizations learn to use evidence-based management?

Nembhard and Tucker (2016) suggest that managers take the following steps:

1. *Frame the use of evidence and changes in decision making as a learning experience.* Efforts to increase evidence-based management decision making will be easier if the move is framed as a learning experience. Doing so gives individuals freedom to make errors and, importantly, encourages people to examine failures to learn from them. Such a frame motivates individuals to engage in activities designed to generate learning, such as pilot tests. Managers can set aside funds to support pilot tests and similar small-scale learning exercises. Promoting evidence-based decision making as an interdependent, team endeavor rather than as an independent, performance task further facilitates learning (Edmondson 2003). As Pfeffer and Sutton (2006) write, "Celebrate and develop collective brilliance."

   Adopting a learning frame, however, can be particularly difficult in the healthcare environment, which today has greater uncertainty than it has had in the past. As a result, strong leadership is essential, particularly to prevent organizations from slipping into the habit of emphasizing performance at the expense of learning (Edmondson 2003).

2. *Foster a culture of psychological safety.* Organizations that want their managers and staff to learn to use evidence in decision making need

to develop cultures that facilitate such learning. Individuals must feel safe to engage in the "risky" activities of pointing out weaknesses and errors; such activities are necessary for learning to occur (Nembhard and Edmondson 2006; Edmondson 1999).

Research shows that organizations and groups with high psychological safety are better able to solve problems by addressing underlying causes (Tucker 2007) and to learn how to adapt new practices to their context (Tucker, Nembhard, and Edmondson 2007). In contrast, organizations that do not provide a culture safe for risk taking will likely find that managers and staff are reluctant to engage in honest discussions about weaknesses in systems and performance—even though such discussions are necessary for evidence-based decision making to take hold.

Of course, changing organizational culture takes time, often years. Leaders can begin the process by displaying the behavior that they hope to develop and providing support to others who follow their example (Schein 1992). As noted previously, validated survey instruments are available to measure the extent to which the organizational culture supports learning (Singer et al. 2012).

3. *Engage in learn-how and learn-why activities.* Studies have shown what types of activities help organizations learn. Structured improvement processes—such as experiments, plan-do-study-act cycles, and the Six Sigma method—are, at their core, efforts to learn how and why certain actions result in better outcomes. These same activities can promote evidence-based management insofar as they focus managers on data and data-driven decision making.

Pfeffer and Sutton (2006) suggest that leaders encourage learning by inviting managers to conduct their own small experiments to test the validity of proposed courses of action. Activities that allow individuals to adapt new management practices to their settings and to learn vicariously from the experiences of others are likely to yield better results.

In other words, individuals need to feel that they have the autonomy to alter evidence-based practices to fit their particular situations (Rogers 2003). Indeed, some managers may prefer to develop evidence for particular decisions using data from their own organizations, rather than draw on evidence that comes from others. Though this approach might be more time-consuming, it may yield better results because individuals tend to adopt—and maintain—solutions that they generate themselves.

4. *Invest in infrastructure and time to support evidence-based decision making.* Organizations and managers need structural support for

engaging in evidence-based decision making. This support includes, for example, processes and infrastructure that enable the creation, storage, and dissemination of information that helps the organization perform better. Just as they should provide funds to support pilot tests, healthcare organizations should set aside funds to invest routinely in support systems for evidence-based decision making. In particular, healthcare organizations and managers need information technology and measurement systems that enable information about performance to be collected, analyzed, and shared. To the extent that such processes occur, learning can happen and be rewarded, providing additional motivation for engaging in evidence-based management.

Considerable attention and resources have been focused on the adoption and use of electronic health records for clinical purposes. However, our efforts to invest in and leverage information systems to support evidence-based management decisions could be expanded. One organization that has had success with such efforts is Intermountain Healthcare, which has been a leader in using information systems that combine clinical, operations, and cost data to make management decisions (James and Savitz 2011). Another example is New York University's Langone Medical Center, which is effectively using a similar integrated information system (Huckman, Sadun, and Norris 2016).

Moreover, we should invest more not only in information technology but also in education and training for managers and staff members. Pfeffer and Sutton (2006) advocate for increasing the amount of resources that organizations devote to the continuing professional education of managers. Similarly, Walshe and Rundall (2001) note that, in healthcare, the uptake of evidence-based medicine has been better than the uptake of evidence-based management in part because medicine has a culture of integrating research and practice, which requires continuing education and training.

5. *Set realistic expectations; performance may get worse before it gets better.* Research shows that learning can produce positive outcomes, such as high rates of improvement and high organizational performance. The same can be true for evidence-based management, as I have argued, for the same reasons. However, positive results may take time, because typically a learning curve exists for the use of evidence in management decisions. The literature on learning organizations indicates that benefits usually emerge after a time of decreased performance, because organizations divert attention and resources to learning activities, which reduces the resources available for routine "production" activities (Levitt and March 1988; Nembhard and Tucker 2011).

Preparing employees and managers for the "worse-before-better" experience is an important aspect of leading any organizational change effort (Kotter 1996)—and certainly for leading efforts to increase the use of evidence-based management. Without this preparation, individuals may become discouraged when they experience decline in performance and thus slow or cease their efforts to change.

Preparing organizations for a long-term endeavor can help manage individuals' disappointment and prevent their retreat. An appropriate expectation might be, for instance, a two- to three-year window to see improvements from evidence-based management. The early months are not a waste, because organizations learn from what does not go well initially. These experiences provide insight into the mechanisms between action and results, and such insight can generate successful outcomes in the future.

6. *Use stable, cross-functional teams as the building blocks for evidence-based management.* Cross-functional teams and team learning are important vehicles for organizational change and thus for developing the practices and culture of evidence-based decision making (Fried, Topping, and Edmondson 2011).

Organizations and managers need to invest in developing the skills, incentives, and rewards for effective cross-functional management teams. Though organizations are recognizing the importance of multidisciplinary clinical teams, we are still some distance from seeing their widespread and effective use; the same certainly holds true for management. Multidisciplinary teams are critical for the success of process improvement and organizational problem solving.

As I stated earlier, evidence-based management has many similarities to process improvement, Six Sigma, and organizational problem-solving approaches. They all focus on overcoming the dysfunctions that come from complex organizational structures, division of labor, and specialization in management. Specifically, they do so by bringing together individuals who, though they have diverse roles, all have some stake in an important work process or decision (e.g., allocating budgets, deciding on opening or closing a service line, dealing with a patient safety or patient satisfaction problem).

7. *Emphasize supportive senior leadership.* All of the efforts and practices described in this section benefit from supportive senior leadership. Leadership has the authority and the influence to shape all elements of organizational design, systems, and culture. These elements should be aligned as much as possible for optimal use of evidence-based

management and organizational learning and performance. Nembhard and Tucker (2016) argue that, if structures and systems are in place to support organizational change but the culture is not receptive (or vice versa), learning is unlikely. This argument highlights the importance of alignment as organizations learn how to engage in evidence-based management.

Leaders have the responsibility to create and align the structures, systems, and culture that are needed to support organizations and managers as they learn to engage in evidence-based decision making. Research shows that support from leadership is necessary because of the risks inherent in identifying organizational weaknesses and experimenting with potential solutions to problems (Kaplan et al. 2012) and because such support influences culture (Vera and Crossan 2004).

To achieve organizational success, leaders should attend to all the items listed in this section. Shortcomings in any of these areas can be an obstacle to the uptake of evidence-based management and decision making. For evidence-based management to take root, organizations need a devoted leadership team. In particular, leaders must allow time for their own and others' reflection, which is critical for learning and easily wanes in high-pressure environments (Ancona et al. 2007). Indeed, I argue that, at least for major decisions (e.g., those that involve significant budget choices or capital allocation), leaders should routinely set aside time for systematic reflection and analysis of the processes involved in decision making. To what extent were the steps of evidence-based decision making followed? Did we ask the right questions? What data or evidence did we use to make the decision?

Conclusions

One can easily criticize the performance of the US healthcare system and healthcare organizations—and, by extension, the managers of these organizations. Of course, bringing change to these organizations is much more difficult. However, we now have a relatively good understanding of factors that inhibit organizational and managerial performance, and we are also developing a much better understanding of how to overcome these barriers. Drawing on advances in the study of organizational learning, and particularly on the excellent work of Nembhard and Tucker (2016), I have discussed several steps that managers can, and should, take to increase the use of evidence-based decision making in their organizations. I conclude with some additional observations about how to begin this journey.

One clear message involves the need to be strategic. Managers need to develop plans—including a vision and strategies to achieve it—for how they will promote evidence-based decision making at the organizational level or even on a smaller scale in units and service programs. The obstacles to success are too great to proceed without a road map.

In fact, practitioners of process improvement methods emphasize the need to ask strategic questions before beginning a project: What is the importance of the clinical process we are aiming to improve? What stakeholders need to be involved? What is the evidence that shows a gap in performance that needs to be closed? Do we have the resources (including political support) for an intervention to improve the process? Even a relatively circumscribed performance improvement project requires strategic thinking and analysis.

The available evidence about promoting organizational learning and evidence-based management indicates that the process needs strong leaders armed with sound strategy. For example, when Intermountain began its effort to improve the quality and cost of its clinical processes, the organization first identified its common procedures and its key measures of cost and quality for those procedures. This work enabled leaders to identify where to allocate scarce resources for improvement projects (James and Savitz 2011).

Walshe and Rundall (2001) provide another powerful example of a large-scale strategy to promote evidence-based management in healthcare—the Center for Health Management Research (CHMR). The CHMR consisted of a partnership among several leading healthcare systems and researchers, and the partners worked together for many years both to identify important management questions for which evidence was needed and to conduct (with the financial support of the participating systems) timely studies to address these questions. This approach promoted evidence-based management in the participating systems and beyond, as the researchers published their findings for others to draw on as well. Centers for health services research exist in many healthcare systems across the nation (e.g., Kaiser Permanente, Henry Ford, Group Health of Puget Sound), but relatively few of their studies focus on management issues (as opposed to clinical or policy matters). We need more efforts like the CHMR.

Clearly, the current environment for healthcare organizations and managers presents a number of challenges and threats to their performance and survival; however, these conditions can also stimulate new efforts for performance improvement. Managers should seize opportunities to move themselves and their organizations to learn how to make evidence-based decisions more routinely.

References

Ancona, D., T. W. Malone, W. J. Orlikowski, and P. M. Senge. 2007. "In Praise of the Incomplete Leader." *Harvard Business Review* 85 (2): 92–100.

Argote, L. 2012. *Organizational Learning: Creating, Retaining and Transferring Knowledge*. New York: Springer.

Barends, E. 2016. "A Reader's Guide to Evidence-Based Management." *Controlling & Management Review* 60 (1): 36–40.

Burns, L. R., J. S. McCullough, D. R. Wholey, G. Kruse, P. Kralovec, and R. Muller. 2015. "Is the System Really the Solution? Operating Costs in Hospital Systems." *Medical Care Research and Review* 72 (3): 247–72.

Burt, R. S. 1992. *Structural Holes: The Social Structure of Competition*. Cambridge, MA: Harvard University Press.

Chan, K. S., E. Chang, N. Nassery, H. Y. Chang, and J. B. Segal. 2013. "The State of Overuse Measurement: A Critical Review." *Medical Care Research and Review* 70 (5): 473–96.

Crossan, M. M., and M. Apaydin. 2010. "A Multi-dimensional Framework of Organizational Innovation: A Systematic Review of the Literature." *Journal of Management Studies* 47 (6): 1154–91.

Damschroder, L. J., D. C. Aron, R. E. Keith, S. R. Kirsh, J. A. Alexander, and J. C. Lowery. 2009. "Fostering Implementation of Health Services Research Findings into Practice: A Consolidated Framework for Advancing Implementation Science." *Implementation Science* 4: 50.

D'Aunno, T., H. A. Pollack, L. Jiang, L. R. Metsch, and P. D. Friedman. 2014. "HIV Testing in the Nation's Opioid Treatment Programs, 2005–2011: The Role of State Regulations." *Health Services Research* 49 (1): 230–48.

Edmondson, A. C. 2003. "Framing for Learning: Lessons in Successful Technology Implementation." *California Management Review* 45 (2): 34–54 .

———. 1999. "Psychological Safety and Learning Behavior in Work Teams." *Administrative Science Quarterly* 44 (2): 350–83.

Fiol, C. M., and M. A. Lyles. 1985. "Organizational Learning." *Academy of Management Review* 10 (4): 803–13.

Fried, B. J., S. Topping, and A. C. Edmondson. 2011. "Teams and Team Effectiveness in Health Services Organizations." In *Shortell and Kaluzny's Health Care Management: Organization Design and Behavior*, edited by L. Burnes, E. Bradley, and B. Weiner, 221–48. Clifton Park, NY: Delmar Cengage Learning.

Gladwell, M. 2005. *Blink: The Power of Thinking Without Thinking*. New York: Little, Brown and Co.

Huckman, R. S., R. Sadun, and M. Norris. 2016. "Weathering the Storm at NYU Langone Medical Center." *Harvard Business School Case* 616-026. Boston: Harvard Business School.

James, B. C., and L. A. Savitz. 2011. "How Intermountain Trimmed Health Care Costs Through Robust Quality Improvement Efforts." *Health Affairs* 30 (6): 1185–91.

Janis, I. L. 1982. *Groupthink: Psychological Studies of Policy Decisions and Fiascoes.* Boston: Houghton Mifflin.

Kahneman, D. 2011. *Thinking, Fast and Slow.* New York: Farrar, Straus and Giroux.

Kaplan, H. C., L. P. Provost, C. M. Froehle, and P. A. Margolis. 2012. "The Model for Understanding Success in Quality (MUSIQ): Building a Theory of Context in Healthcare Quality Improvement." *BMJ Quality & Safety* 21 (1): 13–20.

Kotter, J. P. 1996. *Leading Change.* Boston: Harvard Business School Press.

Lapré, M. A., and I. M. Nembhard. 2010. "Inside the Organizational Learning Curve: Understanding the Organizational Learning Process." *Foundations and Trends in Technology, Information and Operations Management* 4 (1): 1–103.

Levitt, B., and J. G. March. 1988. "Organizational Learning." *Annual Review of Sociology* 14 (1): 319–34.

Meyers, D. C., J. A. Durlak, and A. Wandersman. 2012. "The Quality Implementation Framework: A Synthesis of Critical Steps in the Implementation Process." *American Journal of Community Psychology* 50 (3–4): 462–80.

Nembhard, I. M., and A. C. Edmondson. 2006. "Making It Safe: The Effects of Leader Inclusiveness and Professional Status on Psychological Safety and Improvement Efforts in Health Care Teams." *Journal of Organizational Behavior* 27 (7): 941–66.

Nembhard, I. M., and A. L. Tucker. 2016. "Applying Organizational Learning Research to Accountable Care Organizations." *Medical Care Research and Review* 73 (6): 673–84.

———. 2011. "Deliberate Learning to Improve Performance in Dynamic Service Settings: Evidence from Hospital Intensive Care Units." *Organization Science* 22 (4): 907–22.

Pfeffer, J., and R. I. Sutton. 2006. *Hard Facts, Dangerous Half-Truths, & Total Nonsense: Profiting from Evidence-Based Management.* Boston: Harvard Business School Publishing.

Powell, A. A., H. E. Bloomfield, D. J. Burgess, T. J. Wilt, and M. R. Partin. 2013. "A Conceptual Framework for Understanding and Reducing Overuse by Primary Care Providers." *Medical Care Research and Review* 70 (5): 451–72.

Rogers, E. M. 2003. *Diffusion of Innovations.* New York: Free Press.

Rye, C. B., and J. R. Kimberly. 2007. "The Adoption of Innovations by Provider Organizations in Health Care." *Medical Care Research and Review* 64 (2): 235–78.

Schein, E. H. 1992. *Organizational Cultures and Leadership.* San Fransisco: Jossey-Bass.

Selker, H., C. Grossmann, A. Adams, D. Goldmann, C. Dezil, G. Meyer, V. Roger, L. Savitz, and R. Platt. 2011. *The Common Rule and Continuous Improvement in Health Care: A Learning Health System Perspective.* Washington, DC: National Academies Press.

Singer, S. J., S. C. Moore, M. Meterko, and S. Williams. 2012. "Development of a Short-Form Learning Organization Survey: The LOS-27." *Medical Care Research and Review* 69 (4): 432–59.

Tucker, A. L. 2007. "An Empirical Study of System Improvement by Frontline Employees in Hospital Units." *Manufacturing & Service Operations Management* 9 (4): 492–505.

Tucker, A. L., I. M. Nembhard, and A. C. Edmondson. 2007. "Implementing New Practices: An Empirical Study of Organizational Learning in Hospital Intensive Care Units." *Management Science* 53 (6): 894–907.

Vaughan, D. 1990. "Autonomy, Interdependence, and Social Control: NASA and the Space Shuttle Challenger." *Administrative Science Quarterly* 35 (2): 225–57.

Vera, D., and M. Crossan. 2004. "Strategic Leadership and Organizational Learning." *Academy of Management Review* 29 (2): 222–40.

Vogus, T. J., and K. M. Sutcliffe. 2007. "The Safety Organizing Scale: Development and Validation of a Behavioral Measure of Safety Culture in Hospital Nursing Units." *Medical Care* 45 (1): 46–54.

Walshe, K., and T. G. Rundall. 2001. "Evidence-Based Management: From Theory to Practice in Health Care." *Milbank Quarterly* 79 (3): 429–57.

LEARNING FROM OTHER DOMAINS

by Denise M. Rousseau and Brian C. Gunia

Evidence-based management (EBMgmt) represents a specific area of evidence-based practice (EBP)—one that is relatively new and not yet as thoroughly developed as evidence-based medicine and certain other EBP fields. However, to the best of our knowledge, the critical conditions for the use of evidence-based management resemble those that apply in other areas of evidence-based practice. In this chapter, we look to other domains as we connect basic research findings about evidence-based practice with innovations in teaching and practicing evidence-based management.

Three Conditions: Ability, Motivation, and Opportunities

A chapter in the *Annual Review of Psychology* reports on three critical conditions found in the research literature on evidence-based practice: the practitioner's *ability*, *motivation*, and *opportunities* to engage in EBP-related activities (Rousseau and Gunia 2016). These conditions reflect the general *AMO model* for workplace behavior (Ajzen 1991; Vroom 1964), and they apply in medicine, nursing, policing, and a host of other areas that engage in evidence-based practice. In management, notions of ability, motivation, and opportunity denote the skill of professional managers in making use of both scientific and local evidence (e.g., organizational indicators, big data) in their workplace decisions.

Ability to Practice

Two types of capabilities influence an individual's ability to use evidence in organizations. The first are the *foundational competencies*—the general skills and knowledge needed to engage in all aspects of evidence-based practice. The second are *functional competencies*—the specific skills and knowledge related to the use of particular kinds of evidence.

Foundational Competencies

The foundational competencies include the ability to think critically and apply technical knowledge acquired through education and practice experience (Sackett et al. 2000). Critical thinking makes it possible for practitioners to "think about how they think," recognize their oversights and biases, and cultivate deeper insights into the situations they face. Importantly, critical thinking lowers the likelihood that a manager will stop the search for an appropriate course of action after coming up with a minimally satisfactory answer. Critical thinking encourages the manager not to simply come up with a quick fix but to obtain more complete information that can override the biases driving initial reactions or impulses. In doing so, critical thinking motivates managers to seek both scientific and organizational evidence to answer practice-related questions. Conversely, people who are unable to think critically are inclined toward naive realism and take the information at hand at face value. Insufficient critical thinking leads to a preference for intuitive decisions (Dawes 2008) and a downplaying of opportunities to use high-quality evidence (cf. Highhouse 2008; Lilienfeld, Lohr, and Olatunji 2008).

Another foundational competency for evidence-based practice is *technical expertise*—that is, the domain knowledge specific to a given field. Domain knowledge helps practitioners make appropriate judgments, recognize incomplete information, evaluate evidence quality, and interpret new evidence (Ericsson and Lehmann 1996). Deep domain knowledge also works in combination with critical thinking skills to improve decision quality. Indeed, critical thinking in the absence of domain knowledge may not be particularly helpful. Further, domain knowledge is likely to influence the adoption of evidence-based practice because managers who are well educated in their fields are less likely to hold inaccurate beliefs in the first place. Educated and experienced human resource managers, for example, are less likely than less-trained counterparts to trust their own potentially biased intuitions (Highhouse 2008; Rynes, Colbert, and Brown 2002). In sum, foundational competencies such as critical thinking and technical knowledge are necessary to excel as a practitioner—especially as an evidence-based practitioner.

Functional Competencies

The functional competencies are the specific skills and knowledge related to EBP activities—for instance, acquiring, evaluating, and interpreting evidence. Evidence-based managers need to be able to identify information needs as they arise, translate them into potentially answerable questions, and acquire the evidence needed to find answers. The managers must then critically evaluate the quality and applicability of evidence and use the most appropriate evidence to inform their actions. Still other skills may be necessary depending on the kind of evidence involved. Use of scientific evidence requires familiarity with scientific databases and a sufficient understanding of research design issues to judge evidence quality. Use of organizational evidence requires managers to know how to measure or obtain reliable and valid data on organizational factors and outcomes.

Statistical reasoning is the ability to think about and accurately understand data, from basic observations to numerical indicators, in terms of probability and related statistical concepts. This form of reasoning is particularly important for the acquisition and accurate interpretation of organizational data. If statistical reasoning is lacking, practitioners may tend to rely on organizational data that are most familiar or most consistent with their intuitions. Related to statistical reasoning is the capacity to engage in quantitative analysis of data.

Evidence-based decision processes require a repertoire of capabilities. For familiar or repeat decisions, evidence-based decision making might involve the development of procedures, routines, and checklists that capitalize on what is already known about effective practice (Gawande 2010). From Taylor's Scientific Management to the Toyota Production System, the need to standardize a process in order to improve it has often been noted (Monden 2011; Taylor 1914). A key benefit of standardized procedures is that they facilitate the practitioner's ability to measure outcomes and take action based on feedback. In contrast, for rare but consequential situations (e.g., responses to unanticipated effects of climate change), research on responses to unique events supports the value of learning by doing and experimentation (Weick and Sutcliffe 2011).

The functional skills of acquiring, appraising, and interpreting evidence are of foremost importance in evidence-based practice. Naturally, acquisition of evidence is easiest in areas where evidence has been integrated into systematic reviews and evidence summaries; however, the availability of reviews and summaries tends to be greater in fields with longer EBP experience, and management is not one of those fields. Less systematic attention has been given to the acquisition of local, stakeholder, or experiential evidence, although gathering these forms of evidence via interviews, focus groups, and other methods is typically an important part of the EBP diagnostic process. Acquisition can also entail running local experiments and using in-house databases for monitoring outcomes (Davenport, Harris, and Morison 2010; Kovner, Fine, and D'Aquila 2009). As in the case of scientific evidence, the ability to acquire local evidence depends on the abilities of the practitioner (e.g., analytical ability) as well as on features of the local infrastructure, such as high-quality data and control systems (Davenport, Harris, and Morison 2010) and support from senior leadership for data acquisition (Kovner, Fine, and D'Aquila 2009).

The task of searching academic literatures to locate the best available research evidence is central to the practice of evidence-based management, yet information search is an ill-structured, complex cognitive activity that people typically do not do well (Rynes, Rousseau, and Barends 2014). Although internet search engines such as Google Scholar are powerful supports for evidence-based practice, studies of bibliographic search logs consistently find that queries composed by university and public library patrons are flawed. Many searchers use too few search terms, fail to make proper use of Boolean operators, and misunderstand the system in use. Studies of search training efforts of various types and scales have shown that such training can be effective in promoting evidence-based practice (Goodman, Gary, and Wood 2014).

Many practitioners also have difficulty appraising evidence quality; in fact, some find the appraisal of evidence to be more difficult than finding it in the first place (McCluskey and Lovarini 2005). For scientific evidence, this difficulty persists despite the existence of systematic reviews, because many reviews fail to qualify their conclusions based on evidence quality (Berkman et al. 2013). Guidelines and checklists for appraising research quality have been found to improve the accuracy of scientific evidence appraisals (e.g., Downs and Black 1998; Sackett et al. 2000). Additionally, Eric Barends of the Center for Evidence-Based Management has developed a mobile application, called the CAT (Critically Appraised Topic) app, which helps practitioners recall the critical questions to ask themselves when reviewing evidence of various types. In contrast, little guidance exists for appraising local organizational evidence, practitioner experience, or stakeholder perspectives, leaving such appraisals up to individual judgment.

Having high-quality evidence is not the same as having answers. Practitioners have to deal with any discrepant evidence, in addition to interpreting and applying the available evidence to their own situations. When existing evidence does not correspond to the situations practitioners confront, evidence-based practice becomes more difficult. Additionally, in some cases, the published scientific evidence on interventions may not be detailed enough to guide actual use. Glasziou and colleagues (2008) reviewed 80 studies chosen for their importance to evidence-based medicine and found that only half of the studies' methods sections were clear and comprehensive enough to enable clinicians to reproduce the intervention.

Practitioners have to adapt evidence from the simpler controlled conditions of scientific research to the more complicated conditions of practice. In many cases, they may also need to adapt the best available evidence from an altogether different field or discipline. For instance, patient safety practitioners learn from airline safety research (Denham et al. 2012), and veterinarians regularly adapt findings from human medicine (Roudebush et al. 2004). Scholars have noted, however, that transferring knowledge between disciplines may require a different paradigm than creating new knowledge (Watson and Hewett 2006); it also may require different practitioner skills.

Once a practitioner has acted based on evidence, she must then evaluate the outcome. However, meaningful outcome assessment requires the practitioner to prepare in advance by obtaining a relevant and reliable baseline measure (e.g., pretest measures of infection rates, customer complaints, employee satisfaction, or retention). The need for assessment applies both in the application of scientific and organizational evidence and in circumstances where no evidence was available. In the latter case, the practitioner can complete only the last step of the EBP process: assessing the outcome. Still, by providing the practitioner with feedback, this last phase of the EBP process permits valid learning based on experience. Overall, functional competencies allow practitioners to engage in all relevant aspects of evidence-based practice, from asking questions to assessing outcomes.

Several measurement instruments have been developed to assess the functional competencies of evidence-based managers, at least with regard to the use of scientific evidence. The Fresno test, which assesses how well people perform each component of evidence-based practice rather than relying on self-reports, is widely used in evaluation (McCluskey and Bishop 2009). As EBP becomes more sophisticated within a given discipline, additional functional skills may become important, possibly necessitating practitioner participation in research (e.g., Scurlock-Evans, Upton, and Upton 2014). At the same time, training in evidence acquisition and use is not likely to lead to actual behavior change unless individuals are motivated to do so (McCluskey and Lovarini 2005).

As with any other critical capability, organizations need to track the ability of their managers to exercise evidence-based management's foundational and functional competencies. Tracking enables organizations to assess adequacy, target development, and ensure that people with proper competencies are making the important decisions (Boudreau and Ramstad 2007).

Motivation to Practice

Motivation, the drive to engage in EBP-related behaviors, is a function of three kinds of beliefs (Ajzen 1991; Rousseau and Gunia 2016):

1. *Behavioral beliefs* represent a favorable or unfavorable attitude toward the behaviors.
2. *Perceived behavioral control* reflects an individual's belief that he is capable of the behaviors.
3. *Normative beliefs* reflect perceived social norms regarding the commonality of the behaviors.

The individual's intention to perform a behavior is expected to be strongest when all three beliefs are high.

Behavioral Beliefs

Behavioral beliefs in evidence-based management reflect the extent to which EBP behaviors are seen as beneficial. The appeal of evidence-based practice in general has been linked to beliefs in its benefits (Aarons 2004), and more knowledgeable practitioners are more likely to see evidence-based management as beneficial (e.g., Melnyk et al. 2004). Conversely, where introduction of evidence-based practices costs the manager either economically or psychologically, resistance is more likely (Ajzen 1991). For example, managers tend to resist the introduction of structured hiring practices that simply reduce their control over who gets hired (Bozionelos 2005). For this reason, trying to replace a non-evidence-based practice with an evidence-based practice is easier when the new practice brings the user benefits (Bates et al. 2003).

When leading interventions and change-management efforts, high-level managers often must promote evidence-based practice by driving changes in thinking and behavior (Bates et al. 2003). Consistent with this idea, use of an EBP mentor can improve people's perception of benefits, knowledge, and practice (Melnyk et al. 2004). Additionally, ties to favorable EBP opinion leaders outside the organization increase EBP's perceived benefits and people's openness to innovation—a disposition that contributes to positive EBP attitudes (Aarons 2004). Whatever their source, then, behavioral beliefs that evidence-based practice is beneficial contribute to its active adoption.

Perceived Behavioral Control

Perceived behavioral control reflects the manager's confidence in her ability to manifest EBP behaviors—which differs from actual ability, as discussed previously. Education in evidence-based practice typically increases self-perceived knowledge and skills (e.g., Haas et al. 2012), and ongoing supervisory support following EBP training appears to heighten these effects (Beidas and Kendall 2010). In sum, perceived behavioral control is related to training and support that strengthen practitioners' beliefs in their abilities, thus promoting their self-efficacy as evidence-based practitioners.

Normative Beliefs

Normative beliefs in evidence-based management reflect the extent to which a manager believes that practicing in an evidence-based way is normal or common. Such norms can reflect the manager's education and training, as well as the education and training of coworkers. In work groups that share the belief that evidence-based management is difficult, individuals are less likely to view it as normative (Dalheim et al. 2012). Norms related to evidence-based management, as well as other motivational beliefs, are also shaped by broad organizational and institutional cultures. Leadership support helps to legitimize evidence-based management and promotes its complementarity with practitioner experience (Melnyk et al. 2012). Similarly, the support of professional peers encourages the uptake of innovations generally, and evidence use in particular (Ferlie et al. 2005).

Roles that encourage practitioners to participate in or conduct their own research make evidence-based practice more acceptable (Kothari and Wathen 2013; Melnyk and Fineout-Overholt 2011). In promoting evidence-based management, one difficulty may be that today's practitioners are generally less involved in research than were past practitioners, as observed in organizational psychology (Anderson, Herriot, and Hodgkinson 2001). This decline may be attributed to the greater time and competitive pressures facing today's organizations. Such pressure can discourage activities that are more long-term or developmental in nature. Overall, normative beliefs trace to an array of organizational and institutional factors and—along with behavioral beliefs and perceived behavioral control—can exert a strong influence on the decision to engage in evidence-based practice.

Evidence from a large-scale survey of managers in the Netherlands and the United States (Barends 2015) suggests that educated professional managers do consider scientific research useful in their management practice, at levels at least as high as other sources. However, the problem remains one of ease of access, particularly considering that summaries of scientific findings relevant to managerial practice are not readily available. This lack of readily available information contrasts with the Cochrane Library used by clinicians in medicine and WebMD available to the larger public. Building practitioner capacity to conduct rapid evidence reviews for themselves and developing online summaries of management evidence are important concerns for the future of evidence-based management.

Opportunity to Practice

Opportunity to practice refers to the structural and resource support that an organization provides for EBMgmt activities. Ability and motivation are less likely to lead to actual behavior change if individuals do not also have the wherewithal to practice—including but not limited to access to relevant evidence and the resources (e.g., time, social support) to enable its interpretation and application. A sense that practice conditions interfere with evidence-based practice is often called the "reality of practice" (Novotney 2014). Opportunity to practice is linked to on-the-job autonomy and flexibility, which creates control over one's practice (Belden et al. 2012). It is also linked to the absence of extreme demands such as high time pressure; such demands may increase reliance on intuition (e.g., Dalheim et al. 2012).

Additionally, practitioners sometimes feel that their opportunity to practice is limited because large heterogeneous caseloads can limit the accessibility of relevant evidence and decision supports (Hoagwood et al. 2001). Another constraint on opportunity to practice is a lack of supervisory support (Melnyk et al. 2012). When supervisors are supportive, practitioners can encourage the development of evidence-informed guidelines and protocols, make time at meetings to discuss evidence use, and use evidence in their own decisions. A key facilitator of the opportunity to practice is psychological safety, the shared belief among group members that the setting is safe for risk-taking. Psychological safety increases the likelihood that people will engage in the experiential learning needed to adapt evidence-based practices to the work setting (Tucker, Nembhard, and Edmondson 2007).

As practitioners gain experience with evidence-based practice, they tend to report fewer perceived practice barriers. Specifically, research involving practitioner skill level suggests a link between EBP self-efficacy and the perception that the setting provides opportunities to practice (Melnyk et al. 2004). Additionally, experience with EBP can help individuals and their organizations learn to adapt evidence to practice and develop decision supports that ease evidence use (Zanardelli 2012).

Institutional or infrastructure supports from beyond the immediate work setting also can increase the opportunity for evidence-based practice. The development of online search portals and research databases (e.g., the Cochrane Library of Evidence Summaries) has greatly advanced professionals' access to scientific research. In the early years of evidence-based practice, information in such databases was largely geared toward basic questions about what works. In more recent years, systematic reviews have emerged that use new approaches and address a broader array of questions involving such issues as cost-effectiveness, risks associated with interventions, and implementation concerns (Lavis et al. 2005). This expansion of review topics is aided by the development of practice-oriented research, which investigates the practice conditions that serve as EBP barriers and facilitators (Castonguay et al. 2013). In sum, we are developing a good understanding of the factors that increase opportunity to practice and an appreciation that, without the opportunity to practice, the ability and motivation to practice may not be enough.

New Initiatives that Open Possibilities for Evidence-Based Management

As this review has revealed, practitioners' ability, motivation, and opportunity represent the major facilitators of, and barriers to, EBMgmt implementation. At the same time, scholars have proposed a variety of approaches for surmounting implementation challenges. In this section, we highlight several.

Taking Evidence-Based Management Training Online: Increasing Practitioner Ability and Motivation

In 2014, Eric Barends and Denise Rousseau began collaborating with Carnegie Mellon University's Open Learning Initiative (OLI), a project funded by the Studer Group. OLI develops innovative online courses with the goal of building high-quality training modules based on the latest research on effective learning. As part of this process, OLI conducts original research to improve learning and transform higher education. The core concepts that OLI implements come from Carnegie Mellon's research on cognitive tutoring, a key principle of which is the provision of ongoing feedback to learners as they work through problems. The feedback helps learners identify and correct incorrect assumptions and clarify understanding of important learning principles.

The OLI course "Evidence-Based Practice in Management and Consulting" introduces students to the basic concepts and skills of evidence-based practice. The course's website states (OLI 2016):

> The course is directly relevant to students who would like to improve the quality and outcome of their decision-making. Managers and consultants are required to take action based on their decisions, and such decisions may have profound effects on employees, customers and clients, the organization, and society more widely. But how good are such decisions? How can we ensure that managers and consultants get hold of, accurately interpret, and make use of the best available evidence in their decision making? This course will help students develop the practical skills managers and consultants need to bring evidence-based approaches to their organization. In the process of developing these skills you will also find out a lot about management research.

Topics in the course include critical thinking, identifying and gathering best available evidence, appraisal of the quality of evidence, and applying different forms of evidence to decision making. To date, "Evidence-Based Practice in Management and Consulting" has been used in EBMgmt classes at Carnegie Mellon and elsewhere, with students noting an increase in specific skills (e.g., assessing evidence quality) and increased awareness of opportunities to apply EBMgmt concepts. The CAT app, developed by Barends, supports the critical appraisal of scientific evidence taught in these courses.

The BIG Initiative: Promoting the Opportunity to Practice

One promising program at Johns Hopkins University is the Business in Government (BIG) Initiative, housed at the Carey Business School. The initiative creates a dialogue between the business school and groups within the US federal government about evidence-based principles that help organizations work better. Specifically, it seeks to help governmental organizations, such as executive agencies, learn, access, and implement evidence-based principles while generating novel organizational research and evidence. Although BIG entails multiple activities, one that has shown particular promise for surmounting implementation challenges is the research partnership.

A research partnership starts when a practitioner in a federal government organization identifies a tangible challenge to an organization's effectiveness and describes it to an organizational researcher. The practitioner's description typically uses everyday organizational terms—for instance, motivation is too low, turnover is too high, or a process is too slow. The researcher then works with the practitioner to clarify the problem, obtaining input and buy-in for a study to resolve the problem.

The researcher next identifies an appropriate theoretical framework for addressing the problem, along with one or more interesting and unanswered research questions, answers to which could both solve the problem and provide theoretical insight. The practitioner and researcher discuss and design a relevant research study, which the researcher executes with input from the practitioner. At the end of the study, the researcher shares and summarizes the data with the practitioner, who aids in the interpretation.

As a result of the partnership, the practitioner and the organization have direct evidence that they can incorporate into decision making as appropriate. Assuming novel and interesting results, the researcher also has the opportunity to publish the findings, sanitized of any identifying details. This approach has shown promise for solving diverse issues of organizational effectiveness at a range of federal government organizations.

We believe this approach solves several challenges of ability, motivation, and opportunity and thus merits further attention. In particular, the approach solves problems of ability by outsourcing most research abilities to the researcher. Under the model described, the practitioner is not expected to have many foundational or functional EBP competencies other than critical thinking, domain knowledge, and a basic respect for evidence.

The approach solves several motivational challenges by rooting the process in a real problem that is troubling the practitioner. Motivation to solve such problems tends to be high, so practitioners tend to have positive behavioral beliefs toward changes that will address the issue. We should note, however, that normative beliefs can remain a challenge, because the approach is new and thus not particularly likely to be supported by others in the setting. A major challenge lies with convincing key decision-makers of the approach's legitimacy.

Finally, the BIG approach solves problems of opportunity by placing relatively low demands on the practitioner. In essence, all the practitioner needs to do is clearly identify the problem, obtain internal buy-in for the research study, provide input throughout the process, and promote buy-in of the results at the end. None of these steps is easy or time-free—the steps concerning buy-in can be especially time-consuming—but they require much less effort or time than a full-blown, practitioner-driven effort to implement evidence-based principles on their own. The research partnership model represents one among many ways of surmounting the ability, motivation, and opportunity challenges that stand in the way of EBMgmt implementation.

AMO Lessons from Evidence-Based Policing: It's All About Implementation

Imagine having an evidence base camp, an annual meeting where the leading implementers of evidence-based management could discuss evidence about effective practice and identify important topics for review. This kind of evidence base camp actually does exist in the field of evidence-based policing.

The Eighth Annual Conference on Evidence-Based Policing took place in July 2015 in Cambridge, England. It was organized and led by Professor Larry Sherman, the world-renowned criminologist whose research has led to such important concepts as "crime hot spots," which aim to reduce crime by focusing police efforts on high-frequency locales, and "restorative justice" between offenders and victims, which aims to reduce the likelihood of repeated offense. Sherman has led the movement toward evidence-based policing to improve expertise and effectiveness via experiments and experience (Sherman 2013).

Practitioners and researchers in fields related to crime and policing gathered at the Cambridge conference to share their practices and research into efficacy and implementation. A key point presenters make is that, like people in other professions, police officers generally prefer to rely on experience rather than research; so when research is part of their experience, they are more likely to use it.

Policing as a field has made considerable progress over the past few decades in terms of conducting randomized controlled trials to evaluate effectiveness of policing interventions (Sherman 2013). Peter Neyroud, a former police superintendent completing his doctorate at Cambridge, has identified 107 randomized controlled trials since 1970 dealing with policing interventions (and at least 30 more in the pipeline), which he believes can serve as a good base of knowledge for the field. Neyroud emphasizes that treatment integrity—that is, the extent to which specific procedures are followed—is important to the effects of police practices. An understanding of the "best conditions" or success factors increases the likelihood of desired outcomes; designed treatments are rarely delivered 100 percent.

The Cambridge conference showcased a variety of randomized controlled trials evaluating the effects of innovative policing practices. One, the Philadelphia Policing Tactics Experiment (Groff et al. 2015), examined the effects of three approaches—foot patrol, offender-focused policing, and problem-oriented policing—in hot spots where incidents of crime had been high. Its findings included evidence of a 23 percent reduction in violent crime where offender-focused policing was applied (compared to controls with regular policing tactics). In addition, the community where the policing practices were studied reacted positively to a focus on repeat offenders. This study represents an important example of EBP research because it demonstrates not only what works but also whether one tactic is better than others.

Other randomized controlled trials described at the conference dealt with the use of body-worn cameras. One trial was by Barak Ariel in California, and another was by Paul Drover and Jayne Sykes in the United Kingdom. The body-worn cameras record everything from the officer's perspective, including what the officer says and sees from the very beginning (unlike a bystander's story, in which the outset of an incident is often missed). In addition to talking about findings from the perspectives of the police, police unions, and the public, the researchers emphasized that a good deal of practical attention was given to promoting consistent use of the cameras, including efforts to develop muscle memory for turning the cameras on. To make participating in the experiment easier for busy police officers, the police researchers report avoiding terms such as "treatment" and "control," using "cameras on" and "cameras off" instead.

A common theme across a variety of presenters at the conference involved the conditions that promote the uptake and use of evidence-based policing. Such conditions include the involvement of a respected and powerful advocate, an evolutionary (not revolutionary) perspective to implement practices incrementally, and opportunities presented by external demands. When implementing EBP programs, having an official unit to serve as an organizational or agency resource—responsible for spreading evidence-based practice, supporting research in the organization, and coordinating next steps—was found to be valuable. In addition to providing oversight in the shift toward evidence-based policing, this unit may also invite proposals for projects and lend advice and support.

Presenters at the conference noted the value of in-house peer review in establishing processes for improving research protocols. In this area, an organization might benefit from ties with academics, such as embedded PhD-level criminologists who can review projects and support EBP education. Improved oversight may also help with the assessment of police activity. Police are no different from anybody else and dislike filling out extra forms. Therefore, the idea of designing assessment into the work can constitute the beginning of a more systematic and integrated data warehouse, in which metrics are linked to an organization's existing information-gathering systems.

Training programs are widespread, and they often begin with senior leadership and cascade down. In the United Kingdom, key leaders in policing are selected to complete Cambridge University's master's degree program in evidence-based policing, which has a thesis requirement. Completing the thesis serves as a way of training the trainers, so that graduates are then able to train others to do their own local policing research. Evidence-based policing can be an important part of onboarding efforts; Trinidad and Tobago incorporates 24 hours of evidence-based training for new recruits.

Additional resources to promote evidence-based policing include websites to educate both organization members and the public and ongoing reviews of existing practice to see how they comport with both external and internal evidence. Of course, senior leaders must reward units and individuals for engaging in evidence-based practice. In policing, such rewards are particularly important because they offset people's common tendency to use blame and punishment.

A last lesson from the conference involved the importance of social networks. Evidence-based practice is a social movement, and such movements among professionals rely on their networks (Ferlie et al. 2005). Social networks are highways of change. The Society of Evidence Based Policing (SEBP) grew out of the British EBP movement and encourages broader production, use, and communication of research evidence related to police work (SEBP 2016). Interactions and face-to-face meetings can promote research translation and influence people to work differently.

Conclusion

As a late adopter of evidence-based practice, management can benefit from the lessons learned from the professions already using it as a basic mode for making decisions and solving problems. These lessons reveal the importance of EBMgmt implementation activities that promote the ability, motivation, and opportunity to practice systematic use of quality evidence.

References

Aarons, G. A. 2004. "Mental Health Provider Attitudes Toward Adoption of Evidence-Based Practice: The Evidence-Based Practice Attitude Scale (EBPAS)." *Mental Health Services Research* 6 (2): 61–74.

Ajzen, I. 1991. "The Theory of Planned Behavior." *Organizational Behavior and Human Decision Processes* 50 (2): 179–211.

Anderson, N., P. Herriot, and G. P. Hodgkinson. 2001. "The Practitioner–Researcher Divide in Industrial, Work and Organizational (IWO) Psychology: Where Are

We Now, and Where Do We Go from Here?" *Journal of Occupational and Organizational Psychology* 74 (4): 391–411.

Barends, E. G. 2015. *In Search of Evidence*. Amsterdam, Netherlands: Free University of Amsterdam.

Bates, D. W., G. J. Kuperman, S. Wang, T. Gandhi, A. Kittler, L. Volk, C. Spurr, R. Khorasani, M. Tanasijevic, and B. Middleton. 2003. "Ten Commandments for Effective Clinical Decision Support: Making the Practice of Evidence-Based Medicine a Reality." *Journal of the American Medical Informatics Association* 10 (6): 523–30.

Beidas, R. S., and P. C. Kendall. 2010. "Training Therapists in Evidence-Based Practice: A Critical Review of Studies from a Systems-Contextual Perspective." *Clinical Psychology* 17 (1): 1–30.

Belden, C. V., J. Leafman, G. Nehrenz, and P. Miller. 2012. "The Effect of Evidence Based Practice on Workplace Empowerment of Rural Registered Nurses." *Online Journal of Rural Nursing and Health Care* 12 (2): 64–76.

Berkman, N. D., K. N. Lohr, L. C. Morgan, T. M. Kuo, and S. C. Morton. 2013. "Interrater Reliability of Grading Strength of Evidence Varies with the Complexity of the Evidence in Systematic Reviews." *Journal of Clinical Epidemiology* 66 (10): 1105–17.

Boudreau, J. W., and P. M. Ramstad. 2007. *Beyond HR: The New Science of Human Capital*. Boston: Harvard Business School Press.

Bozionelos, N. 2005. "When the Inferior Candidate Is Offered the Job: The Selection Interview as a Political and Power Game." *Human Relations* 58 (12): 1605–31.

Castonguay, L. G., M. Barham, W. Lutz, and A. McAleavy. 2013. "Practice-Oriented Research." In *Bergin and Garfield's Handbook of Psychotherapy and Behavior Change,* 6th ed., edited by M. J. Lambert, 85–133. Hoboken, NJ: Wiley & Sons.

Dalheim, A., S. Harthug, R. M. Nilsen, and M. W. Nortvedt. 2012. "Factors Influencing the Development of Evidence-Based Practice Among Nurses: A Self-Report Survey." *BMC Health Services Research* 12: 367.

Davenport, T. H., J. G. Harris, and R. Morison. 2010. *Analytics at Work: Smarter Decisions, Better Results*. Boston: Harvard Business Press.

Dawes, R. M. 2008. "Psychotherapy: The Myth of Expertise." In *Navigating the Mindfield: A Guide to Separating Science from Pseudoscience in Mental Health*, edited by S. O. Lilienfeld, J. Ruscio, and S. J. Lynn, 311–44. Amherst, NY: Prometheus.

Denham, C. R., C. B. Sullenberger III, D. W. Quaid, and J. J. Nance. 2012. "An NTSB for Health Care—Learning from Innovation: Debate and Innovate or Capitulate." *Journal of Patient Safety* 8 (1): 3–14.

Downs, S. H., and N. Black. 1998. "The Feasibility of Creating a Checklist for the Assessment of the Methodological Quality Both of Randomised and

Non-randomised Studies of Health Care Interventions." *Journal of Epidemiology and Community Health* 52 (6): 377–84.

Ericsson, K. A., and A. C. Lehmann. 1996. "Expert and Exceptional Performance: Evidence on Maximal Adaptations on Task Constraints." *Annual Review of Psychology* 47: 273–305.

Ferlie, E., L. Fitzgerald, M. Wood, and C. Hawkins. 2005. "The Nonspread of Innovations: The Mediating Role of Professionals." *Academy of Management Journal* 48 (1): 117–34.

Gawande, A. 2010. *The Checklist Manifesto: How to Get Things Right.* New York: Metropolitan Books.

Glasziou, P., E. Meats, C. Heneghan, and S. Shepperd. 2008. "What Is Missing from Descriptions of Treatment in Trials and Reviews?" *BMJ* 336 (7659): 1472–74.

Goodman, J. S., M. S. Gary, and R. E. Wood. 2014. "Bibliographic Search Training for Evidence-Based Management Education: A Review of Relevant Literatures." *Academy of Management Learning & Education* 13 (3): 322–53.

Groff, E. R., J. H. Ratcliffe, C. P. Haberman, E. T. Sorg, N. M. Joyce, and R. B. Taylor. 2015. "Does What Police Do at Hot Spots Matter? The Philadelphia Policing Tactics Experiment." *Criminology* 53 (1): 23–53.

Haas, L. M., D. Peterson, R. Lefevbre, and D. Varvek. 2012. "Evaluation of the Effects of an Evidence-Based Practice Curriculum on Knowledge, Attitudes, and Self-Assessed Skills and Behaviors in Chiropractic Students." *Journal of Manipulative and Physiological Therapeutics* 35 (9): 701–9.

Highhouse, S. 2008. "Stubborn Reliance on Intuition and Subjectivity in Employee Selection." *Industrial and Organizational Psychology: Perspectives on Science and Practice* 1 (3): 333–42.

Hoagwood, K. E., B. J. Burns, L. Kiser, H. Ringeisen, and S. K. Schoenwald. 2001. "Evidence-Based Practice in Child and Adolescent Mental Health Services." *Psychiatric Services* 52 (9): 1179–89.

Kothari, A., and N. Wathen. 2013. "A Critical Second Look at Integrated Knowledge Translation." *Health Policy* 109 (2): 187–91.

Kovner, A. R., D. J. Fine, and R. D'Aquila. 2009. *Evidence-Based Management in Healthcare.* Chicago: Health Administration Press.

Lavis, J., H. Davies, A. Oxman, J. L. Denis, K. Golden-Biddle, and E. Ferlie. 2005. "Towards Systematic Reviews That Inform Health Care Management and Policy-Making." *Journal of Health Services Research & Policy* 10 (suppl. 1): 35–48.

Lilienfeld, S. O., J. M. Lohr, and B. O. Olatunji. 2008. "Encouraging Students to Think Critically About Psychotherapy: Overcoming Naïve Realism." In *Teaching Critical Thinking in Psychology: A Handbook of Best Practices*, edited by D. S. Dunn, J. S. Halonen, and R. A. Smith, 267–72. Oxford, UK: Wiley-Blackwell.

McCluskey, A., and B. Bishop. 2009. "The Adapted Fresno Test of Competence in Evidence-Based Practice." *Journal of Continuing Education in the Health Professions* 29 (2): 119–26.

McCluskey, A., and M. Lovarini. 2005. "Providing Education on Evidence-Based Practice Improved Knowledge but Did Not Change Behaviour: A Before and After Study." *BMC Medical Education* 5: 40.

Melnyk, B. M., and E. Fineout-Overholt. 2011. *Evidence-Based Practice in Nursing & Healthcare: A Guide to Best Practice.* Philadelphia, PA: Lippincott Williams & Wilkins.

Melnyk, B. M., E. Fineout-Overholt, N. Fischbeck Feinstein, H. Li, L. Small, L. Wilcox, and R. Kraus. 2004. "Nurses' Perceived Knowledge, Beliefs, Skills, and Needs Regarding Evidence-Based Practice: Implications for Accelerating the Paradigm Shift." *Worldviews on Evidence-Based Nursing* 1 (3): 185–93.

Melnyk, B. M., E. Fineout-Overholt, L. Gallagher-Ford, and L. Kaplan. 2012. "The State of Evidence-Based Practice in US Nurses: Critical Implications for Nurse Leaders and Educators." *Journal of Nursing Administration* 42 (9): 410–17.

Monden, Y. 2011. *Toyota Production System: An Integrated Approach to Just-in-Time.* Boca Raton, FL: CRC Press.

Novotney, A. 2014. "Educating the Educators." *Monitor on Psychology* 45 (5): 48–51.

Open Learning Initiative (OLI). 2016. "Evidence-Based Practice in Management and Consulting." Carnegie Mellon University. Accessed July 30. http://oli.cmu.edu /courses/free-open/evidence-based-practice-in-management-and-consulting/.

Roudebush, P., T. A. Allen, C. E. Dodd, and B. J. Novotny. 2004. "Application of Evidence-Based Medicine to Veterinary Clinical Nutrition." *Journal of the American Veterinary Medical Association* 224 (11): 1766–71.

Rousseau, D. M., and B. C. Gunia. 2016. "Evidence-Based Practice: The Psychology of EBP Implementation." *Annual Review of Psychology* 67: 667–92.

Rynes, S. L., A. E. Colbert, and K. G. Brown. 2002. "HR Professionals' Beliefs About Effective Human Resource Practices: Correspondence Between Research and Practice." *Human Resource Management* 41 (2): 149–74.

Rynes, S. L., D. M. Rousseau, and E. Barends. 2014. "From the Guest Editors: Change the World: Teach Evidence-Based Practice!" *Academy of Management Learning & Education* 13 (3): 305–21.

Sackett, D. L., S. E. Strauss, W. S. Richardson, W. Rosenberg, and R. Brian Haynes. 2000. *Evidence-Based Medicine: How to Practice and Teach EBM.* London: Churchill Livingstone.

Scurlock-Evans, L., P. Upton, and D. Upton. 2014. "Evidence-Based Practice in Physiotherapy: A Systematic Review of Barriers, Enablers, and Interventions." *Physiotherapy* 100 (3): 208–19.

Sherman, L. W. 2013. "The Rise of Evidence-Based Policing: Targeting, Testing, and Tracking." *Crime and Justice* 42 (1): 377–451.

Society of Evidence Based Policing (SEBP). 2016. "Society of Evidence Based Policing." Accessed June 30. www.sebp.police.uk.

Taylor, F. W. 1914. *The Principles of Scientific Management.* New York: Harper.

Tucker, A. L., I. M. Nembhard, and A. C. Edmondson. 2007. "Implementing New Practices: An Empirical Study of Organizational Learning in Hospital Intensive Care Units. *Management Science* 53 (6): 894–907.

Vroom, V. H. 1964. *Work and Motivation.* New York: Wiley & Sons.

Watson, S., and K. Hewett. 2006. "A Multi-Theoretical Model of Knowledge Transfer in Organizations: Determinants of Knowledge Contribution and Knowledge Reuse." *Journal of Management Studies* 43 (2): 141–73.

Weick, K. E., and K. M. Sutcliffe. 2011. *Managing the Unexpected: Resilient Performance in an Age of Uncertainty.* New York: Wiley & Sons.

Zanardelli, J. 2012. "At the Intersection of the Academy and Practice at Asbury Heights." In *The Oxford Handbook of Evidence-Based Management,* edited by D. M. Rousseau, 191–97. New York: Oxford University Press.

SCIENTIFIC EVIDENCE— EXAMPLES OF PRACTICE

CASE STUDY

THE EVOLUTION OF EVIDENCE-BASED CEO EVALUATION IN A MULTI-UNIT HEALTH SYSTEM

by Lawrence Prybil and Michael Slubowski

Introduction

SCL Health is a faith-based, nonprofit health system based in Denver, Colorado. It owns or manages ten hospitals and sponsors or cosponsors a broad range of other health-related facilities, programs, and services in Colorado, Kansas, and Montana. System-wide revenues in fiscal year 2014 were $2.5 billion. SCL Health has been ranked in the top quintile of US health systems by Truven Health Analytics, based on a combination of clinical and financial measures (Landen 2014).

The SCL Health organizational model includes a system-level board of directors, a chief executive officer (CEO), and corporate staff. Specific responsibilities and decision-making authority are delegated by the SCL Health board of directors to local boards and CEOs. A system-wide mission statement, core values, and policies unify and provide overall direction for the entire organization.

This chapter describes the evolution of SCL Health's approach to establishing performance expectations for the system's CEO and evaluating the CEO's accomplishments in relation to these expectations. It discusses the genesis of an evidence-based approach that worked successfully for several years, factors that disrupted that process for a period of time, and the model that has been reintroduced and now is institutionalized in the system.

Background

For all types of corporate organizations, appointing the CEO, establishing performance expectations, and assessing her level of success in meeting those

Note: This case study builds from the one presented in chapter 12 of the first edition of this book. You are encouraged to review the earlier edition for additional context.

expectations are among a governing board's most fundamental and important duties (Peregrine 2014; NACD 2004). National studies in both the investor-owned and nonprofit sectors show that a large majority of boards evaluate their CEO's performance using some form of preestablished criteria (American College of Healthcare Executives 2013; NACD 2011; Szekendi et al. 2015). However, numerous authorities have expressed serious concerns about the rigor and efficacy of CEO evaluation processes in many organizations (AHA Center for Healthcare Governance 2014; Cohen 2008).

Precisely this situation prevailed within SCL Health—then known as the Sisters of Charity of Leavenworth Health System—during the late 1990s and the early twenty-first century. A form of CEO performance evaluation existed, but it was highly qualitative and conducted in a largely exclusive fashion by the board chair. During this period, the board chair and CEO informally agreed on the CEO's priorities for the coming year. These performance expectations were not linked directly to the system's incentive compensation program for senior managers, other board members had minimal (if any) input in evaluating the CEO's performance, and changes to the CEO's base salary and incentive compensation essentially were determined by the chair in dialogue with the CEO.

Over time, the flaws in this approach became apparent to other board members, and they saw a clear need for change. In 2002, the completion of the board chair's term and the appointment of a new chair, who recognized the problem, created an opportunity for a fresh look at SCL Health's process for CEO performance assessment and expectation setting. This review was timely for several reasons, including the 2002 enactment of the Sarbanes-Oxley Act—which focused national attention on governance in both the investor-owned *and* nonprofit sectors—and growing pressures by the Internal Revenue Service, payers, and the public at large for better governance and more accountability.

Initial Transformation of SCL Health CEO Evaluation Policy and Practices

The new board chair, the board compensation committee, the entire board of directors, and the CEO concurred on the need for an evidence-based and more inclusive approach to setting CEO performance expectations and assessing the CEO's progress in relation to them. They agreed that the new model should engage *all* board members; yield written performance objectives that provide clear, board-approved guidance for the CEO; bring solid, quantitative information into the performance evaluation process; and ensure transparency and accountability. Following best practices in the investor-owned and nonprofit sectors, the board compensation committee, in concert with the CEO and an independent compensation consultant selected by and accountable to the committee, was charged with designing the new model for setting CEO expectations and assessing his performance in achieving them (Prybil et al. 2009).

The new, evidence-based approach was implemented on a pilot basis in fiscal year 2003. With input from all board members, the CEO, and the compensation consultant, the approach was assessed and adopted for ongoing use after the first year's experience. This approach was employed for the following five years, with an annual review and, with minor refinements, annual affirmation by the board of directors.

Disruptions to the System and the CEO Evaluation Process

Fiscal years 2010, 2011, and 2012 represented a period of major challenges and changes for SCL Health. Key issues included the following:

- Dissolution of a joint operating agreement involving an SCL Health hospital and facilities sponsored by another organization in Denver and, subsequently, the acquisition of those facilities by SCL Health—a complicated and contentious process that required much SCL Health board and management time and effort over many months
- The retirement of SCL Health's longtime CEO and the recruitment, after a national search process, of his successor
- A decision by the SCL Health board of directors and management leadership team, after in-depth deliberation and consideration of all plausible alternatives, to divest its facilities in Kansas City to another system
- Relocation of the SCL Health corporate offices and staff from Kansas City to Denver, a location more central to the new mix of SCL Health facilities and with a growing population that provides a range of growth opportunities for the system
- Serious strategic issues and operational problems that resulted in a substantial loss on systemwide operations in fiscal year 2010 and necessitated a fundamental reexamination of SCL Health strategies and a series of operational and management changes

These challenges and changes became the principal focus of the SCL Health board and management team between 2010 and 2012. The system and its leadership were confronted with a series of serious difficulties that threatened their survival. As a result, the formal process of setting CEO expectations and assessing performance in relation to them, which had been developed and employed in earlier years, was simply set aside. Both the board of directors and the new CEO had to devote their time and energy to crisis management, financial turnaround, the integration of newly acquired Denver facilities, and the rapid transformation of the health system from a holding company to an operating company model. During this period, the CEO's priorities were focused on major issues that all parties felt required immediate action. Even during this period, however, the board leadership and the CEO maintained commitment to open dialogue, clarity of priorities, and candor and transparency in addressing both progress and problems.

Reinstituting a Formal CEO Evaluation Process

After the most urgent issues were addressed and the system's overall situation was stabilized, the board of directors and CEO agreed on the need to reinstitute a more formal protocol for setting the CEO's performance expectations and evaluating accomplishments in relation to them. In making and implementing this decision, the board and CEO employed an evidence-based approach (Barends, Rousseau, and Briner 2014; Kovner, D'Aquila, and Fine 2009). They reviewed the reasons that the formal process instituted in 2003 had been set aside for several years, appraised the consequences of that action, and examined current information regarding best practices in CEO performance evaluation. They concluded that the evidence strongly supported developing and reinstituting a formal protocol for establishing the board's expectations for SCL Health's CEO and evaluating his performance in addressing those expectations.

The new protocol was created and adopted in 2013. It was based on principles congruent with those used in building the original approach in 2002. The principles included the following:

- First, with input and consultation with the CEO, the SCL Health board should annually provide the CEO with a written set of personal performance objectives on which the CEO would place special emphasis during the coming year.
- Second, the objectives should be measurable; linked closely to the SCL Health mission, values, and strategic plan; and integrated with the SCL Health incentive compensation plan for the system's management team.

- Third, *all* members of the SCL Health board should have the opportunity to provide input in the process of formulating the CEO's performance objectives and assessing the CEO's success in addressing them.

- Fourth, the board compensation committee, with the advice of the committee's executive compensation consultant, should be responsible for coordinating the performance evaluation process and assembling information for consideration by the board chair and executive committee. The intent is to base the process on fair, objective assessment of the best possible information regarding actual performance in relation to preestablished expectations.

- Finally, all aspects of the CEO evaluation process should be conducted in a spirit of commitment to continuous improvement—in the system's operating performance, in the CEO's personal performance, and in the evaluation process itself. Commitment to evidence-based assessment and ongoing improvement are vital to achieving and maintaining excellence in management and in governance.

Exhibit 8.1 depicts how these principles were operationalized in SCL Health's 2014 CEO evaluation process and timetable. To illustrate the process in greater detail, we focus here specifically on steps 5 and 6. In step 5, the CEO develops and submits a written self-evaluation report to the board chair and the chair of the board compensation committee. This self-evaluation incorporates evidence-based measures from the goals the CEO proposed for 2014 in a previous report, as well as measures that respond to eight areas for improvement identified by the SCL Health board (physician practice performance, revenue cycle, achieving volume projections, leveraging information system investments, solidifying payer partnerships, initiatives to increase patient loyalty, capabilities to manage global payments, and growth of strategic product lines). The CEO includes evidence of accomplishments in relation to each of these goals, including quantitative, qualitative, and other observable measures. A form is then developed with a grid on which each of the board members can assess the CEO's performance against each of these areas for improvement, in step 6.

Both the SCL Health board of directors and the CEO are glad that a formal, evidence-based approach has been reinstituted. They believe it is fair, thorough, and beneficial for the CEO, the board of directors, and the system as a whole. The process can always be improved, and ongoing review and modification when indicated is an integral part of the process (see step 13). The intent is to maintain a CEO evaluation protocol that will continue to meet best-practice standards for nonprofit, tax-exempt organizations and enhance both the CEO's and the system's performance.

EXHIBIT 8.1
SCL Health CEO
Performance
Evaluation
Process,
Timeline, and
Responsibilities
for 2014

Action	Completed by	Date Due
1. Review and discuss outline of SCL Health president/CEO 2014 performance evaluation form, process, and timeline.	Board compensation committee	10/28/14
2. Submit president/CEO's proposed 2015 performance objectives to board chair.	President/CEO	01/16/15
3. Executive committee meets • to determine its assessment of system performance in relation to 2014 performance measures, and • to discuss and approve CEO's proposed performance objectives for 2015. As part of this process, the chair of the board compensation committee and the president/CEO provide input to the executive committee's deliberations.	Executive committee, board chair, chair of compensation committee, president/CEO	02/25/15 (teleconference)
4. Complete and forward to SCL Health chief human performance officer the 2014 system performance results. (Though numbers should be fairly accurate, subsequent audit adjustments are possible.)	Executive vice president and chief financial officer, corporate controller	03/03/15
5. Submit self-evaluation to board chair and the chair of the board compensation committee.	President/CEO	03/06/15
6. Distribute CEO performance evaluation form to SCL Health board members for completion.	Board chair, senior vice president, and chief HR officer	03/06/15
7. Return completed CEO performance evaluation forms to the chair of the board compensation committee.	Board members	03/13/15
8. Board chair, supported by the compensation committee chair, finalizes the CEO 2014 performance evaluation report and distributes summary evaluation report to the executive committee (excluding the CEO).	Board chair, chair of the compensation committee	03/20/15

EXHIBIT 8.1
SCL Health CEO
Performance
Evaluation
Process,
Timeline, and
Responsibilities
for 2014
(Continued)

9. Executive committee meets
  • to discuss CEO 2014 performance,
  • to finalize 2015 CEO performance objectives (up to three),
  • to determine appropriate compensation implications, and
  • to help the board chair prepare for meeting with the CEO.
	Executive committee	03/25/15 (teleconference)

10. Meet with president/CEO to review 2014 performance evaluation, compensation, and 2015 performance objectives.	Board chair	04/03/15
11. Submit to SCL Health senior vice president and chief HR officer the 2014 performance increase, to be effective the first pay period in May 2015.	Board chair	04/07/15
12. Distribute the president/CEO 2014 evaluation report to SCL Health board members.	Board chair	04/30/15
13. Review the 2014 CEO evaluation process and timeline, and identify improvements for the 2015 SCL Health president/CEO evaluation process.	Board compensation committee	As needed

Case Study Questions

1. Why did SCL Health significantly revise the evidence-based CEO evaluation that had served them well before 2010?

2. What are the key changes SCL Health made in the protocol in 2013?

3. What are the key advantages of these changes, and what are the costs and risks in making them?

4. Why don't more hospitals and health systems adopt a protocol similar to the one used by SCL Health?

5. What would have to happen in a local hospital or health system for it to adopt such a protocol?

References

AHA Center for Healthcare Governance. 2014. *2014 National Health Care Governance Survey Report.* Chicago: AHA Center for Healthcare Governance.

American College of Healthcare Executives. 2013. "CEO Research Findings: Employment Contracts and Evaluation." *Healthcare Executive* 28 (1): 100.

Barends, E., D. M. Rousseau, and R. B. Briner. 2014. *Evidence-Based Management: The Basic Principles.* Center for Evidence-Based Management. Accessed June 9, 2016. www.cebma.org/wp-content/uploads/Evidence-Based-Practice-The -Basic-Principles.pdf.

Cohen, K. 2008. *Best Practices for Developing Effective and Enduring Board/CEO Relationships.* Chicago: Center for Healthcare Governance.

Kovner, A. R., R. D'Aquila, and D. Fine. 2009. "Introduction: On the Practice of Evidence-Based Management." In *Evidence-Based Management in Health-care,* edited by A. R. Kovner, D. J. Fine, and R. D'Aquila, xxi–xxvii. Chicago: Health Administration Press.

Landen, R. 2014. "Higher Quality, Healthier Finances." *Modern Healthcare* 44 (1): 14–20.

National Association of Corporate Directors (NACD). 2011. *NACD Public Company Governance Survey.* Washington, DC: NACD.

———. 2004. *Report of the NACD Blue Ribbon Commission on Board Leadership.* Washington, DC: NACD.

Peregrine, M. 2014. *Healthcare Governance Amidst Systematic Industry Change: What the Law Expects.* San Diego, CA: The Governance Institute.

Prybil, L., W. Murray, T. Cotter, and E. Bryant. 2009. "Transforming CEO Evaluation in a Multi-Unit Healthcare Organization." In *Evidence-Based Management in Healthcare,* edited by A. R. Kovner, D. J. Fine, and R. D'Aquila, 153–159. Chicago: Health Administration Press.

Szekendi, M., L. Prybil, D. Cohen, B. Godsey, D. Fardo, and J. Cerese. 2015. "Governance Practices and Performance in US Academic Medical Centers." *American Journal of Medical Quality* 30 (6): 520–25.

9

CASE STUDY

THE HEALTHY TRANSITIONS PROGRAM IN LATE STAGE KIDNEY DISEASE

by Sofia Agoritsas, Steven Fishbane, and Candice Halinski

Introduction

Improved coordination of care and effective management of chronic illness can contribute to significant improvements in patient outcomes. In this chapter, we will highlight a case study involving a kidney-disease-specific care coordination program at Northwell Health, a multihospital integrated healthcare delivery system in New York. With Northwell Health, we used an evidence-based management (EBMgmt) approach to design and implement the pilot program it launched in October 2012. Known as the Healthy Transitions (HT) Program in Late Stage Kidney Disease, the program focuses on appropriate interventions, prevention measures, and preparations for patients choosing an optimal renal replacement therapy (RRT) prior to kidney failure or end-stage renal disease (ESRD). Renal replacement therapies for ESRD may include hemodialysis, which may occur in the hospital, outpatient, or home setting; peritoneal dialysis, which occurs in the home setting; kidney transplantation; and nondialysis therapy or conservative medical management.

The outcomes of the program have exceeded national benchmarks as patients enter dialysis, and the findings have spurred subsequent demonstration projects. The purpose of this case study is to demonstrate how evidence-based management was applied in the design, development, and implementation of the HT Program.

Background

In January 2012, Northwell Health's Executive Administration had the foresight to recognize that dealing with healthcare reform required

Note: This chapter describes one specific program developed at Northwell Health. For information about Northwell's overall approach to evidence-based management, please see the interview with Northwell CEO Michael Dowling presented in chapter 21.

acceptance of responsibility for the clinical and financial outcomes for defined populations, the integration of the fragmented parts of the care continuum, and the development of new care models. The greatest opportunities to improve care exist when (1) the current care model is failing, (2) proven evidence-based interventions can rectify the problems, (3) the population is highly targeted, and (4) the expenditure per patient under the current care model is large enough to support a reallocation of resources for a redesigned care model.

The CEO of Northwell Health, Michael Dowling, asked the leadership from the Kidney and Pelvic Health Service Line to evaluate and address the complex needs of the kidney disease population. Our team, led by Steven Fishbane, MD, identified late-stage chronic kidney disease patients as the population with the greatest opportunity for improvement. We designed the HT Program in Late Stage Kidney Disease, a comprehensive care coordination model, both to better address the complex needs of this chronically ill population and to improve the way care is delivered to these patients as they progress to dialysis. In developing the program, we used both patient-centered medical home (PCMH) and population health management principles.

Chronic kidney disease (CKD) is a condition marked by the presence of kidney damage and the diminished level of kidney function over time. It is categorized into five stages, and the last two—CKD Stage 4 and CKD Stage 5—are the advanced stages prior to kidney failure. Estimated glomerular filtration rate (eGFR) levels are 30 to15 for Stage 4 and 15 to 0 for Stage 5. The lower the eGFR level, the lower the estimated kidney function. At zero, a patient is considered to have complete kidney failure.

Patients with CKD represent 7 percent of Medicare enrollees, yet they consume 22 percent of total expenditures (USRDS 2010). Almost half of all individuals with CKD also have diabetes or cardiovascular disease, or both. CKD incidence has grown as a result of population aging and the epidemics of obesity, diabetes, and hypertension. An estimated 51 million people—about 16 percent of the US population—have CKD, with 8.4 million progressing to late-stage CKD (stages 3–5). In late-stage CKD, patients have (1) double or triple the risk of mortality, (2) a higher risk of hospitalization in the first ten weeks of dialysis, and (3) a diminished quality of life and increased morbidity. Furthermore, an extraordinary surge in total cost of care occurs in the initial year because of poor transitions to dialysis.

A large majority of these dialysis patients—93 percent—begin renal replacement therapy with hemodialysis, compared to 6.1 percent for peritoneal dialysis and less than 1 percent for kidney transplant (USRDS 2011). Very few patients undergo conservative medical management or a nondialysis route.

Applying an Evidence-Based Management Approach

Recognizing the opportunity to improve the care for this vulnerable and complex population, our team used an EBMgmt approach to design and implement the HT Program in Late Stage Kidney Disease.

Step 1: Formulating the Research Question

To obtain stakeholder support, we needed a researchable question that would enable us to supply the best available evidence to Executive Administration. The intervention we wanted to evaluate primarily involved using a patient-centered nurse care coordination model and information technology (IT) to improve outcomes.

Our research question asked whether using a nurse care coordination model would improve outcomes for CKD patients as they transitioned to ESRD. We wanted to reorganize the care model to be more comprehensive, to focus on transitions of care, to use informatics to track patient status, to enhance patient access to care, and to support patient-shared decision making. The increased communication and collaboration would allow providers and patients to take into account the best scientific evidence available, as well as the patient's values, in understanding the disease, knowing the treatment options available, and modifying behavior to reduce complications that may be preventable. The primary interventions center on improved patient education and timely preparation for renal replacement therapies, identifying hospitalization risk, intervening to reduce risk, and improving quality of life.

We considered conducting a pilot that would serve as a proof-of-concept study to assess feasibility, and we requested funding from Executive Administration for three care managers, a nurse manager, and an informatics specialist upon acquiring and assessing the evidence.

Steps 2 and 3: Acquiring and Appraising the Evidence

To best answer our research question, we needed to gather the best available evidence, including empirical evidence and qualitative research, and use information from case reports, scientific principles, and expert opinion. Abundant evidence indicates that the suboptimal outcomes in late-stage CKD are due to pervasive variations in care processes, failure to use evidence-based interventions or treatments, and general fragmentation of care.

Variations in care prior to the onset of dialysis include the following: hospitalizations specific to catheter infection rates, excess intradialytic fluid management, and medication errors; choice of home dialysis alternatives; preemptive transplantation; and inappropriate initiation of dialysis in a hospital setting, where hemodialysis is usually started urgently. These variations will be discussed later in the chapter, when we present the evidence for the seven key clinical focus areas. For each of these variations, we realized that we needed to not only evaluate evidence-based clinical guidelines, but also address how we can support our physicians by using physician extenders to coordinate the complex needs of this population. By evaluating the barriers in the coordination of care for these patients, and by using the best available scientific and experiential evidence, we wanted to understand and expand on the PCMH model using a nephrologist as the primary caregiver and see how nurse care managers could play a key role in patient education and care coordination. To do this, we met weekly with a core design team over the course of six months. We aimed to evaluate and build upon the evidence-based medicine surrounding seven key clinical areas before we implemented the program in October 2012. These focus areas are shown in exhibit 9.1.

Upon the accumulation of the evidence, we understood that an effective program would have to incorporate the synthesis of compiled evidence for each barrier using our nurse care managers to execute key guidelines. This understanding is consistent with Barends's approach to evidence-based management, in which aggregate evidence is compiled in "systematic reviews, synopses, summaries, and evidence-based guidelines" (Barends, Have, and Huisman 2012, 35). The aggregate synthesis of guidelines served as the foundation for our program addressing each of the key focus areas.

The Patient-Centered Medical Home

The patient-centered medical home is an emerging healthcare delivery model that aims to improve patient outcomes and reduce costs, particularly for chronic disease management patients. The model is based on a set of principles approved jointly by the American College of Physicians (ACP), the American Academy of Family Physicians (AAFP), the American Academy of Pediatrics (AAP), and the American Osteopathic Association (AOA) in 2007 (AAFP 2007).

The PCMH model features a team-based delivery approach led by a healthcare provider, intended to provide continuous and comprehensive medical care to patients while maximizing health outcomes (ACP 2006). Focused on continuous quality improvement, the care teams use evidence-based medicine and clinical decision support tools to guide decision making while also ensuring that patients and their families have the education and support to actively participate in their own care. Services are physician directed; however, care coordination is vital to enhanced access to care and self-management support. Care is coordinated across medical specialties, hospitals, nursing home facilities, and also the patient's primary caregiver or family (Cassidy 2010). Care is facilitated by informatics and analytical tools to allow patient tracking, clinical monitoring, specialist follow-up, and population-based decision

1. Excessive use of dialysis catheters and related complications
2. Underuse of arteriovenous fistulas
3. Excessive hospitalizations due to fluid overload
4. Excessive medication errors
5. Inappropriate hemodialysis initiation in a hospital setting
6. Underuse of peritoneal dialysis
7. Preemptive kidney transplantation rate

EXHIBIT 9.1
Seven Key
Clinical Focus
Areas

making. Data sharing among providers allows maximized coordination and management. Access is facilitated by expanded or after-hours access to a physician or practice staff, by telephone or secure e-mail.

As of 2012, evaluations of PCMH models were limited (Williams et al. 2012), although early systematic reviews seemed promising (Peikes et al. 2012). In an Agency for Healthcare Research and Quality (AHRQ) report by Peikes and colleagues (2012), evidence ratings were provided by evaluation design and by outcomes for 14 quantitative analyses. The ratings gave us insight on proven strategies instead of "reinventing the wheel." These programs were not specific to CKD. In our review of the literature and our surveys of CKD PCMH programs across the country, we found that some programs used nurses and ancillary support to assist in CKD patient education; however, scientific evaluations specific to CKD were not available. Multiple programs have used chronic care management models (CCM) instead. Although both PCMH and CCM improvement delivery models are comprehensive and patient-centric and provide continuous care, medical home models expand on access to care. Both use informatics to track patient care. We also found few CKD programs specifically using PCMH or medical home model terminology.

The most lauded medical home model, Geisinger's ProvenHealth Navigator program (Norfolk and Hartle 2013), embeds a care coordinator in a clinic setting and also provides telephonic support (Paulus, Davis, and Steele 2008). Other largely deployed programs in the United States, including Fresenius, primarily include telephonic case management support. DaVita's Village Health Program primarily incorporates telephonic support and some field support, with visits to some patient homes. We were not able to find much evidence in the literature that programs conducted home visits, either to provide education in the home or home care services. This gap in the literature has been validated by a systematic review by Aydede and colleagues (2014), in which 17 studies examined home care interventions among adult CKD patients and assessed the impact on outcomes.

Evidence for the Seven Key Clinical Focus Areas

As mentioned earlier, a multitude of clinical evidence does exist on how to improve many of the key focus areas we identified; however, national averages on quality outcomes remain lower than benchmarks. Our core design team met weekly to understand the key barriers and areas in need of improvement. The team consisted of (1) our medical director, a leading clinical researcher; (2) our administrative director, who had over ten years of executive management experience and multiple years of organizational experience; (3) our clinical director, a nurse practitioner who also had ten years of dialysis nursing experience; and (4) an informatics specialist, who had multiple years of clinical database experience. The team systematically searched for clinical evidence using literature reviews from the latest journals and experience guided from our medical director and clinical director. Because of the team's research backgrounds, we could easily understand prioritization of the validity and reliability of the research. However, we did not systematically prioritize.

The following list provides a brief description of the leading evidence collected and existing gaps in each of the key focus areas:

- *Excessive use of dialysis catheters and related complications.* Dialysis catheters increase the risk of infections, hospitalizations, and death, particularly in the first few months of dialysis (Allon 2004). This risk is widely understood by the nephrology community, yet in the United States, 82 percent of new patients start dialysis with a catheter. National quality and utilization data is publicly reported through the United States Renal Data System (USRDS), the Centers for Medicare & Medicaid Services (CMS) renal data registry for all CKD and ESRD Medicare patients. As alternatives to catheters, appropriate vascular access management and the placement of arteriovenous fistulas (AVFs) are recommended methods for providing long-lasting sites for blood to be removed and returned during hemodialysis.

- *Underuse of arteriovenous fistulas.* AVFs improve patients' experience of care, improve outcomes for the ESRD population, and decrease per capita cost of care. Although the early placement of AVFs in CKD stages 4 and 5 is optimal for patients starting hemodialysis, the procedure is underused. Poor coordination and preparation exist between the patient, the nephrologist, and the vascular surgery team before the onset of dialysis. The Kidney Disease Outcomes Quality Initiative (KDOQI), in collaboration with CMS, has published national guidelines for promoting AVFs, through the Fistula First program (Navuluri and Regalado 2009). KDOQI has also provided evidence-based clinical practice guidelines for all stages of CKD and related complications since 1997. The evidence supports the idea that underuse of AVFs is a correctable problem. The appropriate care model can lead to improvements in communication, follow-up in between doctor appointments, and coordination of a working AVF's maturation. Evidence supports the idea that optimal timing and referral to vascular surgery are dependent on the opinions and choices of patients and physicians (Hassan Murad et al. 2008). Our nurse director was able to recognize from her dialysis experience that the care managers not only assist with coordination but that they also need to assess the maturation of the AVF in defined evaluation periods.

- *Excessive hospitalizations due to fluid overload.* The combination in late CKD of reduced renal salt and water excretion, poor cardiac function, and highly fragmented and episodic medical care lead to frequent hospitalizations for fluid overload. Many times, poor dietary management and lack of symptom awareness limit the patient from proper self-management. Several professional organizations have issued evidence-based guidelines for reducing sodium intake. Potential barriers to patients' compliance with sodium intake guidelines include, but are not limited to, poor knowledge about the sodium content of food (among both patients and providers), complex labeling information, and patient preferences (Wright and Cavanaugh 2010).

- *Excessive medication errors.* Patients with chronic kidney disease on dialysis are prescribed an average of 10 to 12 medications (St. Peter 2010). Medication errors are common in late-stage CKD, as managing daily medications for patients with multiple co-morbidities can be complicated and overwhelming. Common causes contributing to medication errors include missed doses, underdoses, overdoses, therapeutic duplication, polypharmacy, and incomplete medication reconciliation. Past research has found that 20 to 67 percent of prescriptions for late-stage CKD patients contain errors and that 18 percent of all hospital admissions among this group are caused by medication errors, of which 60 percent are preventable (Harchowal 1997). Moreover, hospitalized patients with CKD are at higher risk for adverse consequences of medical care compared with those without the disease (Seliger et al. 2008).

- *Inappropriate hemodialysis initiation in a hospital setting.* Most dialysis starts take place in acute care hospitals (adding costs and risk for nosocomial complications), even though the majority of patients are stable enough to receive their first dialysis treatments in outpatient dialysis centers. Appropriate selection of patients for outpatient dialysis initiation can reduce costs and morbidity.

- *Underuse of peritoneal dialysis.* Many countries outside the United States, particularly the United Kingdom and Canada, have shifted their populations to more cost-effective modalities, such as peritoneal dialysis, which occurs in the home. Hemodialysis, used in outpatient settings three times a week, is still the dominant therapy in the United States. The use of home modalities in the United States, as indicated in USRDS data, is disproportionately low relative to the use of in-center modalities. The National Institute for Health and Clinical Excellence offers guidelines, based on systematic review and informal expert consensus, regarding options and support for peritoneal dialysis as a modality (Centre for Clinical Practice 2011). Although peritoneal dialysis is not the prevailing therapy, it is technically simpler than alternatives. It gives patients greater autonomy and independence, and it is lower in actual cost compared to hemodialysis in most countries. It has also been associated with a slower decline in residual kidney function, compared to hemodialysis. Survival rates are similar between peritoneal dialysis patients and hemodialysis patients. Although the peritoneal dialysis is considered a more favorable option, medical and social contraindications, in addition to issues with caregiver support, may affect whether peritoneal dialysis takes place; such factors need further evaluation (Liebman et al. 2012).

- *Barriers to preemptive kidney transplantation.* Preemptive transplantation requires patients to have a suitable, compatible, and prequalified living donor prior to dialysis. Because the series of preevaluation tests for both the recipient and the donor can take weeks or months, the patient will need time to navigate a complex healthcare delivery system. Kidney transplantation is the preferred treatment for end-stage renal disease because it not only triples the patient's life expectancy, compared with remaining on dialysis, but also improves quality of life. In a survey of nephrologists, preemptive transplantation was considered the optimal treatment modality for eligible patients. Late referral, patient health and insurance status, and delayed transplant center evaluation are perceived as major barriers to preemptive transplantation (Pradel et al. 2008). Our organizational experience included living donor availability as an additional factor.

Step 4: Aggregating the Evidence

The Medical Advisory Board (MAB), a committee of nephrologists participating in the HT Program, was established to contribute insight, scientific direction, and expert opinion on medical conditions and clinical developments. This group was initially responsible for "aggregating" the evidence in our EBMgmt approach, serving as a peer-review expert governance structure to apply programmatic decision making and review the quality data. The MAB includes medical representation from each nephrology practice site involved in the HT Program. The formal infrastructure is vital; it gives value to the physician group as stakeholders, which reinforces their compliance and adherence to program guidelines.

Our initial presentations explained the goals, target, and justification of the program, which were based on our core-team work and evaluation of the evidence. The goals, targets, and justifications are shown in exhibit 9.2. The overall program objective is to rectify fragmented care in late-stage CKD through a nurse care coordination model. The program aims to improve clinical outcomes by reducing risk for mortality and hospitalizations, increase quality of life, and reduce the surge in total cost of care by avoiding unnecessary utilizations (i.e., hospitalizations) in the peridialysis period.

Step 5: Applying the Evidence to the Decision

The HT Program uses an integrated care delivery model to coordinate complex care processes for patients with late-stage CKD. The nephrologist, the nurse care manager, the patient, and other providers use a team-based approach, based on a PCMH model. The care manager tracks and measures outcomes and provides progress updates and additional information, with the aim of achieving broad quality-driven targets.

Six key component areas of the care delivery model were developed based on the evidence compiled. Clinical protocols for workflows related to each program component help reduce variability among providers and care managers. Patient education materials also address each of the key focus areas. A CKD database registry was designed to monitor patient outcomes, with decision support capabilities to evaluate program impact and an ongoing quality management program. Components of the IT system are closely integrated with the electronic medical record and incorporate computerized prompts, population management capabilities (including reports and feedback), specialized decision support, electronic scheduling, and personal health records. All prompts include the metrics related to the seven clinical focus areas. These efforts improve timeliness of care, reduce late-stage disease complications, and decrease unnecessary utilization of services.

The HT nurse care managers work in a hands-on manner with patients and maintain close working relationships with physicians. Enrollment of patients takes place in the clinic setting after the nurse care manager has been initially introduced by the nephrologist. The nurse care manager conducts an initial intake visit in the patient's home (preferably with key caregivers present), focusing on education about kidney disease and dialysis options and creating the patient profile in the HT database management system. The visit includes discussion of advance directives, screening for depression and anxiety, and assessment of the home environment for food quality and safety. After the initial visit, telephone contact with the patient—at least once

EXHIBIT 9.2
Program Goals,
Targets, and
Justifications

Goal	Description/Target	Justification
1. Reduce hospitalizations in late-stage kidney disease.	Reduce mean hospitalization rate compared to national baseline.	Cost of care in late-stage CKD is excessive in large part because of increased and preventable hospitalizations. Such hospitalizations can be related to (1) poor planning for patients initiating dialysis in the hospital rather than in outpatient dialysis settings and (2) complications associated with use of catheter placement rather than timely vascular access placement. Hospitalizations for catheter-related infections cost an average of $23,000 (Ramanathan et al. 2007). Hospitalization reduction efforts can be based on education, dietary support, daily weight management, system management, and infection prevention.
2. Improve education about RRT options (i.e., dialysis, transplantation, or nondialytic conservative therapy).	Provide comprehensive education and management/facilitation services to 100 percent of patients enrolled.	Education is grossly inadequate, resulting in poor patient preparation and excessive and often inappropriate reliance on hemodialysis.
3. Increase RRT modality selection rate prior to ESRD.	Increase rate of enrolled patients who have made RRT modality selection choices to 90 percent.	Inadequate education leads to patients failing to make RRT modality/options selections, which usually results in the urgent start of hemodialysis without an access (i.e., AVF) and the need for catheter placement in a hospital setting.
4. Increase the percentage of patients choosing and preparing for home dialysis modalities and preemptive kidney transplantation.	Increase selection of home modalities and preemptive kidney transplantation from less than 1 percent nationally.	Inadequate education, planning, and facilitation have contributed to underuse of home dialysis and kidney transplantation.

EXHIBIT 9.2

Program Goals, Targets, and Justifications *(Continued)*

5. Increase timely AVF placement prior to ESRD for patients choosing hemodialysis.	Increase percentage of patients starting hemodialysis with AVFs from 20 percent nationally to 60 percent.	The underuse of AVFs is a correctable problem, as evidenced by the Fistula First program. Through the implementation of our Countdown to Fistula guideline, we would be able to improve poor communication resulting from fragmented care and ensure coordination of a working AVF.
6. Improve patient quality of life.	Improve patient quality of life, as measured by the Kidney Disease Quality of Life score, by 25 percent within one year.	Late-stage CKD is a period of confusion and anxiety. Our program aims to create order and improve patient quality of life by supporting the patient.

per month—addresses all aspects of care, including medication reconciliation, reinforcement of education, updating of the risk profile, and answering any questions. Each patient has an individualized plan of care based on the patient's risk profile and needs. The nurse interacts with the patient's physicians and coordinates information between them, helping to facilitate transitions in care.

The program components within the nurse care coordination model build upon the evidence in each of the seven clinical focus areas. The care manager also addresses a variety of other care issues related to this chronically ill population—for instance, management of mental health problems, nutrition, advance directives, and safety of the home environment. A two-week intensive curriculum trains the care managers on these evidence-based concepts, and scripts, guidelines, checklists, and decision support tools are provided. The curriculum was based on the key clinical focus areas and the evidence used to support the program decisions. All the program components aim to improve the healthcare patients receive, support the health of the population, and reduce costs. The standardized evidence-based training materials and pathways were approved by the MAB and have been implemented since October 2012.

The program components are as follows:

1. *Modality selection.* Upon consulting with the nephrologist and determining that a patient is a candidate for renal replacement therapy, the nurse care manager conducts an initial home visit with the patient

and a caregiver. The nurse care manager provides comprehensive education about the RRT treatment options available to all CKD patients (i.e., hemodialysis, peritoneal dialysis, transplantation, nondialysis). Patients and their providers make decisions together about the RRT options, taking into account the best clinical evidence available, as well as the patients' values and preferences.

2. *Low salt every day and Phonelink.* The nurse is able to review and discuss the patient's diet and inspect the patient's refrigerator and cabinets. She teaches the idea of low salt every day (reflecting the need in late-stage CKD for a low-sodium diet) and stresses the importance of dietary consistency. The nurse provides a scale to the patient and teaches the patient about how and when to respond to a change in weight or symptoms. The nurse also teaches the patient how to use the HT Phonelink system to relay daily weights and health status information to the database registry. The patient dials in daily weights, which are captured through an automated daily report and then trended over time for the nurse. Prompts are provided on a report to the nurse care manager if significant changes in weight occur over time. If the nurse sees any significant changes, she calls the patient for an update in his status.

3. *Countdown to Fistula.* The HT Program has developed an intensive, coordinated management intervention: the HT Countdown to Fistula, which builds upon the KDOQI Fistula First program. Countdown to Fistula is a comprehensive stepwise program to ensure AVF placement in all appropriate patients, with coordinated follow-up and failure-recovery processes by the HT nurse care manager. The informatics system also has the ability to prompt the user and generate reports based on the parameters of the Countdown to Fistula program.

4. *Steps to reduce hospitalizations from catheter infections.* The primary cause of excess infections in CKD patients is use of dialysis catheters, so the Countdown to Fistula guideline is critically important. In addition, because staphylococcal skin colonization is common in this population, hygiene, including hand hygiene, will be heavily emphasized for patients who do have catheters. Adult vaccinations are also tracked and actively managed for all patients as a mechanism to reduce hospitalizations.

5. *Hemodialysis safe start.* Working closely with the patient's nephrologist, the HT care manager facilitates education and the timing of having a working AVF in place. The monitoring of patient status over time allows for timely planning in initiating dialysis in an outpatient facility setting. Recent data may indicate that outpatient starts may be as low as 25 percent nationally (Wong et al. 2016).

6. *Medication reconciliation*. All medications are ascertained by direct inspection of actual medication containers in the patient's home. The actual medications taken are reconciled with those on the physician's list in the electronic health record. Medications are also verified monthly over the phone with the patient. Furthermore, nurse care managers have been comprehensively educated on the medications that may be harmful to the patient's renal function.

Step 6: Evaluating the Results

As part of its governance role, the MAB conducts monthly assessments of the program based on the data presented. The core design team, with approvals by the MAB, developed a set of variables for each patient that allow for program operations, clinical quality, processes, and outcomes to be rigorously assessed and managed. These variables are consistent with the data fields identified in the proposed program's clinical and workflow guidelines and are captured in the informatics system. Furthermore, the IT system can aggregate the key demographic and performance indicators onto a program dashboard relating to process, outcomes, intervention effectiveness, provider, and patient satisfaction. The dashboard is evaluated weekly by the core team and monthly by the MAB.

By October 2014, one year after implementation, 161 patients had been enrolled in the program. Modality selection occurred in 88 percent of patients enrolled. Among patients who reached ESRD, through October 31, 2015, 63 percent started ESRD with hemodialysis, 20 percent started with peritoneal dialysis, and 7 percent had a preemptive transplant. Exhibit 9.3 displays our key outcomes from the HT Program, with national averages available for comparison.

Conclusion

Traditional quality improvement efforts have been anchored in lengthy planning that attempts to account for all contingencies at the time of implementation—usually resulting in failed or partial implementation. The HT Program demonstrates not only how an EBMgmt approach was applied to achieve the most effective outcomes, but also how it was instrumental in expanding upon the evidence that currently exists. Through an EBMgmt approach, we were able to (1) prioritize the quality of the research available, (2) more systematically and efficiently understand where gaps in the research exist, and (3) make decisions depending on the availability of the evidence.

In our example, systematic reviews had already been conducted for some of the key clinical focus areas. But despite the abundance of evidence

EXHIBIT 9.3
Healthy
Transition
Program Metrics

Healthy Transition in Late-Stage CKD Metrics (n = 161 patients, CKD Stage 4 and Stage 5) October 15, 2012–October 31, 2015	HT Pilot Oct 2012– Oct 2015	USRDS Data 2011
Hospitalizations (all causes, CKD 4–5, per thousand patient years)	800	1100
Fistula rate at initiation of hemodialysis	63%	18%
Catheter rate at initiation of hemodialysis	37%	82%
Outpatient initiation of hemodialysis	63%	Less than 37% (Crews et al. 2010)
Transplant rate	7%	0.70%
Peritoneal dialysis rate	20%	6%

in some areas, national performance in the related outcomes was poor. We understood that the current care model, with the nephrologist providing sole education and preparation, is limited (consider, for example, the under-utilization of AVFs). This issue was brought to the forefront because of our clinical director's dialysis experience and understanding that the care team needs a structured framework for evaluation. Our framework was known and followed by the care manager, the nephrologist, the vascular surgeon, and the patient. Because of our evaluations and our ability to make the best possible decisions, we achieved a mature fistula rate for patients of 63 percent—compared to the US average of 18 percent—over three years. Furthermore, the majority of these patients had a safe dialysis start in the outpatient dialysis center, rather than one begun in a hospitalization.

Although little prior research had been published specific to CKD, our research question—about using the patient-centered medical home as a mechanism for providing high-quality care across the full range of individuals' health needs—proved effective in our pilot. The innovation in our program stemmed from integrating the synthesis of compiled evidence for nurse care managers to use and tying it to an IT system that would help care managers be more efficient and focus on the identified outcomes.

After three years, our pilot performance metrics demonstrate how the HT Program improves the healthcare that patients receive, supports the health of the population, and reduces unnecessary utilization. They show that our intervention helps patients overcome barriers and facilitates timely treatment options. Aware that we need stronger empirical evidence to validate the findings of our program, we have begun a formal randomized control study that is currently in progress. In May 2014, the program was awarded a Center for Medicare & Medicaid Innovation grant of $2.45 million for further development, multiple-site expansion, and testing.

Case Study Questions

1. What are the key aspects of the CKD care coordination program at Northwell Health?
2. Why did top management adopt these changes?
3. How was an evidence-based process used in designing the intervention?
4. What are the strengths and weaknesses of the approach that the managers used to evaluate the results of the intervention?
5. What are the constraints and opportunities that other large hospitals might encounter in adapting the approach used at Northwell?

References

Allon, M. 2004. "Dialysis Catheter-Related Bacteremia: Treatment and Prophylaxis." *American Journal of Kidney Diseases* 44 (5): 779–91.

American Academy of Family Physicians (AAFP). 2007. "Joint Principles of the Patient-Centered Medical Home." Published March 7. www.aafp.org/dam /AAFP/documents/practice_management/pcmh/initiatives/PCMHJoint .pdf.

American College of Physicians (ACP). 2006. *The Advanced Medical Home: A Patient-Centered, Physician-Guided Model of Health Care.* Accessed July 6, 2016. www .acponline.org/acp_policy/policies/adv_medicalhome_patient_centered _model_healthcare_2006.pdf.

Aydede, S. K., P. Komenda, O. Djurdjev, and A. Levin. 2014. "Chronic Kidney Disease and Support Provided by Home Care Services: A Systematic Review." *BMC Nephrology.* Published July 18. www.biomedcentral.com /1471-2369/15/118.

Barends, E., S. T. Have, and F. Huisman. 2012. "Learning from Other Evidence-Based Practices: The Case of Medicine." In *The Oxford Handbook of Evidence-Based Management,* edited by D. M. Rousseau, 25–42. New York: Oxford University Press.

Cassidy, A. 2010. "Patient-Centered Medical Homes." *Health Affairs.* Published September 14. www.healthaffairs.org/healthpolicybriefs/brief.php?brief_id=25.

Centre for Clinical Practice. 2011. "Peritoneal Dialysis in the Treatment of Stage 5 Chronic Kidney Disease." National Institute for Health and Care Excellence. www.guideline.gov/content.aspx?id=34826.

Crews, D. C., B. G. Jaar, L. C. Plantinga, H. S. Kassem, N. E. Fink, and N. R. Pow. 2010. "Inpatient Hemodialysis Initiation: Reasons, Risk Factors and Outcomes." *Nephron Clinical Practise* 114 (1): c19–c28.

Harchowal, J. T. 1997. "Drug-Related Problems on a Renal Unit." *British Journal of Renal Medicine* 2: 22–24.

Hassan Murad, M., A. N. Sidawy, M. B. Elamin, A. Z. Rizvi, D. N. Flynn, F. R. McCausland, M. M. McGrath, D. H. Vo, Z. El-Zoghby, E. T. Casey, A. A. Duncan, M. J. Tracz, P. J. Erwin, and V. M. Montori. 2008. "Timing of Referral for Vascular Access Placement: A Systematic Review." *Journal of Vascular Surgery* 48 (5): S31–S33.

Liebman, S. E., D. A. Bushinsky, J. G. Dolan, and P. Veazie. 2012. "Differences Between Dialysis Modality Selection and Initiation." *American Journal of Kidney Diseases* 59 (4): 550–57.

Navuluri, N., and S. Regalado. 2009. "The KDOQI 2006 Vascular Access Update and Fistula First Program Synopsis." *Seminars in Interventional Radiology* 26 (2): 122–24.

Norfolk, E., and J. Hartle. 2013. "Nephrology Care in a Fully Integrated Care Model: Lessons from the Geisinger Health System." *Clinical Journal of the American Society of Nephrology.* Published January. http://cjasn.asnjournals .org/content/early/2013/01/17/CJN.08460812.full.

Paulus, R. A., J. Davis, and G. D. Steele. 2008. "Continuous Innovation in Health Care: Implications of the Geisinger Experience." *Health Affairs* 27 (5): 1235–45.

Peikes, D., A. Zutshi, J. Genevro, K. Smith, M. Parchman, and D. Meyers. 2012. *Early Evidence on the Patient-Centered Medical Home.* AHRQ Publication No. 12-0020-EF. Rockville, MD: Agency for Healthcare Research and Quality.

Pradel, F. G., R. Jain, C. D. Mullins, J. A. Vassalotti, and S. T. Bartlett. 2008. "A Survey of Nephrologists' Views on Preemptive Transplantation." *Clinical Journal of the American Society of Nephrology* 3 (6): 1837–45.

Ramanathan, V., E. J. Chiu, J. T. Thomas, A. Khan, G. M. Dolson, and R. O. Darouiche. 2007. "Healthcare Costs Associated with Hemodialysis Catheter-Related Infections: A Single-Center Experience." *Infection Control and Hospital Epidemiology* 28 (5): 606–9.

Seliger, S. L., M. Zhan, V. D. Hsu, L. D. Walker, and J. C. Fink. 2008. "Chronic Kidney Disease Adversely Influences Patient Safety." *Journal of the American Society of Nephrology* 19 (12): 2414–19.

St. Peter, W. L. 2010. "Improving Medication Safety in Chronic Kidney Disease Patients on Dialysis Through Medication Reconciliation." *Advances in Chronic Kidney Disease* 17 (5): 413–19.

United States Renal Data System (USRDS). 2011. *Annual Data Report: Atlas of Chronic Kidney Disease and End-Stage Renal Disease in the United States.* Bethesda, MD: National Institutes of Health, National Institute of Diabetes and Digestive and Kidney Diseases.

————. 2010. *Annual Data Report: Atlas of Chronic Kidney Disease and End-Stage Renal Disease in the United States.* Bethesda, MD: National Institutes of Health, National Institute of Diabetes and Digestive and Kidney Diseases.

Williams, J. W., G. L. Jackson, B. J. Powers, R. Chatterjee, J. Prvu Bettger, A. R. Kemper, V. Hasselblad, R. J. Dolor, R. J. Irvine, B. L. Heidenfelder, A. S. Kendrick, and R. Gray. 2012. *The Patient-Centered Medical Home: Closing the Quality Gap; Revisiting the State of the Science.* Evidence Report / Technology Assessment No. 208. Rockville, MD: Agency for Healthcare Research and Quality.

Wong, S. P., E. K. Vig, J. S. Taylor, N. R. Burrows, C. F. Liu, D. E. Williams, P. L. Hebert, and A. M. O'Hare. 2016. "Timing of Initiation of Maintenance Dialysis: A Qualitative Analysis of the Electronic Medical Records of a National Cohort of Patients from the Department of Veterans Affairs." *JAMA Internal Medicine* 176 (2): 228–35.

Wright, J. A., and K. L. Cavanaugh. 2010. "Dietary Sodium in Chronic Kidney Disease: A Comprehensive Approach." *Seminars in Dialysis* 23 (4): 415–21.

CASE STUDY

EVIDENCE-BASED CRITERIA FOR HOSPITAL EVACUATION, TEN YEARS AFTER HURRICANE KATRINA

by K. Joanne McGlown, Stephen J. O'Connor,
and Richard M. Shewchuk

Introduction

The city of New Orleans, Louisiana, is one of the great traveler destinations in the United States. Known for its history, architecture, cuisine, jazz music, and Mardi Gras, it stands as one of America's most culturally unique cities, earning such nicknames as "The Crescent City," "The City That Care Forgot," and "The Big Easy." It sits six feet below sea level, is in close proximity to the Gulf Coast, and borders Lake Pontchartrain to the northeast. Hurricanes flooded the city in 1915, 1940, 1947, 1965, and 1969 (Leins 2015), but New Orleans went almost 40 years without any direct-hit hurricanes—a streak that contributed to a false sense of security and a decided lack of attention to disaster planning.

In late August 2005, Hurricane Katrina—the sixth strongest Atlantic hurricane on record and the third strongest to strike the United States—took aim at the city. Katrina flooded 80 percent of New Orleans (Leins 2015) and damaged about 70 percent of the city's residences. Although 1.5 million people were evacuated prior to the storm, between 150,000 and 200,000 residents are believed to have remained in the city (Soergel 2015).The city's healthcare system fared well through the hurricane landfall, but it experienced crisis in the aftermath, as levees failed and major breaches allowed water to inundate the city. Before Katrina, the New Orleans metropolitan area was served by 78 state-licensed hospitals, including 23 in Orleans Parish (Marsa 2015). After Katrina, most of the city's hospitals were closed. Only three of Orleans Parish's nine acute care hospitals were operational, with limited capacity (Rudowitz, Rowland, and Shartzer 2006).

Note: This case study builds from the one presented in chapter 18 of the first edition of this book. You are encouraged to review the earlier edition for additional context.

Katrina had a devastating impact on the healthcare infrastructure of New Orleans and on the system's ability to provide care. Delivery of health services was severely hampered by power losses, flooding, and debris. Pre-storm medical issues worsened as emergency medical support disappeared and the seriously ill or injured became nontransportable (Shatz, Wolcott, and Fairburn 2006). Clearly, important aspects of a comprehensive disaster-planning strategy—such as whether to evacuate hospital patients and the process by which evacuations could occur before, during, or after a storm—had not fully been considered.

This chapter examines the evidence informing hospital evacuation in response to a hurricane disaster event. Our question of focus is, What impact did Hurricane Katrina have on statewide hospital evacuation preparedness and planning, and how have the criteria varied in the years following the event? We present hospital lessons learned and examine the evolving evidence. We next categorize more recent hospital evacuation evidence according to the four sources of evidence provided by Barends, Rousseau, and Briner (2014), and we consider the adequacy of this evidence for informing future hospital evacuations during hurricanes. We then call for a more inclusive consideration of the nature of evidence, suggest a more rigorous and systematic approach for decision making, and consider how this approach could be used to build and extend a sufficient body of evidence.

Hospital Evacuation Evidence Pre-Katrina

A new National Response Plan (NRP) became operational throughout the United States in December 2004, with a four-month phase-in period—allowing barely any time for discussion and integration before Katrina hit the Gulf Coast. Based on the previously established National Incident Management System (NIMS), the NRP was designed for all types of hazards, and it provided a framework for US disaster response at all levels. The framework incorporated efforts by the federal, state, local, and tribal governments; the private sector; and nongovernmental organizations. It also defined the roles and responsibilities of key authorities.

As Katrina approached, federal officials used the National Disaster Medical System (NDMS) to help evacuate patients from hospitals. It was the first time the system, which had been established in 1984 (Lister 2005), was used to evacuate such a large number of patients. In 2006, a report about the effectiveness of the NDMS as a plan to evacuate hospital and nursing home patients focused on the people responsible for the decision to evacuate, issues that administrators considered with respect to the evacuation decision, and federal capabilities that supported the evacuation of healthcare facilities (US

Government Accountability Office 2006). Important findings emerged from this report and from other literature about the events in New Orleans.

Despite the prior disaster plans, New Orleans was clearly not prepared for a catastrophic event. In an October 2015 interview, Michael Brown, director of the Federal Emergency Management Agency (FEMA) at the time of Katrina, noted that large-scale FEMA-funded exercises for a potential Category 5 hurricane had been shut down by the agency in July 2005 after finding the City of New Orleans to be "so dysfunctional and so ill prepared that we can't even conduct the exercise" (Ellis 2015). Officials lacked clarity about who actually made evacuation decisions, what issues were considered, and what capabilities were available to support hospital evacuations.

Emergence of Information as Evidence Following Katrina

CEOs of healthcare organizations and other members of the Louisiana Hospital Association evaluated their responses to Katrina (Bovender and Carey 2006; Coombs 2015; Gray and Herbert 2007). They identified practices and procedures in a number of different areas that they considered useful in the evacuation processes. Exhibit 10.1 summarizes the findings.

Shortcomings of planning can be laid at the feet of almost all the hospitals and public authorities who failed to understand what flooding would do to hospitals and to respond quickly and effectively to the conditions at hand. The way hospitals dealt with the adversity is part of the experience that must be remembered in the future (Gray and Herbert 2007). Congressional and White House reports have emphasized the need for better advance planning, communications, coordination, and deployment of resources (US Government Accountability Office 2006; Boland 2006).

From exhibit 10.1, we can summarize four principal lessons:

1. Collaborative planning toward a cohesive, fully integrated, and interoperable plan for response to a major national disaster may best be addressed in concert with all other stakeholders.
2. Development of a healthcare coalition structure and enhancement of public–private partnerships for mutual assistance and collaborative service are imperative for successful response and recovery from catastrophic events.
3. Remaining legal and financial issues continue to hamper reimbursement and create confusion about liabilities after a disaster. Policymakers should bring attention to and address these issues as soon as possible. Continuing to wait for the next large disaster event will only hamper effective response and recovery efforts.

EXHIBIT 10.1
Evidence-Based Action in Key Areas Related to Hospital Evacuation Following Hurricane Katrina

	2005–2010: Immediate Response and the First Five Years Following Katrina	2010–2015: Five to Ten Years Out
Facility evacuation planning, including safety and security issues (This overarching topic includes the other areas listed in this table.)	In discussions about the preparedness of Louisiana hospitals, Anjanette Herbert (2015, personal communication), the director of security, safety, and emergency preparedness at Lafayette General Medical Center and Region 4 hospital emergency preparedness coordinator for Louisiana, states: "We immediately realized evacuation and shelter in place would be our biggest planning concern."	The rights of survivors include "the right to an evacuation that prevents death and assists in recovery" (Campanella and Laska 2015).
	Facilities developed a plan for total facility evacuation. Decision criteria for evacuation were identified and integrated with other area hospitals. These plans included triage and patient prioritization, multiple transport options, and staffing coverage for patients transferred. Hospitals must be part of area-wide disaster and evacuation planning (Gray and Herbert 2007). Planning should account for the possible loss of critical infrastructure.	Louisiana Hospital Association facilities are still addressing issues of evacuation versus shelter in place, and they have accepted a position that the hospital CEO is the *only* decision maker in evacuation issues (Herbert 2015, personal communication).
	Strong arguments were made for evacuation prior to an event (Fox News 2010).	The Joint Commission and the Centers for Medicare & Medicaid Services require that all hospitals have evacuation plans (Powell, Hanfling, and Gostin 2012).
	The need to develop a secure facility in disaster situations was not yet fully acknowledged as of 2005. However, the presence of an armed security force, in light of the looting and gunfire that followed the Katrina landfall, did increase staff's sense of security and willingness to remain on duty.	Joint Commission accreditation standards, updated after Katrina, were designed to enable facilities to function alone for 96 hours. However, these recommendations proved insufficient in 2012's Superstorm Sandy (Powell, Hanfling, and Gostin 2012).
		Two widely cited tools available for decision makers include the *Hospital Evacuation Decision Guide* from the US Department of Health and Human Services (DHHS 2015a) and the *Hospital Assessment and Recovery Guide* (DHHS 2015b; Hassol, Biddinger, and Zane 2013).

	2005–2010: Immediate Response and the First Five Years Following Katrina	2010–2015: Five to Ten Years Out
Current, reliable, and redundant communication	Communication is the most critical factor in determination to evacuate and ease of completion. Newer technology and multiple, redundant systems should have existed for internal and external communication. Hospitals purchased new satellite telephone systems, newer-generation satellite phones, and 800-megahertz radio systems—some prior to landfall of Katrina, others after the event. "Ham radio" operation was established with hospital volunteer operators and hospital-purchased equipment. Healthcare leaders reported that redundant communication systems are required for an effective evacuation (Fox News 2010).	Communication remains the most important function in disasters. Key concerns include establishing regular communication times with other hospitals, partners, and stakeholders and maintaining fastidious communication logs. Planners from the Louisiana Hospital Association and Department of Health asked what information they need to provide the hospitals. According to Herbert (2015, personal communication): "We need to start alerting them when a storm is just leaving Africa. This gives about 10 days to raise the alert—to have it on their radar. If we alert when it is still forming, this gives them a long planning process. The information is there to increase awareness." Louisiana also developed a statewide Emergency Response Network (LERN). A 24-hour call center reaches hospitals throughout the state (Herbert 2015, personal communication). Healthcare leaders identified "providing risk communication" and "sharing information and statistics" in the top three tasks the Centers for Disease Control and Prevention (CDC) should perform in large public health events and disasters (DHHS/CDC 2013, 12). Key information that should be provided by the CDC includes sources for private assets, consistent and timely clinical information and messaging, situational awareness on damage to critical infrastructure, and identity of federal agencies in charge during specific phases of an event (DHHS/CDC 2013).

(continued)

EXHIBIT 10.1
Evidence-Based Action in Key Areas Related to Hospital Evacuation Following Hurricane Katrina *(Continued)*

	2005–2010: Immediate Response and the First Five Years Following Katrina	2010–2015: Five to Ten Years Out
Staffing and processes for patient transfer and routing	A core emergency team and backup team were identified. A new group of nurses was identified to accompany and care for patients evacuated to other hospitals.	What information could an organization share with other healthcare providers during a crisis? It can share information about capacity and availability, alternate care locations, resources, conditions/statuses, needs, contacts, public service announcements by local doctors to the public, and expected delivery times of supplies and resources (DHHS/CDC 2013).
	Major planning was completed with affiliated corporate hospitals.	Organizations should ensure partnerships with area hospitals for mutual assistance and be consistent in assignments and staffing.
	Support emerged for a statewide system of bed tracking, coordinated by the state hospital association.	A statewide bed tracking system is fully functional in Louisiana and coordinated with the federal bed reporting system.
	Unexpected ethical and legal issues related to duty of care arose from the sheltering of patients' family and relatives (Bovender and Carey 2006).	
	Post-Katrina, healthcare leaders recommended that hospitals not be used as shelters (Fox News 2010).	

	2005–2010: Immediate Response and the First Five Years Following Katrina	2010–2015: Five to Ten Years Out
Equipment, supplies, and logistics for mass patient movement	Hospital Corporation of America (HCA) devoted greater attention and planning to food, water, pharmaceuticals, and general supplies in the immediate aftermath of Katrina. HCA established plans among all hospitals at risk for hurricanes to ensure coverage and resupply of critical stores. Agreements were reached with 26 different helicopter services to ensure availability and airlift capacity. Buses and drivers were secured to bring employees to facilities that will receive patients after evacuation. HCA led area preplanning for mass evacuations using military aircraft.	A recommendation stated that all hospitals should have airlift capability, preplanned and coordinated. Hospitals should identify potential disaster suppliers in advance to allow for flexibility in securing resources during a crisis. Increased awareness of the resources available from federal, state, and local entities is important; however, organizations should build plans for self-sufficiency (DHHS/CDC 2013).
Infrastructure upgrades and protection	In Katrina's aftermath, generators were water-proofed, and sensors for rising waters were installed. Emergency generators were purchased for operating an elevator and providing air conditioning to intensive care units. One hospital was digging a well and installing a backup fuel supply line.	Hospitals were urged to elevate generators to proactively prepare facilities for flooding; increase the number of emergency electrical outlets; prepare for loss of critical infrastructure; and ensure ability to operate separate from municipal water, sewer, and power, which can easily fail.

(continued)

EXHIBIT 10.1
Evidence-Based Action in Key Areas Related to Hospital Evacuation Following Hurricane Katrina *(Continued)*

	2005–2010: Immediate Response and the First Five Years Following Katrina	2010–2015: Five to Ten Years Out
Improved staff training and education	The Metropolitan Hospital Council (MHC) and the state conducted numerous drills and exercises, which translated into continual staff education to ensure preparedness for disaster response. Hospital personnel should have proper training, and they should know and understand the disaster plan. This training should be required of all physicians to obtain privileges to practice at a hospital (Pau 2013).	Quinlan, Thomas, and Guthrie (2006) of Ochsner Health System suggested that healthcare leaders should practice gratitude to all who served the health system. Herbert (2015, personal communication) recommends: "Start with Basic Incident Command courses. This is exposure to the language and concepts. It's free and available to all. Check your own Department of Homeland Security or public health department for free courses."
Interagency and hospital coordination in patient care delivery	Louisiana's statewide hospital regionalization concept, with hospitals reporting and communicating into a central statewide command center, was crucial for patient flow and treatment. MHC's effort to integrate area hospitals through exercises and planning continues. Many interim and alternate facilities emerged to meet healthcare needs. The Louisiana Hospital Association (2014) published a "Hospital CEO Hurricane Checklist" to assist with planning.	Growth in partnerships and improvement of the wellness and healthcare services available to communities are important (Coombs 2015). Hospitals should make greater use of public–private partnerships—the most successful options for the future—and build collaborative efforts toward worst-case scenarios. Hospitals in New Orleans and elsewhere in Louisiana have developed a strong coalition structure for future collaborative services (Herbert 2015, personal communication). Standardization between states is important. Many healthcare systems work across state borders and face variances in the rules and processes needed to request government assistance during and after emergencies (DHHS/CDC 2013).

	2005–2010: Immediate Response and the First Five Years Following Katrina	2010–2015: Five to Ten Years Out
	Herbert (2015, personal communication) describes Louisiana hospital planning post-Katrina: "All state, federal, and private partners participated. We know it worked. During 2008, Hurricane Gustav, the largest evacuation in the US history was held when we evacuated the full (Gulf) coastal region, then reassessed after the emergency."	Greater executive attention to disaster preparedness is vital, especially in regions of the country without disaster coalitions or cooperatives (DHHS/CDC 2013).

The partnerships that were most critical and constructive when responding to a disaster were federal, state, and local public health; local emergency medical services; other regional hospitals; and critical suppliers, including electrical and utility companies (DHHS/CDC 2013).

Herbert (2015, personal communication) describes Louisiana hospital planning post-Katrina: "Our success? We have strong coalitions. We now have regular meetings. We formed to plan, train, and respond together. (Our) coalitions are gaining their strength." |
| **Medical records information sharing and coordination** | Lack of electronic medical records systems at the time of Katrina prevented information from reaching the receiving hospitals, and no repository was safe from the storm.

Medical records have been restructured to allow remote access to critical patient information. A summary sheet of recent care delivery can be generated on demand at certain New Orleans hospitals to accompany patients being evacuated.

Electronic medical records should accompany all patients (Fox News 2010). | Consensus of a number of healthcare leaders is that the identification of patients, their destination, and summaries of their condition are imperative in the evacuation process. |

(continued)

EXHIBIT 10.1
Evidence-Based
Action in Key
Areas Related
to Hospital
Evacuation
Following
Hurricane
Katrina
(Continued)

	2005–2010: Immediate Response and the First Five Years Following Katrina	2010–2015: Five to Ten Years Out
Pet care	Pet care provision proved important for ensuring that staff would report to work in disasters. Mass pet care has aspects of both "art" and "science." Having designated staff to care for pets and a safe, remote location for improved pet care are important.	A number of veterinary organizations and FEMA have since published extensive guidelines for pet care preparedness for disasters. Many New Orleans healthcare executives have advised against accepting pets into the hospital environment in disaster situations—both for the safety and welfare of human patients and for the provision of ideal pet health.
Financial and legal issues	Large storms can completely alter the demographic base of a city and bring about additional financial hardships for people seeking care. In the first two years after Katrina, federal reimbursement issues remained unresolved. The financial crisis facing the city, and each facility, was great.	Healthcare executives experienced in disaster leadership identified the following financial and legal liabilities post-disaster: Communication with FEMA for claims settlement is difficult and time consuming. Insurance carriers will often not reimburse voluntary evacuations as they would mandatory government-ordered evacuations. Executives take on tremendous financial risk in ordering a voluntary evacuation. Facilities incur significant expense when caring for displaced populations—primarily uncompensated care. Reimbursement for alternate care sites and care performed in nontraditional environments remains controversial. Financial losses must have thorough documentation, including photo documentation (DHHS/CDC 2013). Regarding decisions to evacuate or shelter in place, Powell, Hanfling, and Gostin (2012, 2570) state:

2005–2010: Immediate Response and the First Five Years Following Katrina	2010–2015: Five to Ten Years Out
	"The Secretary of Health and Human Services should consider issuing an early public health emergency declaration to reduce legal concerns and regulatory constraints."
	A report from Marsh (2015) highlighted the impact of hurricanes on insurance issues and healthcare: "Changes over the past ten years in property insurance, claims, analytics, risk engineering, and crisis management were all influenced by Hurricanes Katrina and Ike, Superstorm Sandy, and other events, in the US and globally. . . . Individual insureds can hopefully use such lessons (learned) as they prepare to respond to catastrophes and increase their organization's resilience."
	Decisions in areas of insurance reinstatement, replacement, and mitigation often led to confrontation across issues of reconstructive alternatives, use protocols, and partial payments (Marsh 2015).
	Potential claims issues raised by Katrina and other disasters included business interruption, deductibles, service interruption, civil authorities for ingress/egress (when the government shuts down an area), and loss payment plans (Marsh 2015).

4. Communication remains an important aspect of disaster preparedness, successful response, and recovery.

To Evacuate or Not?

Gray and Herbert (2007, 293) state that "the evacuation of large numbers of severely ill patients will always be difficult, dangerous, and costly in both economic and human terms." The process of evacuation must be preplanned, the resources required must be readily available, and the actions must be possible under the evolving circumstances. Receiving facilities must be identified, capable, and ready to receive an influx of transferred patients. Staffing must be available to provide care for those awaiting transport, those in transit, and those newly arrived who are creating a "surge capacity" challenge for the host facility. "The calculus for whether to evacuate is complex, involving the cost and risk of evacuation, the certainty and anticipated severity of the event, and the time available for action" (Gray and Herbert 2007, 293). If evacuation occurs but turns out to be unnecessary, the adverse consequences could be great.

Hospitals at the time of Katrina were generally unprepared for the loss of essential services and shortages of food, water, and supplies, and they were unable to be self-sufficient for a week. When Katrina hit, the severity and location of impact was uncertain, as a need for evacuation had not presented itself before.

Perspectives at Ten Years Out

Jack Bovender, Jr., CEO of HCA during Katrina, cited *preparation of the facility* and *personal preparation* as the top two issues among the many lessons learned from the flooding and evacuation of the Tulane University Medical Center (Bovender and Carey 2006). This position was supported by a preponderance of literature calling for greater preparedness of communications and systems, infrastructure hardening, multiple transportation options, and improved coordination for evacuation. Later literature, about a decade out, emphasized partnerships and collaborative relationships among hospitals and healthcare entities through coalition building.

Infrastructure hardening—a term now more commonly used in the computing industry—involves strengthening a system and protecting against potential attack or harm. A 2001 *Newsweek* article following the September 11 terrorist attacks stated that the cost to harden the US transportation, communication, and energy infrastructure to provide state-of-the-art homeland defense could be half a trillion dollars and that "ongoing personnel costs could be staggering" (Fineman 2001). In Katrina, both the citywide infrastructure and the internal infrastructures of healthcare facilities were found to be weak and vulnerable to "attack" from natural disasters.

As new policies and regulations developed nationally in the post-Katrina period, a painful realization emerged: Reimbursement systems for care delivery during disasters were slow and fraught with problems. The Joint Commission and the Centers for Medicare & Medicaid Services (CMS) emphasized adequate disaster planning and functioning as part of a fully integrated emergency management system; such emphasis was an important development for the majority of hospitals and healthcare systems, though many commented that the expectation level for adequate planning was woefully low. Accrediting organizations have since placed greater emphasis on the role and responsibility of senior leadership in oversight and engagement in their facilities' planning and preparedness efforts (Joint Commission 2013).

In introducing new and revised requirements for emergency management oversight, effective January 2014, The Joint Commission (2013, 14) wrote, "Research indicates that hospitals plan and respond more effectively when accountability for hospitalwide emergency management is assigned to leadership at a high level of the organization." The revised elements of performance from The Joint Commission provide a clearer description of leadership-level oversight and the expanded requirements of senior hospital leadership. Larger health systems—which have more ample budgets and more trained emergency management personnel—reported more sophisticated and interoperable planning efforts. Many of the larger providers were committed to sending at least senior management for healthcare emergency management training at the US Department of Homeland Security (DHS) training center—funded by taxpayer dollars.

A final area that requires focus is the need to more collaboratively address the many difficult decisions, such as facility evacuation, that must be made in advance of a disaster or catastrophic event.

Disasters—and Their Research—Are Different

In the 1980s, the field of disaster research was evolving, and it comprised primarily narratives, stories, and interviews. The field changed significantly, however, when two leaders of the World Association of Disaster and Emergency Medicine (WADEM), Dr. Marvin Birnbaum and Dr. Knut Ole Sundnes, identified the need for a more empirical model for moving the global science of disaster research forward.

Published under the oversight of WADEM's Task Force on Quality Control of Disaster Management (TFQCDM), the *Health Disaster Management: Guidelines for Evaluation and Research in the Utstein Style* introduced a structural framework for investigations into the medical and public health aspects of disasters (TFQCDM/WADEM 2002). The framework included a standardized, universal set of definitions; a conceptual model for disasters; and descriptions of basic societal functions bound together by a coordination and control function. The guidelines also provided a disaster response template and two research templates to be used in designing, conducting, analyzing, and reporting research and in evaluations of interventions aimed at preventing hazards from becoming disaster events.

This dynamic document, through validation and modification from field experience and testing, provides reliable methods for the standardization of evaluations and research of the medical and public health aspects of disaster medicine and practice. Since its publication, the work has been successfully implemented by researchers globally in a desire to normalize descriptors, standardize processes, and validate outcomes.

Evidence from Four Categories

A question raised in the first edition of this book, in the chapter titled "Evidence-Based Criteria for Hospital Evacuation: The Case of Hurricane Katrina" was, "Did (Tulane University Hospital and Clinic) have an efficacious, systematic, and evidence-based plan for evacuation in the event of a disaster, and if so, what were the performance criteria for evacuation, and how were they applied?" (McGlown, O'Connor, and Shewchuk 2009, 221). For this chapter, the new question becomes, "What impact did Hurricane Katrina have on evacuation preparedness and planning, and how have the criteria varied over the past ten years?"

Barends, Rousseau, and Briner (2014, 11) write: "A fundamental principle of evidence-based practice is that the quality of our decisions is likely to improve the more we make use of *trustworthy* evidence—in other words, the best available evidence." This statement begs the question: "How well can the evidence you have be trusted?"

Barends, Rousseau, and Briner (2014) identify four sources of evidence: scientific evidence, organizational evidence, experiential evidence, and stakeholder evidence. In reviewing the evidence that has emerged since 2005, we encountered difficulty fitting Katrina and its aftermath to existing models. However, a look at each of the four sources of evidence helped us better define the unique characteristics of evidence-seeking for disaster situations. Descriptions of the four sources of evidence follow, accompanied by our observations and commentary:

1. *Scientific evidence* is scholarly, research-based, and published in academic journals. Prior to 2005, few peer-reviewed articles on actual hospital evacuation had been published in the United States. One of the first, in 1999, addressed the evacuation of the Veterans Affairs

Hospital in Denver, Colorado. Since 2005, a large number of articles have explored the aftermath of Katrina, and many have focused on issues that affected healthcare (e.g., legal cases, regionalization, mental and public health issues of displacement, sociological impacts on survivors). Few of them, however, addressed hospital evacuation. The published scientific literature has been overwhelmingly narrative, with interviews and data collected from people who lived, worked, or managed through a disaster weather event. Their collective voice is truly powerful evidence for situations of this nature.

2. *Organizational evidence* is found in the organization itself. It includes the organization's operation and performance data, business and financial measures, customer satisfaction, and employee information. Evidence stems from both "hard numbers" (e.g., staff turnover rates, medical errors, productivity levels) and "soft numbers" (e.g., perceptions of the organization's culture, attributes, or problems). As Barends, Rousseau, and Briner (2014, 14) point out, "Sometimes there is very little or no quality evidence available." In those cases, we have "no other option but to work with the limited evidence at hand and supplement it through learning by doing." Some decisions may have no scientific or organizational evidence available at all. Following a disaster, organizational evidence (the "hard numbers") informs the impact and guides administrative decision making toward a long-term response and recovery effort. Such an effort may even restructure the healthcare delivery system completely from what existed previously.

    If the evidence seems to be missing, it may actually be there. Possibly, it has simply not been recognized or accepted, and thus it has not been gathered or widely disseminated to make a significant difference in the healthcare preparedness arena. These conditions are changing, as more experts in healthcare disaster research contribute to the existing literature and assist in building a stronger base of disaster-related evidence.

3. *Experiential evidence* stems from professional experiences and the judgments of managers, consultants, business leaders, and other practitioners. These data accumulate over time. Tacit knowledge, or reflecting on the outcomes of similar actions taken in similar situations, is especially valuable, as is the revelation of specialized knowledge acquired through repeated experience and practice (Barends, Rousseau, and Briner 2014).

    We submit that experiential evidence is just as important when it comes from the experiences of the victims, or those affected by a disaster, as when it comes from those who responded or led organizations in the event. A wealth of experiential evidence was gathered following Katrina. Postevent assessments, the identification of issues and solutions for future improvement, and personal reflections from leaders, workers, victims, and survivors formed a large part of the evidence gathered throughout New Orleans, Louisiana, and the Gulf states. Organizations conducted exercises to check preparedness and response improvement, strengthened interoperable communication systems, and hardened infrastructure.

4. *Stakeholder evidence* comes from sources internal to the organization—such as employees, managers, and board members—as well as from external sources, such as suppliers, customers, the government, and the public. A disaster response most likely elicits a greater volume of stakeholder evidence than other types of evidence. All individuals affected by the event—patients, families, relatives, healthcare workers, care providers, first and continuing responders, and special service providers, such as helicopter pilots—were stakeholders, as were the people who provided the facility health administration leadership and the emergency management response at the parish, local, state, FEMA region, and federal levels. Additional stakeholders include politicians, media representatives, government officials (at all levels), vendors and suppliers, contractors, legal counsel, and many more.

The disaster field does not claim abundant evidence. Barends, Rousseau, and Briner (2014, 13) state that, in clinical or managerial evidence-based decision making, "The need to make an immediate decision is generally the exception rather than the rule." However, decision making in disasters often must be immediate. The disaster field does not lend itself to double-blinded, randomized studies under controlled circumstances. Disaster researchers can preplan a study for a specific event, more often than not facing reality that the event never occurs or that a different variation emerges. Furthermore, decision making in disasters must usually be informed, logical, and possible for situations that exist at a particular moment. Disasters either escalate or deescalate; they are rarely static. Our best evidence, derived from work prior to an actual event, will guide rational decisions among stakeholders as the event constantly changes. We acknowledge that, even under the best circumstances, evidence is not conclusive. "In most cases evidence comes with a large degree of uncertainty. Evidence-based practitioners, therefore, make decisions not based on conclusive, solid, up-to-date information, but on probabilities, indications, and tentative conclusions" (Barends, Rousseau, and Briner 2014, 14).

Quinlan, Thomas, and Guthrie (2006, 28) recounted the sage advice that Warner L. Thomas, the CEO of the Ochsner Health System, provided to hospital CEOs: "Catastrophe requires that we throw out old assumptions and think anew." For leaders, "the basics of making a good decision are unchanged: Get on site, look around, and ask questions. . . . Remote management is contrary to good leadership and good stewardship" (Quinlan, Thomas, and Guthrie 2006, 28–29). "As always, management by walking around was the gold standard and served us well" (Quinlan, Thomas, and Guthrie 2006, 27).

Assessment of Evidence-Based Management: Broad Versus Narrow Construal of Evidence

Evidence-based management evolved on the heels of the evidence-based medicine movement. Physicians, as scientists, tend to have a narrower, positivistic conceptualization of what constitutes evidence, and they more easily incorporate into their clinical decision making findings that fit that conceptualization. Healthcare managers, on the other hand, work in complex environments that require them to make decisions under conditions of greater uncertainty and ambiguity, and with more "confounders" in place. Decisions must be made when evidence is incomplete or noninforming. These managers have to act according to the adage of "knowing what to do when you don't know what to do."

Within the context of hospital disaster preparedness, evidence-based decision making is even more difficult, because situations take on greater complexity than they typically do in the context of clinical medicine. The dynamism and uncertainty associated with disaster situations—coupled with the significance of decision outcomes in terms of broad infrastructural, economic, political, and societal ramifications, including the real potential for loss of life on a large scale—contribute to that complexity.

Extreme weather events, such as hurricanes, change the decision-making process itself and are often associated with panic situations (Withanaarachchi and Setunge 2014). Decisions change in response to the form and scale of the disaster. Thus, the decision-making process must be flexible and able to react to the unexpected (Lahidji 2004).

Decision-making processes employed during hurricanes can be used iteratively to identify gaps in the evidence base. Decisions have resulting outcomes, which in turn can be used to inform the evidence. This quasi-experimental research design approach, when coupled with systematically curated and widely disseminated information, can contribute to a better developed evidence base.

Our construal of evidence needs to be broader, organized, and curated in such a way that it can be effectively used in decision making. However, the literature addressing how decisions are made in evidence-based management is sparse. Kovner and Rundall (2009, 64) write:

The multiple ways in which research evidence assists the decision-making process are poorly understood. Many users demand that the available evidence have immediate, instrumental use for a particular decision, but often the available research evidence cannot be used in that way. Rather, the evidence is better used to increase the decision maker's enlightenment regarding the decision issue by increasing the manager's understanding of the nature of a problem; opening up communication among managers and other stakeholders; enabling the managers to generate creative solutions; and enhancing the manager's ability to estimate the likely effects of each alternative solution to a problem. These are important, but underappreciated, contributions of the evidence-based approach to decision making.

It Can Happen Again: Hospital Evacuation Planning

Rachael McWhorter met with her host and state emergency manager, Mitch Brown, in New Orleans to facilitate a symposium for the Louisiana Hospital Hurricane Preparedness Summit, a day-long event held ten years after Katrina. Participants examined and reflected on the current state of hospital hurricane preparedness and the evidence available to assist hospital and governmental leaders in making decisions on whether to evacuate. Rachael was slated to facilitate a consensus panel representing three different groups, or "voices," each with strong leadership input into the future direction of evacuation planning and preparedness for the parish and state. The three groups were hospital and healthcare administrators, members of the Regional Planning Commission, and parish emergency managers.

Participants in the summit had received, two weeks earlier, a report from Rachael that detailed the growing body of hospital evacuation evidence and the lessons learned from immediately after the storm to ten years after the event. The report included a summary of the table shown in exhibit 10.1.

A Systematic Decision-Making Exercise

In addition to presenting and reviewing the state of evidence, Rachael engaged the participants in a systematic decision-making exercise. She instructed participants to consider the available evidence, as well as their own knowledge and expertise in evacuation planning, to address the goal of the summit: *optimal regional hospital evacuation during a hurricane*. The exercise was based on a multicriteria decision-making (MCDM) framework using the analytic hierarchy process (AHP). MCDM has been used to assist decision makers in areas such as "financial analysis, flood risk management, housing evaluation, disaster management, and customer relationship management" (Umm-e-Habiba and Asghar 2009, 321). AHP was created by

Saaty (1980) to analyze complex decisions in which the perspectives of multiple stakeholders must be incorporated. The process helps people clarify a problem or issue they are facing, as well as the criteria (objectives or attributes) and options (strategies or alternatives) relevant to achieving a goal. The criteria can be provided in advance or developed through a consensus process with expert key informants to "increase transparency, dialogue, and ownership of the process and outcome" (Bharwani et al. 2013, 1). Similarly, the options for achieving the goal can be provided in advance or developed through a consensus process.

In reviewing the issues identified in exhibit 10.1, the group agreed on the following criteria as the most important for groups with the goal of improvement:

1. Engaging in collaborative planning
2. Developing healthcare coalitions and enhanced public–private partnerships
3. Addressing legal and financial issues concerning reimbursement and policy

Ensuring internal and external communications, Rachael developed these criteria in an AHD model and challenged the group to identify options for addressing the criteria. The groups were engaged in the exercise, for the process held promise of finally "weighing" the value of the decisions reached. It also clearly illustrated the order of importance for funding and action required to identify and implement a strong statewide strategy to prepare for potential hospital evacuations in the future.

The options selected for consideration in decision making for evacuation were as follows:

1. Economic cost of evacuation
2. Ability to manage patient safety during evacuation
3. Ability to control the timing and implementation of evacuation
4. Sheltering in place (the risk of not evacuating)

When the criteria and options were identified in an appropriate hierarchical framework, participants performed a system of pairwise comparisons in which each criterion was compared against every other criterion with respect to perceived value or importance to the goal. This approach provided a scaling/weight of the relative importance of the criteria. Each option was then compared with every other option with respect to each weighted criterion to derive a value or weight for the option relative to the specific criterion. The pairwise comparison among options was repeated for each weighted criterion.

Measuring Performance and Evaluating Progress

Representing the state emergency managers, Mitch Brown presented the National Planning Scenarios (NPS) and explained the rationale for using them as the basis of future exercises for hurricane preparedness and response. In March 2006, the federal interagency community developed 15 all-hazards planning scenarios to be used in national, state, and local homeland security preparedness activities (FEMA 2009). The scenarios are planning tools representative of a range of potential terrorist attacks and natural disasters, and they are scalable to all government and response levels. The scenarios are the first step in the capabilities-based planning process used by the US Department of Homeland Security (DHS 2005).

Mitch described Scenario #10, "Natural Disaster / Major Hurricane," in which a Category 5 hurricane hits a major metropolitan area with sustained winds of 160 miles per hour and a storm surge more than 20 feet above normal. Massive evacuations are required, and low-lying escape routes are inundated by water, starting five hours before the eye of the hurricane reaches land (DHS 2005). This scenario is similar to the events of Katrina, with the exception that, unlike in Katrina, evacuation in the scenario is mandated 48 hours prior to landfall, with mass evacuations and evacuation routes overwhelmed at 24 hours out. The detail and impact provided allow parish and state officials to test against the scenario, to alter variables from the final number identified, and to evaluate their performance to measure improvement in preparedness. Scenario #10, Mitch explained, is the scenario that should, and must, be used in planning the exercise series for the parish and state.

Continuing a step further, Mitch informed the planning commissioners and healthcare administrators of a well-developed and mandated federal exercise program, complete with processes for conduct and evaluation of exercises to ensure improvement over time. This program, the Homeland Security Exercise and Evaluation Program (HSEEP), "provides a set of guiding principles for exercise programs, as well as a common approach to exercise program management, design and development, conduct, evaluation, and improvement planning" (DHS 2013, Intro-1).

Rachael then proceeded to introduce the additional steps for evidence validation that would allow this group to personalize the issues, identify potential solutions, and prioritize actions to be included in future exercises. With the four key criteria identified and the process for exercise and evaluation determined and agreed upon, planning could continue.

The AHP approach produces various statistics that can be used to examine where panelists have disagreements or lack consistency in how criteria or alternatives are compared. These statistics can provide additional insights for refining the model or identifying additional or different criteria with respect to the goal. Moreover, different elements of the hierarchy—either the criteria or the options—can be respecified at different levels within the model.

Exhibits 10.2 and 10.3 represent examples of an AHP for optimal regional hospital evacuation during a hurricane. It is a multicriteria analytic framework, developed from lessons learned through the Katrina experience and input from knowledgeable key informants, that becomes a consensus statement of evidence for hospital evacuation decision making during a disaster such as a hurricane.

Such a framework can be used to guide the hospital evacuation decision. In the future, after a new hurricane-related hospital evacuation, the framework can be updated and improved through incorporation of new lessons learned and input from expert key informants. Of course, such a decision framework must operate in accordance with the legal command structure of FEMA, where the hierarchy of decision making runs from the local level to the county, state, FEMA regional headquarters, and federal levels. This hierarchy can be considered a behavioral facilitator as well as a constraint to the AHP framework. However, many decision-making processes that feature hierarchy and centralization are being augmented by more decentralized emergency management systems (Kapucu and Garayev 2011). These new systems of emergency management involve collaborative decision making that blends and incorporates the resources, capabilities, and leadership of various programs, government agencies, and organizations to achieve a common goal. The Emergency Management Assistance Compact (EMAC), for instance, is a multistate mutual aid agreement that encourages resource provision during and after disasters (Kapucu and Garayev 2011). Collaboratives

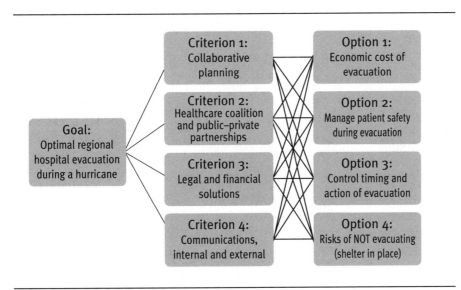

EXHIBIT 10.2

Example of an Analytic Hierarchy Process for Evacuation Options During a Hurricane Event

EXHIBIT 10.3
Hypothetical
Example
of Analytic
Hierarchy
Process Results
from Summit
Participants
for Hospital
Evacuation
Decisions

Goal	Criteria	Global Priorities	Option 1	Option 2	Option 3	Option 4
Optimal regional hospital evacuation during a hurricane	Criterion 1: Collaborative planning	27.1%	0.0216	0.1046	0.1128	0.032
	Criterion 2: Healthcare coalitions and public–private partnerships	35.2%	0.216	0.086	0.034	0.016
	Criterion 3: Legal and financial solutions	15.3%	0.0695	0.0294	0.0141	0.04
	Criterion 4: Communications, internal and external	22.4%	0.071	0.045	0.035	0.073
		100%	37.81%	26.5%	19.59%	16.1%

such as EMAC function when they are well coordinated and when decision making is rapid and effectual. Collaboration fulfills a key aspect in attaining positive outcomes during a hurricane.

In sum, the AHP process provides several conclusions and recommendations related to hospital evacuation:

1. The process points out gaps in our understanding of the evidence to help guide hospital evacuations.
2. It provides a model that can be tested, using quasi-experimental type data, to build a positivistic research base.
3. The hospital evacuation model can be replicated in different areas.
4. The process involves critical stakeholders who have a vested interest in the results; by incorporating their views, it offers an organically derived model.
5. The information is systematized and framed in such a way that it can be used as evidence in the process. Thus, information that is systematized, framed, curated, and archived with metatags (e.g., information from the summit and other similar activities) is recommended. If little progress is observed with respect to specific parts of the model, these areas require greater focus.

6. If ever a case demanded "big data in real time," hospital evacuation prior to and during a hurricane is it. Once a hospital is in the path of a hurricane, the collaboration of stakeholders organized in consort with the Emergency Operations Center—who are all in this together—need to be updated on results of real-time sensitivity analyses. If the results indicate a high probability of evacuation, nearby hospitals need to fully prepare for the evacuation and reception of patients. This type of preparation incurs additional costs, but peer pressure from consortium stakeholders can help hospital administrators justify their wise decisions by reiterating the longer-term cost savings, such as lower insurance premiums.

Future Direction in the Use of Evidence in Practice

Evidence should inform massive public policy changes. A system of public–private cooperation must be developed to marshal the tremendous capabilities of the private sector. Leveraging the existing capabilities of the private sector and focusing on rapid command and control techniques in the government levels is a feasible alternative (Quinlan, Thomas, and Guthrie 2006).

We believe that in the more dynamic, emerging fields—such as disaster management—a "new type of evidence" must accept the following ideas as reality:

1. Forecasts or risk assessments based on the aggregated experiences of many people may be more accurate than forecasts based on one person's personal experience; however, one person's personal experience in a disaster is still valid and valued information.
2. Professional judgments based on hard data or statistical models may be no more accurate than judgments based on individual experience.
3. Knowledge derived from scientific evidence is as important as the opinions of experts; both are part of a "new equation" for examining evidence in dynamic environments.
4. A decision based on the combination of critically appraised experiential, organizational, and scientific evidence yields better outcomes than a decision based on a single source of evidence.
5. Evaluating the outcome of a decision improves both organizational learning and performance, especially in novel and nonroutine situations.

We call for a volume of robust and varied studies based on a multi-criteria decision-making approach that can produce a hierarchical ranking of options or strategies to address objectives designed to contend with the primary aim of a disaster research study. Through multiple iterations and examinations of outcomes, vetted by sensitivity analyses, a basic collection of decision-making tools will stand ready for use in future disaster events—and for enhancement as each new postevent evaluation leads to more informed evidence for improvement.

Integrating the Evidence in Hospital Practice

Healthcare was a central priority during the response and recovery phases of Katrina. The hurricane demonstrated that new plans and tactics must be implemented (Boland 2006) and that "providers in the region have the opportunity and obligation to redesign healthcare for the area" (Quinlan, Thomas, and Guthrie 2006, 27).

As Shatz, Wolcott, and Fairburn (2006, 555) write, "the hurricane of 2005 demonstrated how extensive (these) preparations should be and the cost of inadequate preparation. . . . Proper planning and effective drills can mitigate the extent of damage to structures and human life, and when necessary, effective evacuation of at-risk areas is crucial. In the end, nature is much too powerful a force for us to fight—we can only be prepared to respond to and bend with the potentially devastating forces directed our way."

The Politics of Disaster Management

Of all the articles taking a retrospective look at Katrina ten years later, few focused on the concerns of, or actions related to, *healthcare* issues in disaster planning, evacuation, and disaster response. Disaster-related healthcare concerns represent a national challenge and require action at multiple levels of government and civil authority. Though some pieces are in place, a collaborative and comprehensive approach to address such issues does not yet exist. Disaster planning and preparedness is primarily government-funded, and little effort or money is allocated to address healthcare-specific disaster preparedness.

A 2015 article in the *Natural Hazard Observer* stated that Katrina highlighted serious problems in the nation's ability to respond to disasters—including gaps in emergency management planning, evacuation failures, and social vulnerability issues (Natural Hazards Center 2015).

Powell, Hanfling, and Gostin (2012) compare lessons from Katrina to those from the mass hospital evacuations across New York City related to the landfall of Superstorm Sandy in October 2012. On the positive side, New York hospitals had more detailed emergency plans and better positioned backup generators and fuel pumps that were protected from a flood of 12 feet. As a result of Katrina, hospitals were better able to manage evacuations, receive patients, and prepare for surge capacity. "What seemed to be missing, however, were clear and consistent criteria to guide evacuation decisions" (Powell, Hanfling, and Gostin 2012, 2569). "In the aftermath of Sandy, hospitals were unable to ensure continuity of operations, which is a hallmark of successful disaster plans" (Powell, Hanfling, and Gostin 2012, 2570). The authors support local and regional planning by healthcare coalitions as the best way to promote situational awareness for member organizations through the collection, aggregation, and dissemination of incident information. This integrated planning should prevent the kind of fragmented decision making that occurred in Katrina. "Coordinated plans and integrated decision making will go a long way to mitigating the potential dire consequences that could arise during future forced healthcare facility evacuations" (Powell, Hanfling, and Gostin 2013, 1586).

Hassol, Biddinger, and Zane (2013) and Powell, Hanfling, and Gostin (2013) observe that CMS and The Joint Commission today require that all hospitals have evacuation plans, but they note that the plans provide little or no guidance for making the critical decision of whether to evacuate or shelter in place. The US Department of Health and Human Services has funded the development of two tools to assist senior administrators with this decision: the *Hospital Evacuation Decision Guide* (DHHS 2015a) and the *Hospital Assessment and Recovery Guide* (DHHS 2015b). The first helps leaders identify "harbingers requiring an evacuation" and prioritize considerations to be addressed prior to evacuation. It also distinguishes between preevent and postevent evacuations. The latter document is a 45-page checklist covering 11 separate areas of hospital infrastructure to be evaluated prior to safe reoccupancy of an evacuated and damaged hospital (Hassol, Biddinger, and Zane 2013, 1585–86).

Better Model Development and the Cost–Benefit of Disaster Planning

The losses experienced by the healthcare facilities in Louisiana and across the Gulf states beg the questions: What has to happen for successful local and regional plans for disasters? And are there models of what different kinds of planning cost?

Leading current texts in the field of urban economics, the discipline that lies at the intersection of geography and economics, fail to list *disaster*, *emergency*, or *catastrophe* in their indexes (O'Sullivan 2012; Arnott and McMillen 2008). Some response, however, can be found from the planning profession and from national and global industry and insurers/reinsurers in robust model revisions, data analytics, and forecasting analyses.

Local, regional, and state planning should have left healthcare systems better prepared for the catastrophic events of Katrina. However, Marsh (2015, 3), a global insurance leader, reported that "initial loss estimates from

Katrina missed the mark by a long shot in part because the data loaded into the models was inadequate, incomplete, inaccurate, or miscoded." Models at the time had "overestimated the impact of pure wind damage and underestimated the damage from flooding and storm surge. As a result, initial damage estimates identified only about one-fourth of the total damage" (Marsh 2015, 3–6). "While computer catastrophe (CAT) models were in use at the time, they proved to be greatly out of line with actual losses. . . . Katrina thus became a turning point for the insurance industry on many fronts, including CAT modeling, property policy wording, claims handling, and crisis management" (Marsh 2015, 3).

After every major hurricane event, the insurance industry continues to learn and refine models and projections. The National Response Framework (NRF) defines how federal agencies will respond to emergencies. Updates to the NRF in 2006 were based on the collective experiences in responding to hurricanes Katrina, Wilma, and Rita in 2005, and primary improvements focused on communication and coordination among government agencies (Marsh 2015, 12). Hurricane Ike, which struck in 2008 and persisted inland, reinforced the idea that hurricane preparedness should "not be limited to just coastal locations" (Marsh 2015, 6). An additional observation from Ike was that, "for properties that complied with the latest building codes, damage was minimal" (Marsh 2015, 6). Superstorm Sandy led to yet further iterations in model development.

Toward Resilience in Planning and Preparedness

Perhaps nowhere has the reevaluation of goals and methods happened as quickly as in planning efforts. Before Sandy, the key word was *green*. But in the wake of Sandy, a new term has triumphed: *resilience* (Marshall 2013). "In this new context, things that were once considered outlandish or politically impossible, like giant storm gates across harbors, are now on the table. There are data now, not just speculation, about how high floodwaters can go and the damage they can cause" (Marshall 2013, 38).

"That the term *resilience* was heard less before Sandy than afterward doesn't mean it was ignored. In New York City's *PlaNYC*, released in 2011, the chapter on addressing climate change states that FEMA's flood maps are outdated, that insurance regulations need to be revised, and that critical infrastructure should be protected" (Marshall 2013, 38). "As planning and rebuilding proceed in the Northeast under the new banner of resilience, it is federal money that is making it possible. The funds highlight how US disaster response has become not just emergency rebuilding, but the default mechanism for long-term planning" (Marshall 2013, 39).

"In the immediate rebuilding effort, FEMA is primarily operating through its disaster relief fund and its policies for getting the money. In

September 2011, it published the National Disaster Recovery Framework, which requires states to have hazard mitigation plans. Just over a year later, Sandy certainly tested the model. . . . For longer term planning, the Army Corps of Engineers is playing a leading role" (Marshall 2013, 39).

The insurance industry, the livelihood of which depends on disaster analysis and production, warns that we will see these severe events—and worse—in the future. Swiss Re, one of the largest reinsurance companies in the world, insures insurance companies. Because it operates globally, its models take into account patterns, both natural and human, across the world. Remarking that Superstorm Sandy was not a surprise, the company states, "Sandy was nothing more than a reminder. There are worse ones out there" (Marshall 2013, 40–41).

Federal policies build in disincentives for cities or states to prepare for disaster, and federal policies on funding are not ideal (Marshall 2013). The federal government is concerned with disaster preparedness, but action occurs too slowly to be taken as serious assistance. For example, in 2012, in response to a year of extreme weather events, bipartisan legislation supporting local efforts to plan for natural disaster resilience was introduced in the US Congress. The Strengthening the Resiliency of Our Nation on the Ground (STRONG) Act would form an interagency working group to provide a strategic vision of extreme weather resilience and develop a National Extreme Weather Resilience Action Plan. Its aim is "to minimize the economic and social costs resulting from losses of life, property, well-being, business activity, and economic growth associated with extreme weather events by ensuring that the United States is more resilient to the impacts of extreme weather events in the short- and long-term, and for other purposes" (GovTrack.us 2016). However, three years after the proposed bill was introduced, it has only been assigned to a committee that "will consider it before possibly sending it to the House or Senate as a whole."

The rule proposed by CMS concerning emergency preparedness planning for all providers and suppliers that accept Medicare and Medicaid funds includes the following eight highlights (Herman 2014):

1. A facility's preparedness program should address four core elements: risk assessment/planning, policies and procedures, communication plans, and training/testing.
2. Preparedness efforts should take an "all-hazards" approach.
3. Facilities should be required to meet several checkpoints in risk assessment and planning (e.g., alternative care sites).
4. Facilities should be required to meet certain minimum standards for staff and patients (e.g., amount of food and drink on hand, alternative sources of energy).

5. Hospitals should have established communication plans and ways for employees, physicians, other institutions, and volunteers to share information (within the bounds of the Health Insurance Portability and Accountability Act).

6. Hospitals should review and update preparedness programs annually.

7. Guidelines for general acute care hospitals also would apply to critical access hospitals.

8. Ambulatory surgery centers would not be required to meet all the expectations of the general acute care hospitals.

Industry experts are awaiting release of a federal rule, under development since 2007, that would make emergency preparedness a condition for participation in Medicare and Medicaid for a wide range of healthcare institutions. The rule would cover the basics for healthcare preparedness and potentially affect more than 68,000 providers. The proposed rule has been described as an "urgent public health issue"; however, it has not been delayed by opposition from many of the groups it seeks to serve. The solution "could be to create incentives for providers demonstrating preparedness, like higher Medicare reimbursements, increased credit ratings, and lower insurance premiums" (Fink 2016). A few positive outcomes would be a welcome change for a beleaguered healthcare industry currently expected to undertake costly preparedness activities for accreditation and compliance as an "unfunded mandate."

Next Steps for Healthcare Managers and Leaders

This case study could not possibly include all the issues that arise in a mass casualty or catastrophic event. Therefore, we encourage further investigation into related areas of emergency management, preparedness, and response that are as integral to a successful planning effort as the issues we have discussed here. A multitude of books, white papers, and articles have been generated throughout the nearly 40-year history of emergency management as a profession. This literature addresses key areas that presented critical issues for healthcare leaders prior to and during Katrina. In particular, we invite readers to investigate further the following four areas:

1. *Ethics in disaster.* A variety of ethical concerns—including "failure to prepare" and failure in duty of care—have been raised with regard to the care of patients during disasters and dire circumstances, and some have led to civil charges against physicians, nurses, and healthcare providers. Sheri Fink's (2013) book *Five Days at Memorial* investigates

patient deaths at a New Orleans hospital during Katrina. Records and accounts of the actions of Dr. Anna Pou and colleagues are considered critical study for all healthcare executives.

2. *The role of the military in disaster response.* The public has come to expect the military to respond to disasters and to provide aid in crisis; however, such tasks do not represent the military's primary mission. Under many circumstances, a military response may not be possible, desirable, or feasible. Readers are also encouraged to investigate the role of the National Guard, the conditions for activation in disasters (federally declared or not), and the way that the military sectors, and their vast resources, fit within the National Response Plan.

3. *Basic knowledge.* The healthcare executive must possess basic knowledge across a number of areas:

    - Disaster finance issues, such as what to know and document before and during a disaster for maximum reimbursement and protection after the event; preparedness, including cash on hand, cash burn, and ability to conduct business with no power; and preevent mitigation and postevent recovery

    - Federal funding and emergency preparedness monies to the states, and how the granting of funds differs for not-for-profit and for-profit entities

    - The National Response Framework, the National Incident Management System, and the Hospital Incident Command Systems

    - Inclusion of all responders in a collaborative and fully integrated model for response and recovery, at all levels, in all-hazards events

4. *Research and policy development.* Healthcare leaders should investigate who pays for model research and development, how to bring innovative ideas to the emergency management market, and how to move from proposals to action.

Case Study Questions

1. What is the question that the authors seek to answer in this case study? How does this question differ from the question asked in the case ten years previously?

2. How trustworthy is the scientific, organizational, experiential, and stakeholder evidence that the authors gathered in this chapter?

3. What would have to happen to improve the trustworthiness of the evidence?

4. What are the strengths and weaknesses of the improvement recommendations made by the authors?

5. What would have to happen for these recommendations to be implemented, and by whom would they be implemented?

References

Arnott, R. J., and D. P. McMillen (eds.). 2008. *A Companion to Urban Economics.* Hoboken, NJ: Blackwell Publishing.

Barends, E., D. M. Rousseau, and R. B. Briner. 2014. *Evidence-Based Management: The Basic Principles.* Center for Evidence-Based Management. Accessed June 9, 2016. www.cebma.org/wp-content/uploads/Evidence-Based-Practice-The-Basic-Principles.pdf.

Bharwani, S., C. Varela-Ortega, I. Blanco, P. Esteve, E. Juarez, G. Trombi, M. Moriondo, M. Bindi, T. Devisscher, R. Taylor, and P. Watkiss. 2013. *Analytic Hierarchy Process (AHP). Decision Support Methods for Adaptation.* MEDIATION Project, Briefing Note 7. Published May. www.mediation-project.eu/platform/pbs/pdf/Briefing-Note-7-LR.pdf.

Boland, R. T. 2006. "Can It Get Any Worse?" *Frontiers of Health Services Management* 23 (1): 31–34.

Bovender, J. O. Jr., and B. Carey. 2006. "A Week We Don't Want to Forget: Lessons Learned from Tulane." *Frontiers of Health Services Management* 23 (1): 3–12.

Campanella, R., and S. Laska. 2015. "Katrina: Ten Years Later." Paper presented at the annual meeting of the Natural Hazards Conference, Boulder, CO, July.

Coombs, B. 2015. "Ochsner: Hospital Powerhouse Forged in the Wake of Katrina." *CNBC Online.* Published August 27. www.cnbc.com/2015/08/26/ochsner-hospital-powerhouse-forged-in-the-wake-of-katrina.html.

Ellis, R. 2015. "Hurricane Katrina Teaches Former FEMA Chief Resilience." *NewsOK.* Published October 4. http://newsok.com/hurricane-katrina-teaches-former-fema-chief-resiliences/article/5451187.

Federal Emergency Management Agency (FEMA). 2009. "National Planning Scenarios Fact Sheet." Accessed July 15, 2016. www.fema.gov/media-library-data/20130726-1914-25045-8890/hseep_apr13_.pdf.

Fineman, H. 2001. "A President Finds His True Voice." *Newsweek.* Published September 23. www.newsweek.com/president-finds-his-true-voice-152099.

Fink, S. 2016. "Can Health Care Providers Afford to Be Ready for Disaster?" *New York Times.* Published February 13. www.nytimes.com/2016/02/14/sunday-review/can-health-care-providers-afford-to-be-ready-for-disaster.html.

———. 2013. *Five Days at Memorial: Life and Death in a Storm-Ravaged Hospital.* New York: Crown Publishers.

Fox News. 2010. "Hurricane Katrina's Deadly Legacy at Memorial Medical Center." Published August 27. www.foxnews.com/health/2010/08/27/hurricane -katrinas-deadly-legacy-memorial-medical-center.html.

GovTrack.us. 2016. "H.R. 2227: STRONG Act." Accessed July 19. www.govtrack .us/congress/bills/114/hr2227.

Gray, B. H., and K. Herbert. 2007. "Hospitals in Hurricane Katrina: Challenges Facing Custodial Institutions in a Disaster." *Journal of Health Care for the Poor and Underserved* 18 (2): 283–98.

Hassol, A., P. Biddinger, and R. Zane. 2013. "Hospital Evacuation Decisions in Emergency Situations." *Journal of the American Medical Association* 309 (15): 1585–86.

Herman, B. 2014. "8 Things to Know about CMS' Emergency Preparedness Rule." *Becker's Hospital Review.* Published January 7. www.beckershospitalreview.com /strategic-planning/8-things-to-know-about-cms-emergency-preparedness -rule.html.

Joint Commission. 2013. "New and Revised Requirements Address Emergency Management Oversight." *Perspectives* 33 (7): 14–15.

Kapucu, N., and V. Garayev. 2011. "Collaborative Decision-Making in Emergency and Disaster Management." *International Journal of Public Administration* 34 (6): 366–75.

Kovner, A. R., and T. G. Rundall. 2009. "Evidence-Based Management Reconsidered." In *Evidence-Based Management in Healthcare*, edited by A. R. Kovner, D. J. Fine, and R. D'Aquila, 53–77. Chicago: Health Administration Press.

Lahidji, R. 2004. "Lessons Learned." In *Large-Scale Disasters: Lessons Learned*, 9–23. Paris, France: Organisation for Economic Co-operation and Development.

Leins, C. 2015. "U.S. News Quiz: 10 Years Later, 10 Questions about Katrina." *US News and World Report.* Published August 28. www.usnews.com/news/articles /2015/08/28/us-news-quiz-10-years-later-10-questions-about-katrina.

Lister, S. A. 2005. "Hurricane Katrina: The Public Health and Medical Response." CRS Report for Congress. Published September 21. http://fpc.state.gov /documents/organization/54255.pdf.

Louisiana Hospital Association. 2014. "Hospital CEO Hurricane Checklist." Updated August. www.lhaonline.org/resource/resmgr/HHS/CEO_Checklist _2014.pdf.

Marsa, L. 2015. "Top-Notch Community Health Care Emerges in New Orleans from Hurricane Katrina's Rubble." *USA Today.* Published August 29. www .usatoday.com/story/news/2015/08/28/community-healthcare-emerges— hurricane-katrina-rubble—new-orleans/71331792/.

Marsh. 2015. "10 Years After Hurricane Katrina: Lessons in Preparedness, Response, and Resilience." *Insights.* Published August. www.marsh.com/us/insights /research/katrina-lessons-in-risk-management-and-resiliency.html.

Marshall, A. 2013. "After Sandy: New Money, New Rules." *Planning* 79 (7): 37–41.

McGlown, K. J., S. J. O'Connor, and R. M. Shewchuk. 2009. "Evidence-Based Criteria for Hospital Evacuation: The Case of Hurricane Katrina." In *Evidence-Based Management in Healthcare*, edited by A. R. Kovner, D. J. Fine, and R. D'Aquila, 219–32. Chicago: Health Administration Press.

Natural Hazards Center. 2015. "Disaster News Redux: A Katrina Round Up." Published September 4. https://hazards.colorado.edu/article/disaster-news-redux-5.

O'Sullivan, A. 2012. *Urban Economics*, 8th ed. New York: McGraw-Hill/Irwin.

Pau, A. M. 2013. "Ethical and Legal Challenges in Disaster Medicine: Are You Ready?" *Southern Medical Journal* 106 (1): 27–30.

Powell, T., D. Hanfling, and L. O. Gostin. 2013. "In Reply." *Journal of the American Medical Association* 309 (15): 1586.

———. 2012. "Emergency Preparedness and Public Health: The Lessons of Hurricane Sandy." *Journal of the American Medical Association* 208 (24): 2569–70.

Quinlan, P. J., W. L. Thomas, and R. D. Guthrie. 2006. "Perspectives." *Frontiers of Health Services Management* 23 (1): 25–30.

Rudowitz, R., D. Rowland, and A. Shartzer. 2006. "Health Care in New Orleans Before and After Hurricane Katrina." *Health Affairs* 25 (5): w393–w406.

Saaty, T. L. 1980. *The Analytic Hierarchy Process: Planning, Priority Setting, Resources Allocation*. New York: McGraw-Hill.

Shatz, D. V., K. Wolcott, and J. B. Fairburn. 2006. "Response to Hurricane Disasters." *Surgical Clinics of North America* 86 (3): 545–55.

Soergel, A. 2015. "From Resilience to Resurgence After Katrina." *US News and World Report*. Published August 28. www.usnews.com/news/articles/2015/08/28/new-orleans-economic-resurgence-after-hurricane-katrina.

Task Force on Quality Control of Disaster Management / World Association of Disaster and Emergency Medicine (TFQCDM/WADEM). 2002. *Health Disaster Management: Guidelines for Evaluation and Research in the Utstein Style*. Madison, WI: WADEM.

Umm-e-Habiba and S. Asghar. 2009. "A Survey on Multi-criteria Decision Making Approaches." In *International Conference on Emerging Technologies, 2009*, 321–25. Islamabad, Pakistan: IEEE Inc. Islamabad Section and National University of Computer and Emerging Sciences.

US Department of Health and Human Services (DHHS). 2015a. *Hospital Evacuation Decision Guide*. Accessed July. http://archive.ahrq.gov/prep/hospevacguide.

———. 2015b. *Hospital Assessment and Recovery Guide*. Accessed July. http://archive.ahrq.gov/prep/hosprecovery.

US Department of Health and Human Services / Centers for Disease Control and Prevention (DHHS/CDC). 2013. "Healthcare Executives and Disasters: A Stakeholder Meeting." Meeting summary, November 5.

US Department of Homeland Security (DHS). 2013. *Homeland Security Exercise and Evaluation Program (HSEEP)*. Published April. www.fema.gov/media-library-data/20130726-1914-25045-8890/hseep_apr13_.pdf.

———. 2005. "National Planning Scenarios: Executive Summaries." Accessed via Texas A&M International University July 15, 2016. http://cees.tamiu.edu/covertheborder/TOOLS/NationalPlanningSen.pdf.

US Government Accountability Office (GAO). 2006. "Disaster Preparedness Preliminary Observations on the Evacuation of Hospitals and Nursing Homes Due to Hurricanes." Briefings for Congressional Committees, GAO-06-443R. Published February 16. www.gao.gov/new.items/d06443r.pdf.

Withanaarachchi, J., and S. Setunge. 2014. "Influence of Decision Making During Disasters and How It Impacts a Community." In *The Proceedings of the 10th International Conference of the International Institute for Infrastructure Resilience and Reconstruction (I3R2)*, edited by R. R. Rapp and W. Harland, 176–88. West Lafayette, IN: Purdue University.

CASE STUDY

INTEGRATED CHRONIC CARE MANAGEMENT AND THE USE OF EVIDENCE IN DECISION MAKING

by Kyle L. Grazier

This chapter advances our understanding of how evidence-based management, generally, and evidence-based decision support, specifically, address a complex chronic condition and the way that condition is treated and managed in successful healthcare services delivery systems. A case study in the first edition of this book examined a chronic care management model for depression treatment. Drawing from and expanding on that case study, this chapter illustrates the key principles and processes of evidence-based management:

1. *Asking—translating a practical issue or problem into an answerable question.* How can people with chronic behavioral health conditions, whose medical and social needs require considerable resources, access and receive care needed over a sufficient time to improve outcomes?

2. *Acquiring—systematically searching for and retrieving the evidence.* Because our question includes clinical, social services, and management aspects, acquisition of evidence relies on access to multiple sources of information, such as literature; interviews with managers, clinicians, patients, and families; and observation of management practices.

3. *Appraising—critically judging the trustworthiness and relevance of the evidence.* We use quantitative and qualitative methods to assess the validity and reliability of the data.

4. *Aggregating—weighing and pulling together the evidence.* We assess all forms of inquiry and the results of inquiry, including evidence from the literature, interviews, and observations.

5. *Applying—incorporating the evidence into the decision-making process.* The findings are incorporated into the decision-making process

Note: This case study builds from the one presented in chapter 15 of the first edition of this book. You are encouraged to review the earlier edition for additional context.

using standard work models, Lean processes, or other team-based, collaborative modes of problem identification, countermeasure identification, and pilot testing.

6. *Assessing—evaluating the outcome of the decision taken.* Rapid cycle testing, communication models, and other mechanisms can help us assess the quality of the processes and the measurement and analysis of outcomes.

Background

The original case study from the first edition of this book described the development, implementation, and evaluation of a chronic care management model of depression treatment within primary care group practices of an academic health center (Grazier 2009). In this chapter, the components of that piloted and tested model have been extended to include mental health and substance use disorders—the prevalence and incidence of which also have a large and tested research base—as the targeted chronic conditions. The setting for the model in the original case—physician primary care practices embedded in an academic health system—has also been changed to a metropolitan safety-net hospital and system, known in the case as City Health. The case was based on more than 100 interviews with managers, leaders, patients, judges, prisoners, teachers, providers, and board members of the entity and other affiliated and nonaffiliated organizations, as well as other stakeholders.

Behavioral health disorders afflict millions of Americans and individuals across the globe. The question to be answered in this case is *How can an evidence-based management model address the needs of this population within the US public health and healthcare system?* The organization featured in this case used its mission, vision, values, and leadership to evolve an organizational structure based on evidence to provide an answer.

The Organization: City Health

City Health and Hospital Authority is the largest safety-net provider in the state. At the core of City Health's multilayered mission is the delivery of high-quality acute, maintenance, and preventive care to all city and county residents, regardless of their ability to pay. Although it is the public health entity of the city government, City Health controls the operation, funding, and initiatives of its integrated structure, which comprises the following: a 500-bed hospital with a Level 1 academic trauma center; a 911 medical response system; the City Public Health Department; an 8-clinic network of family health centers; a 12-clinic network of school-based health centers; a regional poison and drug center; 24/7 NurseLine (telephone advice service); City CARES (residential detox facility); Correctional Care (facility for prisoners); and City Health Medical Plan, Inc. Health information technology supports this integrated framework.

Like many metropolitan areas in the United States, City Health's home city is a melting pot of people and, by extension, social and health services needs. The city's population is 40 percent Latino and 10 percent African American. Minority groups make up 70 percent of City Health's patient population, and 30 percent of the minority population speaks no English. Although the city has been successful in reducing the number of homeless residents in the last ten years, its efforts have been stunted by recent economic hardship in the region.

Annually, City Health spends more than $106 million serving the homeless population, admits more than 27,000 "detoxifying public inebriates," provides care to more than 14,000 patients with chronic mental illness, and handles more than 75,000 visits from people with substance abuse issues and more than 162,000 visits from prisoners. City Health cares for one-third of the city's population annually, and 37 percent of the city's children.

Integration of Primary Care and Depression Management as an Effective Model

Depression is the most common mental illness in the United States. An estimated 6.6 percent of Americans suffer from a major depressive disorder each year, but only 51.2 percent of this group currently receives treatment. Only 21.7 percent are adequately treated (Grazier et al. 2014).

The primary goal of integration is the provision of comprehensive care. Three models prevail: Integration can consist of (1) mental health care delivery being ingrained in primary care protocols, (2) the colocation of mental health specialists within primary care settings, or (3) team approaches in which mental health providers lend their expertise to primary care providers.

Through a systematic search of the literature on the integration of primary care and depression screening, treatment, and payment, we concluded that sufficient evidence exists to support integration (Butler et al. 2011; Horvitz-Lennon, Kilbourne, and Pincus 2006). However, despite the prevailing consensus about their value, such models have not seen widespread adoption (Barbui and Tansella 2006). Thus, the objective of our work was to examine the barriers to the adoption of depression and primary care (DPC) models in the United States (Grazier et al. 2014).

Applying Evidence-Based Management

A systematic review of the healthcare academic practice through MEDLINE, PsycINFO, and gray literature shed considerable light on the barriers to the integration of depression and primary care. The authors identified several major issues that appear to inhibit the use of the available evidence in decision making, and they arranged the issues into core categories: vulnerable populations with special needs, patient and family factors, provider factors, treatment issues, organizational factors, and financing/payment issues (Grazier et al. 2014). Given the extent of research available, the importance of the topic, the identification of effective solutions, and recognition of the reasons for lack of progress, what more do we need to understand about the problem to carefully articulate it and its components and to pursue effective solutions?

Asking the Answerable Question

Depression is a serious chronic condition that afflicts millions of individuals across the globe (Kessler et al. 2003). The original case from the first edition described the development, implementation, and evaluation of a chronic care management model of depression treatment within primary care group practices of an academic health center. In this expanded study, the components that were previously piloted and the model that was tested have been identified in several health delivery systems, including a regional behavioral health authority, a county health department, a major statewide not-for-profit integrated delivery system, and a metropolitan safety-net hospital and healthcare system. To provide illustrations of the model and the decision making based on the available evidence, this discussion will focus on the metropolitan safety-net system.

The question: *How does the senior management team use evidence to make the decisions that will result in good outcomes for the people with chronic mental health needs?*

Acquiring: Systematically Searching for and Retrieving the Evidence

Because the target population was considered a high priority, the system assembled work groups to gather evidence from the scholarly and gray literature about models for chronic care management. Other teams interviewed a sample of workers in the system, in addition to patients and families. Qualitative interviews identified a set of key themes, such as patient flow, financial support, care management, postvisit patient coaching, and inclusion of families in decision making. Quantitative evidence included a series of systematic reviews and meta-analyses available in the literature and the results of pilot testing processes in the institution (Whitebird et al. 2013).

Appraising the Trustworthiness and Relevance of the Evidence

The scholarly literature on these topics is robust and includes a number of systematic reviews and meta-analyses (Katon et al. 2010). Multiple peer-reviewed articles provide rigorous evidence on components of the models for chronic disease management, specifically for mental health conditions. Interviews followed standard qualitative protocols for these populations and settings (Hedrick et al. 2003).

Aggregating: Weighing and Pulling Together the Evidence

Because of the complexity of patients and families, extrainstitutional needs, and the safety-net management system itself, aggregating the data and interpretations required a multiple-day retreat. The key teams that had collected the data and assessed the validity participated, along with management leadership from across the organization and from social services and county agents.

Applying the Evidence and Assessing the Outcome of the Decision Taken

At the retreat, leadership was presented with the data and interpretations. Following presentation and discussion, the retreat moved specifically to determining how these findings would inform decisions. Leadership and senior management used the major findings to initiate a team-based process to "simulate" a subsystem within the institution. The process began with patient flow diagrams, which originated within a patient's home, intersected with social services, and continued through to the institution, stemming from the evidence on the importance of continuity of contact and care.

Given the evidence from the literature about barriers to the uptake of collaborative care or integrated models, the clinical managers and administrators discussed how obstacles such as physician culture and lack of reimbursement might need to be overcome prior to implementation (Bao et al. 2011a; Compton 2012; Unützer et al. 2006). As a chief of medicine noted, "Our docs are paid on the basis of units of service; if you pull our patients out of our service, our performance metrics will fall." This and similar comments led to a discussion about whether standard fee-for-service models for mental and medical care support this type of collaborative, and verifiably superior, method of delivering care (Bao et al. 2011b).

The data collection team illustrated other financial models, such as a bundled payment for patients admitted into the program, and additional metrics to recognize when providers were using endorsed protocols for referrals and collaborations.

Conclusion

This process of evidence-based management and decision support resulted in a six-month pilot program, requiring measurement of processes and outcomes, analysis, and expansion to a second-stage program that was larger and longer.

Assignment

Consider how you might respond to the following letter from City Health's CEO to the senior leadership team:

Dear colleagues,

You have performed admirably as City Health moves to this next stage in our quest for integration of critical behavioral health and primary care services across our network of services for our patients and their families. The work teams explored the evidence along several dimensions and presented to you at the leadership retreat their data, analyzed and arrayed in multiple models. What I need from you in the next 30 days is a comprehensive, cohesive strategy statement and work plan for implementing the necessary changes. This plan should be short and succinct. It should provide me and the board with a vision, consistent with City Health's vision, for the strategy and measurable goals. A timeline for implementation must also be driven by the evidence, associated with validated metrics to be collected at baseline, and consistent with the schedule you propose. The proposed model must be backed by a full evaluation plan, so we can monitor our progress and outcomes and know if and where we succeeded, slowed, or failed.

Please gather soon so that the strategy statement and work plan are ready for our board meeting two months hence.

Sincerely,
Your beloved CEO
City Health and Hospital Authority

Case Study Questions

1. Assuming you are the manager of a large health system, how would you use the author's recommendations?
2. As CEO, how would you translate the issue of better coordination of chronic behavioral health care into an answerable set of questions?
3. How would you develop metrics and accountability for coordination of chronic behavioral health conditions?

References

Bao, Y., G. S. Alexopoulos, L. P. Casalino, T. R. Ten Have, J. M. Donohue, E. P. Post, B. R. Schackman, and M. L. Bruce. 2011a. "Collaborative Depression Care Management and Disparities in Depression Treatment and Outcomes." *Archives of General Psychiatry* 68 (6): 627–36.

Bao, Y., L. P. Casalino, S. L. Ettner, M. L. Bruce, L. I. Solberg, and J. Unützer. 2011b. "Designing Payment for Collaborative Care for Depression in Primary Care." *Health Services Research* 46 (5): 1436–51.

Barbui, C., and M. Tansella. 2006. "Identification and Management of Depression in Primary Care Settings: A Meta-review of Evidence." *Epidemiologia e Psichiatria Sociale* 15 (4): 276–83.

Butler, M., R. L. Kane, D. McAlpine, R. Kathol, S. S. Fu, H. Hagedorn, and T. Wilt. 2011. "Does Integrated Care Improve Treatment for Depression? A Systematic Review." *Journal of Ambulatory Care Management* 34 (2): 113–25.

Compton, M. T. 2012. "Systematic Organizational Change for the Collaborative Care Approach to Managing Depressive Disorders." *American Journal of Preventive Medicine* 42 (5): 553–55.

Grazier, K. L. 2009. "Using Evidence in Integrated Chronic Care Management." In *Evidence-Based Management in Healthcare*, edited by A. R. Kovner, D. J. Fine, and R. D'Aquila, 181–88. Chicago: Health Administration Press.

Grazier, K. L., J. E. Smith, J. Song, and M. L. Smiley. 2014. "Integration of Depression and Primary Care: Barriers to Adoption." *Journal of Primary Care and Community Health* 5 (1): 67–73.

Hedrick, S. C., E. F. Chaney, B. Felker, C. F. Liu, N. Hasenberg, P. Heagerty, J. Buchanan, R. Bagala, D. Greenberg, G. Paden, S. D. Fihn, and W. Katon. 2003. "Effectiveness of Collaborative Care Depression Treatment in Veterans' Affairs Primary Care." *Journal of General Internal Medicine* 18 (1): 9–16.

Horvitz-Lennon, M., A. M. Kilbourne, and H. A. Pincus. 2006. "From Silos to Bridges: Meeting the General Health Care Needs of Adults with Severe Mental Illnesses." *Health Affairs* 25 (3): 659–69.

Katon, W. J., E. H. Lin, M. Von Korff, P. Ciechanowski, E. J. Ludman, B. Young, D. Peterson, C. M. Rutter, M. McGregor, and D. McCulloch. 2010. "Collaborative Care for Patients with Depression and Chronic Illnesses." *New England Journal of Medicine* 363 (27): 2611–20.

Kessler, R. C., P. Berglund, O. Demler, R. Jin, D. Koretz, K. R. Merikangas, A. J. Rush, E. E. Walters, and P. S. Wang. 2003. "The Epidemiology of Major Depressive Disorder: Results from the National Comorbidity Survey Replication (NCS-R)." *Journal of the American Medical Association* 289 (23): 3095–105.

Unützer, J., M. Schoenbaum, B. G. Druss, and W. J. Katon. 2006. "Transforming Mental Health Care at the Interface with General Medicine: Report for the President's Commission." *Psychiatric Services* 57 (1): 37–47.

Whitebird, R. R., L. I. Solberg, K. L. Margolis, S. E. Asche, M. A. Trangle, and A. P. Wineman. 2013. "Barriers to Improving Primary Care of Depression Perspectives of Medical Group Leaders." *Qualitative Health Research* 23 (6): 805–14.

ORGANIZATIONAL EVIDENCE

12

ENGINEERING, EVIDENCE, AND EXCELLENCE: THE KAISER PERMANENTE EXAMPLE

by Jed Weissberg and Patrick Courneya

Introduction

Value in healthcare is a framework that can drive care transformation toward excellence (Porter 2009). For those of us who manage any aspect of healthcare, achieving high value for patients in all settings must be our central focus (Porter 2009; Porter, Pabo, and Lee 2013). Value is generated when effective care is provided efficiently and measured by the health outcomes achieved per dollar spent. It is distinct from cost reduction without regard to outcomes, which generates false "savings" from shifting costs and restricting services, and from process of care measurement (Porter 2010).

Value is created by providers' combined efforts over the entire cycle of care, irrespective of organizational unit boundaries, and is most reliably measured at the population level (Porter 2010). The scale and integration of our care delivery system at Kaiser Permanente are ideal for engineering care in pursuit of value. Moving toward a value-based system requires that we design standardized and consistent care processes that yield continuous improvement in effectiveness, efficiency, and the degree to which our efforts align with our patients' goals and desires. Readily available data must be available to point the way to excellence in these dimensions.

At Kaiser Permanente, engineering care to transform delivery is one of our founding principles, dating back to the 1940s. Dr. Sidney Garfield (1945), cofounder of Kaiser Permanente, noted that the basic structure of healthcare delivery, which he described as "chaotic," consisted of solo practices receiving fee-for-service reimbursement (see exhibit 12.1). The predominant delivery structure changed slowly until recently. Between 1988 and 2012, the proportion of physicians who were self-employed decreased from 75 percent to 53 percent—a decrease of 22 points over 24 years (Pope and Schneider 1992; Kane and Emmons 2013). However, following the Affordable Care Act of 2010, the proportion of self-employed physicians shrank by 18 percentage points over two years, reaching 35 percent in 2014.

EXHIBIT 12.1
"Chaotic"
Healthcare,
Then and Now

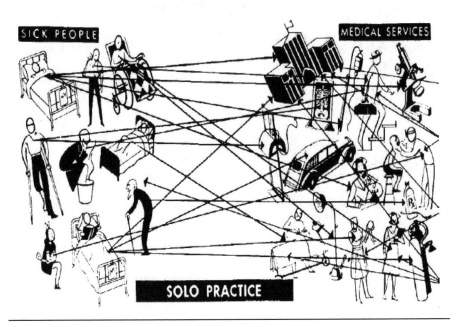

1945

SICK PEOPLE

MEDICAL SERVICES

SOLO PRACTICE

Source: Garfield (1945). Reprinted from "The Plan That Kaiser Built," *Survey Graphic*, December 1945, p. 480.

The percentage of physicians participating in accountable care organizations increased from 3 percent in 2011 to 30 percent in 2014 (Peckham 2015).

Decades before healthcare reform spurred broad efforts to improve care quality and value, Dr. Garfield envisioned a healthcare delivery system that used clinical evidence (e.g., health assessments, laboratory tests, radiography, electrocardiograms) to tailor care to patients' individual needs: illness care, wellness care, and preventive maintenance. The use of paramedical staff would save time for physicians, and a computer center would regulate the flow of patients and information between care units and coordinate the entire system (see exhibit 12.2). This vision provides an example of a learning healthcare system, information rich and patient centered. Evidence is continually refined as a byproduct of care delivery, and the just-in-time availability of evidence and current clinical information to physicians and patients transforms interactions from reactive to proactive (see exhibit 12.3). Consistent with Dr. Garfield's vision, Kaiser Permanente today exemplifies a learning healthcare organization (Schilling et al. 2011). However, all learning is in service of transforming care. Our goal is action, not reflection. We are a learning *and doing* healthcare organization.

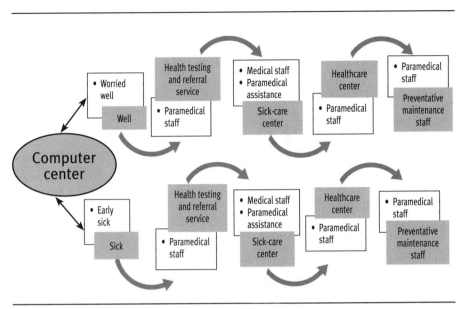

EXHIBIT 12.2
Sidney
Garfield's Vision
of a Better
Healthcare
System

Source: Garfield (1970).

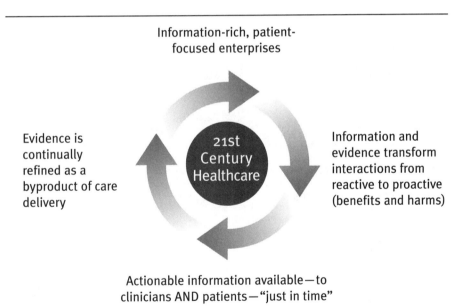

EXHIBIT 12.3
A Learning
Healthcare
Organization

Source: Clancy (2009).

Engineering the Care Delivery System

Kaiser Permanente is the nation's largest not-for-profit health plan and integrated care delivery system, as shown by the figures in exhibit 12.4. Learning in service of care transformation occurs at all organizational levels. A ten-year

EXHIBIT 12.4
Scope and Scale
of Care at Kaiser
Permanente

Members	10 million
Regions	Seven in eight states and the District of Columbia
Physicians	17,790
Employees	177,445
Medical office buildings	621
Hospitals	38
Ambulatory surgery centers	13
Annual activity	
New members enrolled	510,000
Incoming advice and appointment center calls answered	59.3 million
Members using My Health Manager online	4.4 million
Lab test results viewed online each month	2.9 million
Outpatient physician office visits	40.2 million
Prescriptions filled	72.8 million
Mammograms performed	1 million
Colorectal cancer screenings	1.7 million
Surgical procedures performed	224,940
Infants delivered	98,000

partnership with the Institute for Healthcare Improvement has enabled us to design our own model for rapid performance improvement and to train thousands of staff members in its use. Throughout our organization, mentors and improvement advisers assist leaders and frontline team members as they integrate performance improvement into their daily work.

Widespread use of plan-do-check-act (PDCA) cycles fosters innovation to address local problems or improvement opportunities reflected in care and outcome variations. Operational data is pivotal to all phases of care transformation, from identifying improvement opportunities to assessing the impact of PDCA cycles to ensuring sustainability over time. Learnings are shared throughout Kaiser Permanente to discover and disseminate best practices, aiding us as we seek to drive out unwarranted variations in effectiveness, quality, safety, efficiency, and member experiences of care.

Scale Demands Design: The Northern California Appointment and Advice Call Center

The Permanente Medical Group (TPMG) is the physician-led organization providing medical services for Kaiser Permanente Northern California (KPNC) members under a mutually exclusive contract with the Kaiser Foundation Health Plan (KFHP in Northern California). At a 1996 TPMG board meeting, the executive medical director at the time announced that KPNC was creating centralized phone services. The response around the table was tepid, at best. Centralizing phone services required shifting resources and administration to an unknown approach with an uncertain outcome. However, the executive medical director pointed out that KPNC had been trying to improve telephone service to members for several years without achieving its goals. He believed that centralizing and standardizing telephone services would accomplish what individual departments and medical centers could not. Certainly, no one else in the room—and perhaps not even he—foresaw the care transformation that would result.

Three physical call centers were created, each serving distinct geographic areas but operating under a single administration (Conolly et al. 2005). Within a few years, the call centers supported nearly all primary care departments in the Northern California region and subsequently expanded to include numerous additional departments and services. In 2007, after leadership again noted variations in service levels, the three centers were consolidated into a single virtual entity, the Kaiser Permanente Northern California Appointment and Advice Call Center (AACC). Members reach the AACC by calling the department phone number at the medical center where they receive care. In supported departments, calls are routed to the AACC and initially answered in an average of 40 seconds by the next available teleservice representative. Teleservice representatives follow highly structured, physician-approved scripts and transfer some calls to registered nurses (RNs), who advise callers using advice and triage protocols.

The Northern California AACC handles more than a million telephone calls from members each month. Of these, 75 percent are to schedule appointments, obtain information (such as confirming appointment times or obtaining lab results), or leave messages for providers. The balance—approximately 250,000 calls each month—come from patients who require triage or would benefit from advice. Advice RNs resolve approximately 80 percent of calls by providing guidance to patients, enabled by immediate access to KP HealthConnect, our systemwide electronic health record. In the remaining calls, nurses consult with emergency physicians or, in selected situations, use protocols to direct patients to call 911. Care engineering includes empowering teleservice representatives and adding physicians to call center staffing. Representatives screen all incoming calls and respond directly to patient requests for lab results when those results are normal, which has led to a substantial decrease in advice nurse phone calls and reduced demands on highly skilled RN staff. After screening, representatives transfer patient calls to nurses or, in specific instances, directly to physicians.

Approximately 11,000 calls each month are related to urinary tract infections (UTIs). AACC advice nurses evaluate each case and treat uncomplicated cystitis, representing 50 percent of UTI-related calls, over the phone. The value of this approach is evidenced in an increased proportion of patients receiving prescriptions for guideline-recommended antibiotic therapy, higher patient satisfaction, avoidance of unnecessary urinalyses and office visits, and decreased overall treatment costs. Telephone treatment of uncomplicated cystitis is not associated with increased rates of hospitalization, office or emergency department (ED) visits, or total courses of antibiotics (Vinson and Quesenberry 2004).

The AACC treats 48 minor conditions by phone, including conjunctivitis, vaginitis, swimmer's ear, nausea and vomiting (including during pregnancy), coughs lasting longer than ten days, and new and restart prescriptions for birth control pills. During flu season, prophylactic and therapeutic oseltamivir phosphate (Tamiflu) is also available through the clinical call center.

Physicians at seven Kaiser Permanente EDs staff the call center remotely in 6- to 18-hour blocks using a virtual private network. Each physician typically handles 10 to 12 calls per hour, and they report enjoying the break from the hands-on practice of emergency medicine. Physician staffing expanded from a single physician available to consult with call center RNs for a few hours a day during the week to the current level of full-time coverage by 215 physicians in rotation. Two to nine physicians are available 24 hours a day, seven days a week, with staffing determined by call volume trends. Physicians now both consult with call center advice RNs and speak directly with patients.

In one specific example, the call center in 2012 began transferring phone calls from patients older than age 35 with chest pain directly to physicians, who perform an assessment to address three questions: (1) Does the patient need to be seen in the ED? (2) How far is the patient from a Kaiser Permanente ED, and can he or she get there safely? (3) Should the patient call 911, or should the physician arrange for an ambulance? In one year, physician phone staffing decreased by 80 percent the number of patients with chest pain who were inappropriately sent to the ED by AACC staff members. In addition, patients who were quickly triaged and then spoke directly to physicians were more likely to go to the ED when instructed. Call center physicians also speak directly with all members assessed by advice RNs as needing an immediate ED visit. The ability of physicians to conduct more detailed triage reduced by 36 percent the use of ambulances and ED visits, primarily during weekdays when physicians could instead triage patients to an immediate office visit. The practice of transferring phone calls directly to emergency physicians was subsequently extended to patients with abdominal pain and is being expanded to those with shortness of breath.

Since mid-2010, the contribution of the call center has caused ED patient loads to steadily decrease. In 2015, less than 8 percent of patients seen in the ED were referred there by a call center provider, compared to 14 percent five years earlier. Over the same period, the proportion of patients referred to the ED from the call center with the most acute medical needs increased from 80 to 85 percent, and the percentage of patients referred by the clinical call center to nonemergent care who visited the ED within 12 hours also decreased. Strikingly, less than 1 percent of all calls to the clinical call center resulted in a referral to the ED.

On an ongoing basis, the AACC monitors aggregate and physician- and patient-level quality and service processes and outcomes. The goal is to get the right patient to the right level of care at the right time, avoiding both under- and overutilization of services. For example, the call center identifies and reviews the records of all patients who received advice or referral to a physician office or telephone visit from the AACC but were seen in the ED or admitted as an inpatient within 48 hours. A group comprising Kaiser Permanente ED physician liaisons, call center medical directors, quality directors, and reporting staff convenes regularly to ensure that metrics address strategically important processes and outcomes and to develop new metrics for evolving programs and workflows as needed.

Care engineering is directed under the ongoing oversight of a medical director within The Permanente Medical Group. The medical director works collaboratively with an administrator, supported by an analytic team and groups of clinical subject matter experts.

Evidence Leads to Excellence

Evidence is critical as we seek continual improvement in healthcare effectiveness and efficiency. However, to create maximum value, evidence must have certain characteristics. It must be as current as possible, constituting real-time or near-real-time data whenever feasible. It must align with our organizational improvement priorities, because measurement and management are inextricably linked. It must be readily available—to our healthcare providers, patients, and managers—precisely when they need it and in forms that present the most relevant information for each user group.

In 2003, Kaiser Permanente decided to purchase a suite of software applications from Epic Systems and deploy a programwide electronic health record (EHR) (Weissberg 2009). Twelve years later, KP HealthConnect allows clinicians and employees to manage the healthcare and administrative needs of 9.6 million members in seven regions in a seamless and integrated way (Chen et al. 2009). Multiple functionalities in the EHR, such as point-of-care clinical decision support, computerized physician order entry, and panel management tools, contribute to quality and efficiency (Feldstein et al. 2010; Zhou et al. 2010; Zhou et al. 2011). All seven Kaiser Permanente regional health plans are among the top 6 percent of private health plans identified by the National Committee for Quality Assurance (NCQA) for 2014–2015. Three are among the top 2 percent (NCQA 2015b).

However, our vision for the EHR also included the potential to mine clinical data to identify emerging ways to increase value for patients by improving effectiveness and efficiency. In some cases, existing functionalities of the EHR cannot support the level of evidence we need, and we must make additional investments to augment it.

Evidence Leading to Excellence: Southern California Regional Outpatient SureNet

The goal of the Kaiser Permanente Southern California Regional Outpatient SureNet is to prevent patient harm resulting from diagnostic errors. Each of the steps in the diagnostic process is associated with specific failure modes, and the potential harm resulting from these failures ranges from unnecessary testing to death (see exhibit 12.5). The SureNet model allows for the design of corrective actions that are maximally effective and efficient—and for the specification of evidence necessary to support them. Achieving the ideal state of zero errors depends on people factors, team work processes, and technology.

SureNet systematically identifies regional members who have experienced inadvertent lapses in care (Danforth et al. 2014; Graber et al. 2014; Kanter et al. 2013). A small, centralized team with a carefully defined clinical scope and capacity then intervenes before harm reaches the patient, using automated electronic tools to consistently track selected abnormal lab test results for all members. For example, early detection and treatment of chronic kidney disease (CKD) is associated with slowed progression of disease and reduced mortality (Black et al. 2010; Lee et al. 2012; Martinez-Ramirez et al. 2006). The SureNet team identifies members with an abnormal serum creatinine that was not repeated within 90 days of the original test date and verifies the member list with a regional nephrologist. A pending order for a

EXHIBIT 12.5
Why Diagnostic
Errors Occur
and the
Resulting
Potential Harm

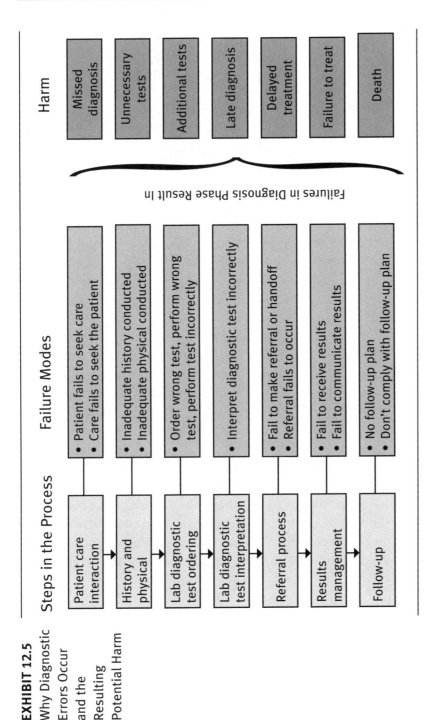

Source: Adapted in part from Gandhi et al. (2006).

repeat lab test is created in each patient's EHR for cosign by the patient's primary care provider. After cosigning is verified by the regional team, the patient is mailed a letter with instructions to go to the lab for repeat testing (Sim et al. 2015).

Other abnormal diagnostic tests monitored by the outpatient SureNet include Pap smears, prostate-specific antigen levels, and fecal occult blood with no record of a colonoscopy. The team also follows patients with selected diagnoses to ensure proper follow-up. For example, the SureNet team began identifying patients with an abdominal aortic aneurysm (AAA) diagnosis. Each month, in a process similar to that described above, the team creates a pending order for an ultrasound in the charts of members who are overdue for screening, the primary care physician cosigns it, and the radiology department contacts the member to schedule an appointment. Since the project began in 2012, 2,062 of 9,404 patients with an AAA diagnosis—22 percent—have been identified as overdue for follow-up and referred for ultrasound imaging.

In addition to diagnostic detection and tracking, the regional SureNet team also focuses on medication safety by monitoring selected medications and identifying potentially harmful medication interactions (see exhibit 12.6). For example, the regional SureNet identified 8,310 members with a history of dementia or falls who were taking a tricyclic antidepressant or sleep medication. A pharmacist on the team collaborated with physicians and primary care providers to complete conversions to appropriate medications or discontinuations in 5,548 members, a relative risk reduction of 67 percent. In another example, the SureNet team has identified patients taking both gemfibrozil and a statin medication, which increases the risk of rhabdomyolysis. Since 2012, the team pharmacist has identified 3,498 members taking both medications and collaborated with primary care providers to convert 3,047 members to a safer alternative or discontinue the use of gemfibrozil—a relative risk reduction of 87 percent.

Since its inception, SureNet in Southern California has launched a new project every two months and currently has a portfolio that includes 31 diagnostic tests and medication safety projects. The program has successfully identified 5 million outpatient safety hazards and facilitated 2.17 million interventions. Projects under development for future implementation include diagnostic follow-up and tracking for elevated thyroid-stimulating hormone, lung nodules, rapid change in CKD stage, breast masses, and melanoma. Medication safety projects under development are related to hormone replacement therapy, colchicine, niacin, phenytoin, and chronic myeloid leukemia treatment.

SureNet projects related to abnormal lab tests and medication safety are proposed by Kaiser Permanente Southern California quality leaders or

EXHIBIT 12.6
Medications
and Medication
Interactions
Monitored
by the Kaiser
Permanente
Southern
California
Regional
Outpatient
SureNet

- Acetaminophen overuse
- Amiodarone (preventive monitoring plan)
- Digoxin: high-dose conversion in the elderly
- Digoxin annual monitoring: serum potassium and creatinine
- Diuretics annual monitoring: serum potassium and creatinine
- Diuretics: medication-induced hyponatremia
- Ethambutol: optic nerve monitoring
- Isoniazid: serum alanine aminotransferase
- Interacting statin combinations: gemfibrozil and amiodarone
- Medication-induced hyperkalemia
- Metformin: vitamin B12 monitoring
- Nonsteroidal anti-inflammatories in Stage 4–5 chronic kidney disease or renal replacement therapy
- Plaquenil: retinal monitoring
- Tricyclic antidepressants or sleep medications and falls

Source: Spence et al. (2011).

clinical experts on the basis of clinical evidence and the potential to improve outcomes. Project proposals pass through several development and approval processes. After the regional medical director of quality and clinical analysis approves an initial project proposal, a panel of subject matter experts and stakeholders (SMES) and leadership convenes. The panel's task is to obtain targeted clinical direction and fully design project elements to identify potential harm and intervene to prevent it. The SMES panel also ensures that projects are coherent and practical from the standpoint of frontline care providers. Projects undergo several iterations in the SMES panel before an approval round by involved medical programs and health plan administrators. Before project launch, an announcement e-mail is sent to all frontline physicians potentially affected by implementation. The SMES panel addresses any feedback generated by the e-mail announcement and provides final approval for project launch.

In 2013, Kaiser Permanente national leadership determined that spreading SureNet from Southern California to all regions was a strategic priority. Leaders within each region independently identified opportunities and developed programs to improve quality and safety. In early 2015, 40 programs to monitor abnormal diagnostic tests and selected conditions and to improve medication safety were operational programwide, and more were in the development or planning stages. Programs common to all regions included tracking patients with positive fecal immunochemical tests and abnormal prostate-specific antigen (PSA) and Pap smear results to ensure appropriate follow-up, as well as monitoring digoxin and amiodarone medication safety.

Tracking the effectiveness of SureNet throughout Kaiser Permanente ensures that patients targeted by outreach efforts receive appropriate follow-up and monitoring. Before programwide SureNet implementation, regions outside Southern California had conducted outreach programs to address diagnostic failures, but their effectiveness was inconsistently assessed. Detailed mapping of data tables in Clarity, the enterprise data warehouse, to regional versions of the EHR is required to replicate the functionalities supporting the Southern California Regional Outpatient SureNet. This effort is under way, and early results confirm the potential of SureNet to improve care programwide. In Kaiser Permanente Northwest, 1,648 positive fecal immunochemical tests were monitored in the first ten months of the program; 634 patients without evidence of appropriate follow-up received targeted outreach, and 12 cases of colorectal cancer were identified. In the Northwest and Hawaii regions, 818 abnormal results were monitored in the first 15 months of separate regional programs to track PSA results; 657 patients received targeted outreach to ensure appropriate care, and 71 cases of prostate cancer were identified.

Evidence Leading to Excellence: OpQ

Excellence in operations requires data-driven management. The OpQ project in Kaiser Permanente Northwest revolves around a web-enabled tool that provides vital operational and performance data in near real-time. Based on proprietary technology and data flows, OpQ displays up-to-date organization-specific metrics reflecting Kaiser Permanente's operational standards and targets. With data refreshed every 15 minutes, OpQ identifies and tracks operational, service, and patient safety gaps to help frontline managers proactively manage office visit access and service quality, ED utilization, patient calls and e-mails, and wait times. A monthly release cycle ensures that information provided through OpQ keeps pace with organizational changes. End users can include facility, patient care, and nursing managers; medical assistant leads; medical chiefs; and case and population care managers.

OpQ supports quality, service, efficiency, and provider satisfaction. Quality data available through the primary care dashboard—shown in exhibit 12.7—include the proportion of visits with recorded blood pressure (first and repeat are measured separately), allergies, current medications, weight, respirations, tobacco use, and, in pediatrics, height and head circumference. Staff in clinical work areas can also view clinical quality measures on a screen as they come in (see exhibit 12.8). Inpatient and ED follow-up visit rates are also displayed in the overview screen. Service-related data include appointment utilization, wait times, and response times to patient telephone calls and

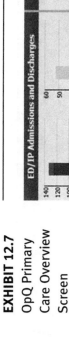

EXHIBIT 12.7
OpQ Primary
Care Overview
Screen

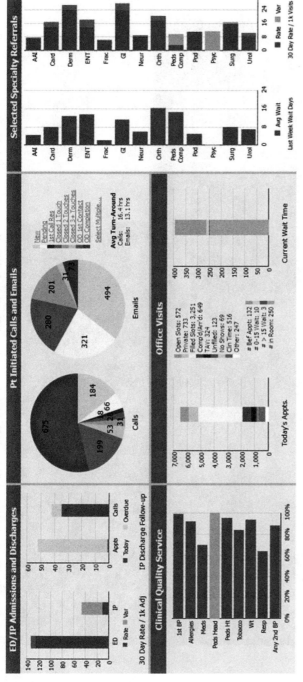

Source: OpQ screen-shot image reproduced with permission from Kaiser Permanente. © 2016 Kaiser Permanente.

EXHIBIT 12.8
Real-Time
Clinical Quality
Surveillance
in OpQ

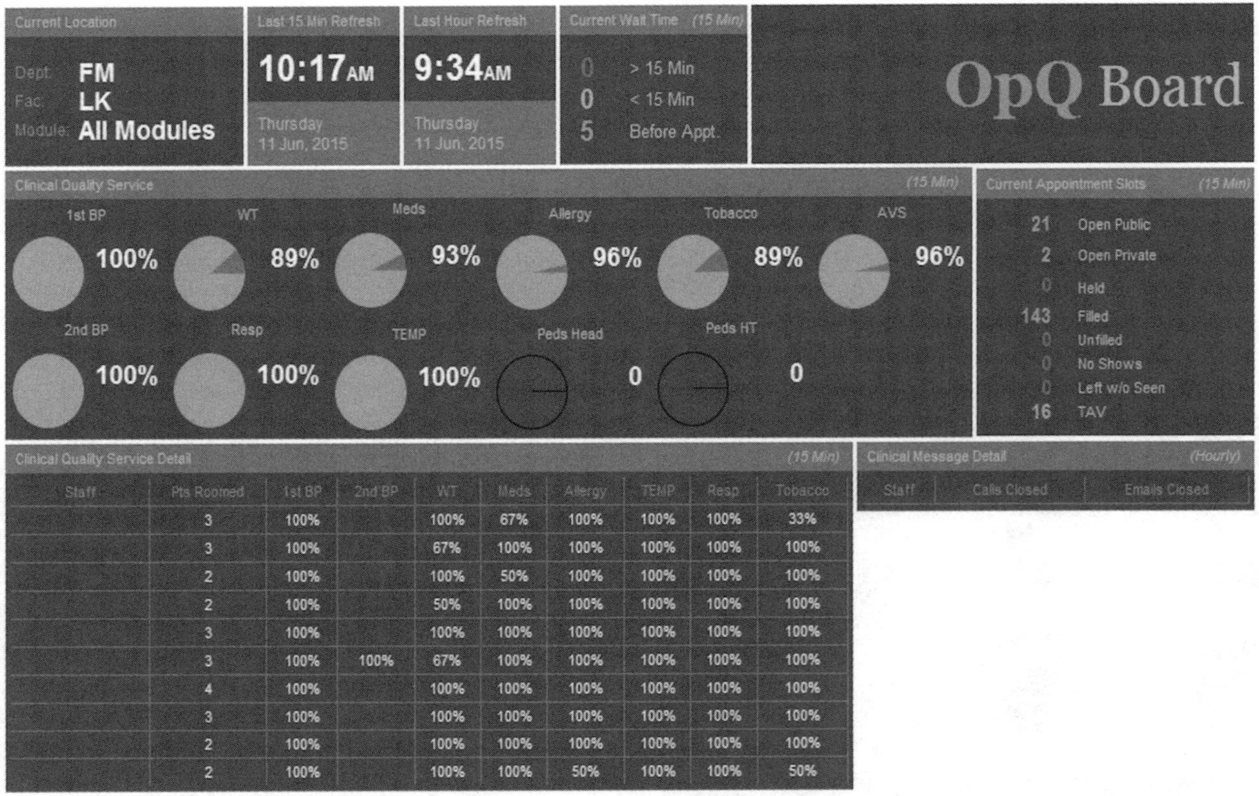

Source: OpQ screen-shot image reproduced with permission from Kaiser Permanente. © 2016 Kaiser Permanente.

EXHIBIT 12.9
OpQ Visit View

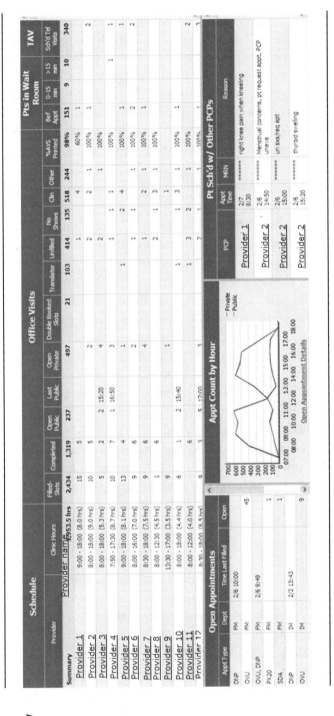

Note: Provider names have been deleted.

Source: OpQ screen-shot image reproduced with permission from Kaiser Permanente. © 2016 Kaiser Permanente.

secure messages. More detailed information is displayed on screens that drill down into ambulatory care visits (see exhibit 12.9), patient phone calls and messages by provider, support staff performance on clinical quality measures, and ED visits and inpatient admissions by facility and provider. Additional data available on OpQ specialty care views include the number of incoming referrals per provider, the number of referrals that were appointed within specific time frames, and the response time to the member after the referral was received. Operational efficiency is promoted by, for example, the ability to proactively assign staff to areas with the highest need. Provider satisfaction is promoted because data allow frontline staff to drive improvement in quality and service metrics.

Data can be used to take action in key ways. During morning team huddles, for instance, the number of urgent patient phone calls can drive temporary reassignment of a medical assistant to cover a higher-than-usual number of appointments. During check-in, reception staff can advise patients if a short wait to be roomed is expected and offer the option of visiting the coffee shop. At a desktop computer, medical assistants (MAs) and licensed vocational nurses, who may triage secure messages for physicians, can view incoming message volumes; for example, if four new messages come in near the end of their shift, they can prioritize accordingly to ensure a prompt response from the physician. In the exam room, abnormal blood pressure readings are highlighted in OpQ, prompting the MA to retake blood pressures, confirm current medications with patients, and update the medication list in KP HealthConnect. Throughout the day, ambulatory care managers can check appointment utilization and wait times, response times to telephone calls and secure messages from patients, and quality of care indicators for support staff.

OpQ has been available to all primary care facilities in Kaiser Permanente Northwest since October 2011. Between June 2012 and October 2013, OpQ rolled out to 38 subspecialty areas. By December 2014, the proportion of regional members seen in primary care with a recorded second blood pressure check, respiratory rate, tobacco use review, or medication review had increased by 2 to 52 percentage points. Substantial improvements also occurred in response times to patient-initiated telephone calls and secure messages. Other projects, such as the implementation of a medical home model of care and access improvement work, may have contributed to these gains, and the unique contribution of OpQ cannot be quantified. However, ambulatory care staff, managers, and senior directors agree that readily available, real-time operations data are a pivotal enabler of improved quality and service.

During the active development phase, monthly meetings with primary and specialty care operational leaders provided governance and prioritization of enhancements. A monthly meeting of a smaller group of "super users" during this phase focused on maximizing primary care performance and incorporating OpQ into standard workflows. Ongoing oversight occurs through analytic services in partnership with operations management.

Evidence Leading to Excellence: On the Horizon

SureNet and OpQ exemplify Kaiser Permanente's dedication to using data to improve care for large populations. Two additional initiatives exemplify the organizational commitment to expanding the reach of evidence.

The first example pertains to CKD, which affects one in ten US adults (National Center for Chronic Disease Prevention and Health Promotion 2014). In the absence of an acute insult, CKD typically progresses to the end stage at a rate that allows for advance planning of renal replacement therapy by hemodialysis, peritoneal dialysis, or a preemptive renal transplant. However, a substantial percentage of patients progressing to end-stage renal disease (ESRD) experience a suboptimal start by beginning hemodialysis as inpatients, using a central venous catheter instead of a mature, surgically placed arteriovenous fistula, or both (Chiu, Alam, and Iqbal 2012). Suboptimal starts are associated with increased morbidity, hospitalization, and mortality (Mendelssohn, Malmberg, and Hamandi 2009).

In 2013–2014, an interregional workgroup of nephrologists developed and implemented interventions to increase "optimal starts" for ESRD through Kaiser Permanente. In addition, they proposed an optimal starts quality measure to the National Quality Forum, a rigorous evidence-based process that takes into account the value and scientific merit of the proposed measure and its intended use for accountability applications (e.g., public reporting) and performance improvement. In 2015, the measure was endorsed by the National Quality Forum, expanding the reach of Kaiser Permanente's evidence-based initiative (National Quality Forum 2015). (See the case study in chapter 9 of this book for a detailed discussion of another evidence-based initiative addressing CKD.)

The concept of evidence driving excellence is most familiar in the context of primary care, in which disease registries enable improved health for large populations. A recent project at Kaiser Permanente brought the benefits of disease registries to specialists managing complex and uncommon conditions (Herrinton et al. 2015). A platform comprising staff, technology, structured collaboration, and EHR data was used collaboratively by experts in specialty medicine and information technology. Specialty department chiefs generated clinical questions and specified diagnostic codes, operational definitions of tests and therapies, and other required parameters. Information technology experts used the information to write queries and extract and process data. Medical specialists then interpreted data to answer the clinical questions.

Examples of clinical issues that were addressed included surveillance of surgical site infection after cataract surgery; identification of patients with gout who were missing lab testing for uric acid levels; identification of pediatric oncology patients who would soon be transferring to adult cancer care, to allow for transition planning; and appropriateness of medical genetics testing. Extending the benefits of evidence-based management to providers outside primary care and to new populations of patients is a natural progression in using evidence to drive excellence.

Kaiser Permanente has made substantial progress toward optimal relationships between system design and evidence in pursuit of excellent care. However, substantial potential remains unrealized; the current agenda includes strengthening organizational capacity for rapid spread of best practices and enabling deeper digital connection between patients and care providers through the use of smartphones, video visits, virtual care, and patient-generated data. Kaiser Permanente's robust and forward-looking strategy to expand the availability of relevant, real-time evidence and integrate it into insightful system design aims to enable better healthcare decisions wherever they are made—in living rooms, exam rooms, and the board room.

Conclusion

The programs described in this chapter are just a sample of the initiatives implemented at Kaiser Permanente in pursuit of high-value care. Pivotal to all of them are the physicians and employees who integrate system design and redesign into their daily work in pursuit of excellence for our members. System-level care engineering supplements their high levels of professionalism and diligence, and their dedication and enthusiasm are inspiring.

Although the examples described in this chapter occurred within our integrated care delivery system, several forces have converged to enable similar initiatives in other settings. These forces include the advent of meaningful use under the Health Information Technology for Economic and Clinical Health Act of 2009, the increasing proportion of hospitals and medical practices using EHRs, and the widespread electronic resulting of lab data and pharmacy dispensings captured by large chains and pharmacy benefits management programs (Centers for Medicare & Medicaid Services 2010; Charles et al. 2013; Hsaio and Hing 2013). The broad availability of the types of data that enable SureNet makes possible the community-wide integration of patient-centered safety nets, built around clinical needs and exemplifying high-value healthcare.

The uses of data described here illustrate the care coordination promised by the structural and functional aspects of patient-centered medical homes (National Committee for Quality Assurance 2015a). Clinicians must operate at the "top of their licenses"; so, too, must we optimize the role of technology to support care coordination. Technological approaches to performing repetitive and time- and attention-intensive tasks free clinicians to do what they do best: care for patients. The safety, quality, efficiency, and service gains we describe can be replicated elsewhere through care engineering supported by evidence, resulting in operational systems such as clinical call centers and electronic safety nets. When these systems are widely available, we can expect to see dramatic reductions in the slips, misses, and lapses that currently characterize many healthcare failures. This is an essential first step in moving toward high-value healthcare.

References

Black, C., P. Sharma, G. Scotland, K. McCullough, D. McGurn, L. Robertson, N. Fluck, A. MacLeod, P. McNamee, G. Prescott, and C. Smith. 2010. "Early Referral Strategies for Management of People with Markers of Renal Disease: A Systematic Review of the Evidence of Clinical Effectiveness, Cost-Effectiveness, and Economic Analysis." *Health Technology Assessment* 14 (21): 1–184.

Centers for Medicare & Medicaid Services. 2010. "Medicare and Medicaid Programs: Electronic Health Record Incentive Program, Final Rule." Published July 28. www.gpo.gov/fdsys/pkg/FR-2010-07-28/pdf/2010-17207.pdf.

Charles, D., J. King, M. F. Furukawa, and V. Patel. 2013. "Hospital Adoption of Electronic Health Record Technology to Meet Meaningful Use Objectives: 2008–2012." Office of the National Coordinator for Health Information Technology. Published March. www.healthit.gov/sites/default/files/oncdata brief10final.pdf.

Chen, C., T. Garrido, D. Chock, G. Okawa, and L. Liang. 2009. "The Kaiser Permanente Electronic Health Record: Transforming and Streamlining Modalities of Care." *Health Affairs* 28 (2): 323–33.

Chiu, K., A. Alam, and S. Iqbal. 2012. "Predictors of Suboptimal and Crash Initiation of Dialysis at Two Tertiary Care Centers." *Hemodialysis International* 16 (Suppl. 1): S39–S46.

Clancy, C. M. 2009. "A Learning Health Care System for Cancer Care." Agency for Healthcare Research and Quality. Presented at the National Cancer Policy Forum, Washington, DC, October 5.

Conolly, P., L. Levine, D. J. Amaral, B. H. Fireman, and T. Driscoll. 2005. "TPMG Northern California Appointments and Advice Call Center." *Journal of Medical Systems* 29 (4): 325–33.

Danforth, K. N., A. E. Smith, R. K. Loo, S. J. Jacobsen, B. S. Mittman, and M. H. Kanter. 2014. "Electronic Clinical Surveillance to Improve Outpatient Care:

Diverse Applications Within an Integrated Delivery System." *EGEMS* 2 (1): 1056.

Feldstein, A. C., N. A. Perrin, R. Unitan, A. G. Rosales, G. A. Nichols, D. H. Smith, J. Schneider, C. M. Davino, Y. Y. Zhou, and N. L. Lee. 2010. "Effect of a Patient Panel-Support Tool on Care Delivery." *American Journal of Managed Care* 16 (10): e256–66.

Gandhi, T. K., A. Kachalia, E. J. Thomas, A. L. Puopolo, C. Yoon, T. A. Brennan, and D. M. Studdert. 2006. "Missed and Delayed Diagnoses in the Ambulatory Setting: A Study of Closed Malpractice Claims." *Annals of Internal Medicine* 145 (7): 488–96.

Garfield, S. R. 1970. "The Delivery of Medical Care." *Scientific American* 222 (4): 15–23.

———. 1945. "The Plan That Kaiser Built." *Survey Graphic* December: 480.

Graber, M. L., R. Trowbridge, J. S. Myers, C. A. Umscheid, W. Strull, and M. H. Kanter. 2014. "The Next Organizational Challenge: Finding and Addressing Diagnostic Error." *Joint Commission Journal on Quality and Patient Safety* 40 (3): 102–10.

Herrinton, L. J., L. Liu, A. Altschuler, R. Dell, V. Rabrenovich, and A. L. Compton-Phillips. 2015. "Big Data, Miniregistries: A Rapid-Turnaround Solution to Get Quality Improvement Data into the Hands of Medical Specialists." *Permanente Journal* 19 (2): 15–21.

Hsaio, C.-J., and E. Hing. 2013. "Use and Characteristics of Electronic Health Record Systems Among Office-Based Physician Practices: United States, 2001–2012." Hyattsville, MD: National Center for Health Statistics.

Kane, C. K., and D. W. Emmons. 2013. *New Data on Physician Practice Arrangements: Private Practice Remains Strong Despite Shifts Toward Hospital Employment.* Chicago: American Medical Association.

Kanter, M. H., G. Lindsay, J. Bellows, and A. Chase. 2013. "Complete Care at Kaiser Permanente: Transforming Chronic and Preventive Care." *Joint Commission Journal on Quality and Patient Safety* 39 (11): 484–94.

Lee, B., M. Turley, D. Meng, Y. Zhou, T. Garrido, A. Lau, and L. Radler. 2012. "Effects of Proactive Population-Based Nephrologist Oversight on Progression of Chronic Kidney Disease: A Retrospective Control Analysis." *BMC Health Services Research* 12: 252.

Martinez-Ramirez, H. R., B. Jalomo-Martinez, L. Cortes-Sanabria, E. Rojas-Campos, G. Barragan, G. Alfaro, and A. M. Cueto-Manzano. 2006. "Renal Function Preservation in Type 2 Diabetes Mellitus Patients with Early Nephropathy: A Comparative Prospective Cohort Study Between Primary Health Care Doctors and a Nephrologist." *American Journal of Kidney Diseases* 47 (1): 78–87.

Mendelssohn, D. C., C. Malmberg, and B. Hamandi. 2009. "An Integrated Review of 'Unplanned' Dialysis Initiation: Reframing the Terminology to 'Suboptimal' Initiation." *BMC Nephrology* 10: 22.

National Center for Chronic Disease Prevention and Health Promotion. 2014. "National Chronic Kidney Disease Fact Sheet, 2014." Centers for Disease Control and Prevention. Accessed May 20. www.cdc.gov/diabetes/pubs/pdf /kidney_factsheet.pdf.

National Committee for Quality Assurance (NCQA). 2015a. "Patient-Centered Medical Home Recognition." Accessed June 19. www.ncqa.org/Programs/Recognition /Practices/PatientCenteredMedicalHomePCMH.aspx.

———. 2015b. "Private Health Plan Rankings 2014–2015." Accessed May 21. www .ncqa.org/ReportCards/HealthPlans/HealthInsurancePlanRankings /PrivateHealthPlanRankings20142015.aspx.

National Quality Forum. 2015. "NQF-Endorsed Measures for Renal Conditions, 2015." Published December. www.qualityforum.org/Projects/n-r/Renal _Measures/Final_Report.aspx.

Peckham, C. 2015. "Medscape Physician Compensation Report 2015." MedScape. Published April 21. www.medscape.com/features/slideshow/compensation /2015/public/overview#page=18.

Pope, G. C., and J. E. Schneider. 1992. "Trends in Physician Income." *Health Affairs* 11 (1): 181–93.

Porter, M. E. 2010. "What Is Value in Health Care?" *New England Journal of Medicine* 363 (26): 2477–81.

———. 2009. "A Strategy for Health Care Reform—Toward a Value-Based System." *New England Journal of Medicine* 361 (2): 109–12.

Porter, M. E., E. A. Pabo, and T. H. Lee. 2013. "Redesigning Primary Care: A Strategic Vision to Improve Value by Organizing Around Patients' Needs." *Health Affairs* 32 (3): 516–25.

Schilling, L., J. W. Dearing, P. Staley, P. Harvey, L. Fahey, and F. Kuruppu. 2011. "Kaiser Permanente's Performance Improvement System, Part 4: Creating a Learning Organization." *Joint Commission Journal on Quality and Patient Safety* 37 (12): 532–43.

Sim, J. J., M. P. Rutkowski, D. C. Selevan, M. Batech, R. Timmins, J. M. Slezak, S. J. Jacobsen, and M. H. Kanter. 2015. "Kaiser Permanente Creatinine Safety Program: A Mechanism to Ensure Widespread Detection and Care for Chronic Kidney Disease." *American Journal of Medicine* 128 (11): 1204–1211.e1.

Spence, M. M., J. K. Polzin, C. L. Weisberger, J. P. Martin, J. P. Rho, and G. H. Willick. 2011. "Evaluation of a Pharmacist-Managed Amiodarone Monitoring Program." *Journal of Managed Care Pharmacy* 17 (7): 513–22.

Vinson, D. R., and C. P. Quesenberry Jr. 2004. "The Safety of Telephone Management of Presumed Cystitis in Women." *Archives of Internal Medicine* 164 (9): 1026–29.

Weissberg, J. 2009. "Electronic Health Records in a Large, Integrated Health System: It's Automatic. . . . NOT! At Least, Not Yet." National Quality Measures Clearinghouse, Agency for Healthcare Research and Quality. Published August 3. www.qualitymeasures.ahrq.gov/expert/expert-commentary .aspx?id=16458.

Zhou, Y. Y., M. H. Kanter, J. J. Wang, and T. Garrido. 2010. "Improved Quality at Kaiser Permanente Through E-mail Between Physicians and Patients." *Health Affairs* 29 (7): 1370–75.

Zhou, Y. Y., R. Unitan, J. J. Wang, T. Garrido, H. L. Chin, M. C. Turley, and L. Radler. 2011. "Improving Population Care with an Integrated Electronic Panel Support Tool." *Population Health Management* 14 (1): 3–9.

BIG DATA AND EVIDENCE-BASED MANAGEMENT AT LYNDON B. JOHNSON GENERAL HOSPITAL

by Jessie L. Tucker III

Introduction

Named for the late Texas legend, former president, and champion for Medicare and Medicaid, Lyndon B. Johnson (LBJ) General Hospital opened on June 2, 1989. It was designated as the first Level III trauma center in Texas in 1996 and has since grown to become one of the busiest Level III trauma centers in the United States (Harris Health System 2016). Providing the full array of community hospital services, LBJ—part of the Harris Health System—operates 258 inpatient beds for the underserved of Harris County in Houston, Texas. Exceeded only by Los Angeles County in California, Harris County has the second highest number of uninsured people in the nation, at 1.2 million (US Census Bureau 2011). With 64 percent charity, 22 percent Medicaid, 9 percent Medicare, and 5 percent insured, LBJ also has one of the worst payer mixes in the nation.

Given the varied patient population served by the hospital, LBJ is challenged to sustain optimal quality, financial viability, and patient experience. Poverty, patient noncompliance, medical illiteracy, homelessness, high rates of mental illness, and language and custom barriers all contribute to a difficult and complex care environment. In addition, Affordable Care Act (ACA) initiatives and value-based purchasing penalties carry an adverse financial impact for less-than-optimal quality.

Avoiding poor clinical outcomes is a key concern of LBJ's leadership and frontline teams. Given the significant positive evidence from the field, the hospital has employed several big data analytic strategies to more efficiently and effectively use limited resources to provide high-quality care.

Note: For additional discussion about big data, please see the interview with John Billings presented in chapter 24.

Big Data and Analytics—Current and Emerging Evidence-Based Solutions

A significant amount of organizational, experiential, and stakeholder evidence indicates that the use of business intelligence produces better performance through a broader understanding of value opportunities (Bottles, Begoli, and Worley 2014; Davenport, Barth, and Bean 2012; Ferguson 2014; Fogarty and Bell 2014; Gandomi and Haider 2015; Hamad et al. 2015; Harrison and Lambiase 2007; Hood, Lovejoy, and Price 2015; Sharma, Mithas, and Kankanhalli 2014; Wyber et al. 2015). This body of work, which is growing exponentially, provides current and future promise for everything from predictive analytics for readmission, emergency department presentation, and patient compliance, to efficiency, revenue cycle, and supply chain excellence.

Big data analytics can be defined as "the sophisticated and rapid analysis of massive amounts of diverse information" for timely decision making to improve outcomes (Roski, Bo-Linn, and Andrews 2014, 1115). Sources of big data can be structured (e.g., discrete fields in an electronic medical record) or unstructured (e.g., free text, audio, images). Sources also include claims and costs, spending and lifestyle, pharmaceutical information, remote devices, wireless monitoring devices, home health monitoring, cell phone data, and telemedicine. Because it avoids the errors involved in sampling, the comprehensive approach of big data analytics provides deeper insights that lead to more evidence-based decisions.

Applying Evidence-Based Management

Step 1: Formulating the Research Question

With clinical, operational, and financial evidence-based practice as a guiding principle, Harris Health's and LBJ's leaders have consistently used best practice literature as a source of ideas. Given the quality, financial, operational capacity, and value opportunities available to the system and the hospital, the Harris Health System CEO in the spring of 2015 solicited input for numerous systemwide initiatives led by the system's operational executive vice presidents (EVPs). In response, the LBJ EVP/administrator (CEO), vice president of operations (COO), chief of the medical staff, and chief nursing officer chartered emergency department and inpatient teams led by medical, nursing, case management, rehabilitation, administrative, and information technology (IT) staff. These groups were asked to review available LBJ information and data from several big data analytic sources, consult with patients for stakeholder evidence, consider relevant literature, and acquire experiential evidence from their counterparts in other hospitals. They sought applicable solutions to the following question: *How can LBJ's patient safety, throughput, operational efficiency, and financial solvency be improved?*

The following sections provide a sample of the many initiatives and projects that resulted from the work of countless members of the multidisciplinary teams.

Steps 2, 3, and 4: Acquiring, Appraising, and Aggregating the Evidence

In attempting to collect evidence and to identify and quantify the current state, the LBJ medical and leadership team critically reviewed the system's and hospital's financial, operational capacity, quality, and external opportunities.

Financial Challenges

Like many county systems and hospitals, Harris Health and LBJ rely on a number of funding streams, including revenue from paying patients, insurers, Harris County, the state of Texas, and the federal government. Since 2013, several factors have produced significant financial strain on the system's $1.3 billion budget: (1) an assessed property tax reduction of 2 cents per $100, equating to a total reduction of $73 to $80 million; (2) a decision by the state not to distribute over $230 million to the state's trauma centers, equating to a total reduction of over $8 million; (3) the decision by the state to negotiate a Medicaid waiver (worth $30 million to the system but expiring in 2016) but not participate in Medicaid expansion, costing the system $87 million; (4) the Affordable Care Act's programmed decrease of disproportionate share funds for hospitals treating a high number of Medicaid and uninsured patients; (5) Medicaid reimbursement rates that rank among the lowest in the country, covering only 58 percent of hospital costs; and (6) marked net increases in pharmaceutical costs, especially for oncological drugs, outpacing the normal rate of inflation.

These financial challenges threatened to force the closure of facilities, reductions in services, and the elimination of programs for the underserved individuals of Harris County. Additionally, two medical schools staff the system's many facilities, and the schools could face unpalatable financial shortfalls. The challenges could also create operational and financial strain on private hospitals that would be asked to care for more indigent patients in their emergency departments with little to no reimbursement. As the nation's busiest Level III trauma center in a city that is already short of trauma centers per capita, any reduction in trauma services at LBJ could be catastrophic.

Operational Capacity Limitations

Operating 258 inpatient beds and bassinets, LBJ accommodates more than 79,000 emergency department visits annually. With inpatient medical/

surgical unit occupancy over 120 percent and emergency department occupancy over 250 percent five to six days per week, LBJ struggled to meet patient demand. Managing the mismatch between needed and available resources, and the inherent bottlenecks and inefficiencies of operating above capacity (Rabin et al. 2012), are a constant challenge.

Quality of Care

Harris Health System earned a Leapfrog Group Hospital Safety Score grade of *C*, meaning that the system clearly has opportunities for improvement. Based largely on Centers for Medicare & Medicaid Services claims data, Hospital Safety Score metrics identified below-average performance on hospital-acquired pressure ulcers (HAPU), central line–associated bloodstream infections (CLABSI), postoperative pulmonary embolisms (PE), deep vein thrombosis (DVT), and several other metrics. The system also did not fare as well as desired on Healthgrades, *US News and World Report*, and *Consumer Reports* assessments. Outcomes suggested that Harris Health had several opportunities related to surgical procedure complication, condition, treatment, mortality, patient satisfaction, and other quality measures.

Given that nearly 20 percent of Medicare patients were readmitted within 30 days at a cost of $17 million (Shulan et al. 2013), readmission and medical error penalties provide a secondary financial incentive to improve quality (Postel et al. 2014).

Industry Shifts from Volume to Value

As many payment systems continued to migrate toward ensuring value and focusing less on volume, Harris Health and LBJ needed to adapt. Value-based care (VBC) presents a shift from the traditional fee-for-service (FFS) reimbursement methodology to reimbursement models that are more closely based on the return on investment for quality, patient experience, and other clinical outcome measures. VBC has by no means become the norm, given the highly profitable nature of current FFS payment structures; however, VBC is becoming increasingly prevalent as patients, payers, governments, employers, and others demand explanations for non-outcomes-based cost variances. Requirements and pressures from the ACA and accountable care organization projects, flush with data, are also facilitating the shift to VBC. In Harris County, taxpayers, the government, employers, and patients expect a cost-effective, value-based return on their investment.

Faced with the aforementioned financial, capacity, quality, and value challenges, the leadership of Harris Health and LBJ developed a number of system, hospital, and clinic initiatives. With an emphasis on immediate and sustained improvement, these initiatives leveraged several big data sources, analytics tools, and vendors to address process improvement opportunities.

Step 5: Applying the Evidence in Decision Making

In choosing foundations for hospital goals and benchmarks, the LBJ team focused on the Institute for Healthcare Improvement (IHI) Triple Aim (i.e., to improve patient experience, health of populations, and cost per capita) and the Robert Wood Johnson Foundation population health outcomes model. These models are shown in exhibits 13.1 and 13.2.

The intent of the leadership team was to address the daunting financial challenges without sacrificing clinical quality, patient experience, and efficiency outcomes. As a result, several big data tools and analytical approaches were employed to sustain the desired delicate value balance.

Big Data Sources and Tools

As part of the Hospitals & Health Networks "Health Care's Most Wired" list since 2011 and an Epic inpatient client since 2009, Harris Health and LBJ have increasingly leveraged available comprehensive data sources. Truven Health Analytics, University Health Consortium (UHC), and Action OI data and tools—introduced to the system in 2012—have provided a broader, more comprehensive access to comparative data from other teaching hospitals and systems. These tools provide population-level, big data analytic opportunities that avoid the parametric limitations of sampling.

Davenport, Barth, and Bean (2012) differentiate nonparametric big data analysis from traditional parametric sample-data analysis in three ways: (1) a proactive focus on processes and flows, and not only retrospective analyses; (2) a reliance on data scientists and product and process developers, rather than data analysts; and (3) a view of analytics as something to be integrated into core business, operational, and production functions and not just

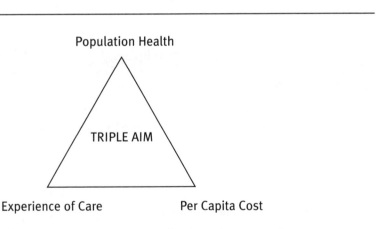

EXHIBIT 13.1
The IHI Triple Aim

Source: Adapted from the Institute for Healthcare Improvement (2016).

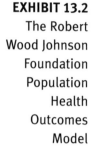

EXHIBIT 13.2
The Robert
Wood Johnson
Foundation
Population
Health
Outcomes
Model

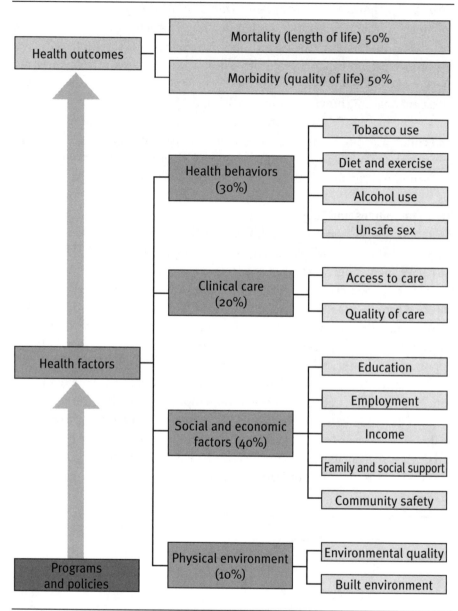

Source: Adapted with permission from the Robert Wood Johnson Foundation (2016).

as an IT function. As a result, internal data scientists employed by the system use ACL Analytics to scour the mountains of available data.

Using data envelopment analysis (DEA), Harrison and Lambiase (2007) identified marked efficiency advances in teaching hospitals that used big data analytic tools. By putting information into the hands of decision makers at all levels, these tools provide guidance in how limited resources can be arrayed to optimize outcomes (Hogarth and Soyer 2015). Truven Health Analytics, UHC, Action OI data, and Global Healthcare Exchange (GHX) are a few of the big data analytic resources used by Harris Health and LBJ. In addition, by joining forces with GHX, Harris Health was able to use GHX's expertise in supply chain management to increase operational efficiency and improve cost effectiveness.

Published Best Practices

Periodicals such as *Health Care Finance News* and *Becker's Hospital Review*, by highlighting evidence-based big data analytic successes from hospitals around the country, served as a rich source of improvement ideas for Harris Health and LBJ. Although finding organizations with similar payer mix, patient population, and capacity constraints was difficult, sufficient generalizable evidence from the field existed to assist in developing action plans. Additionally, leaders were asked to solicit ideas and input from peers in the field and from their clinical and administrative professional organizations.

Solutions

The LBJ team began the journey to improvement by setting initial goals dealing with clinical outcomes, process efficiency, and patient experience. Accepting that these initial goals were only the beginning, the team focused first on a number of emergency department, hospital operational, and patient satisfaction measures.

Action OI is an invaluable tool that compares hospitals to selected peer groups in the industry's largest database of client-supplied data. It enables organizations to assess employed resources and subsequent clinical, efficiency, and financial outcomes to help identify potential improvement opportunities in areas such as mortality, safety, effectiveness, efficiency, and productivity. Providing full-time equivalent (FTE) and dollar opportunities in a host of areas, the database presents important information about productivity and its subsequent financial impact. By systematically reviewing all LBJ departments and services and comparing them to their peers in Action OI, LBJ's leadership tailored the annual budget build around moving 75th percentile (bottom 25th percent) performers to the 50th percentile, 50th percentile performers into the top 25th percentile, and sustaining current top 25th percentile performers. The reviews produced several opportunities that were carefully considered by the medical, clinical, and ancillary teams to determine where productivity could be improved; layoffs were not an option chosen by the system.

After identifying the departments and services that performed worse than the 50th percentile, the directors of those areas were charged with researching the quality, efficiency, and productivity aspects of top-performing peers. Sources of data included Action OI expert suggestions, published peer-reviewed and trade literature, and poster presentations from professional meetings, among other sources. Information garnered from this in-depth query of Action OI best performers was then introduced in various forums to vet proposals for protocol, structure, and process changes. Once accepted as pilots or permanent changes, these opportunities were implemented and monitored to ensure that desired outcomes were achieved.

Given the complexity of LBJ's patients, aggressive case management is essential from a quality, efficiency, and compliance perspective. Most patients are lower income, have lower health literacy, and present complex and challenging social situations. Every inpatient is reviewed by the case management department upon admission to ensure that InterQual criteria are met. In instances where questions arise, case managers speak directly to the medical staff to clarify the accuracy of documentation. Although most of LBJ's patients are self-pay and indigent, this practice ensures accurate billing and assists with preventing readmissions penalties for patients with Medicare.

An additional cost-effective big data opportunity stemmed from the partnership with GHX, whose focus on increasing operational efficiency and driving down costs provided a comprehensive review of every phase of supply chain operations. By mapping processes, identifying duplicative efforts, providing feedback about purchasing, and sharing industry best practices, LBJ leveraged GHX's expertise in every aspect of the supply chain. The automation of many supply chain processes provided decision makers with timely information and helped in the management of significantly constrained and limited resources.

An additional tool, ACL Analytics, supplied comprehensive audit and risk analysis information for decision making. Employed data scientists provided decision makers with valuable retrospective audit and prospective modeling information. In analyzing all data without the limitations of sampling, anomalies and patterns were revealed. As an internal auditing effort, Harris Health and LBJ reviewed timekeeping, accounting, financial, bed utilization, and supply chain data to optimize limited resources, minimize compliance and legal risk, and quickly identify potential areas of concern.

Step 6: Evaluating the Results

Although the selected goals and targets were not lofty when compared to those of nonpublic hospitals, they were significant when compared to those of other public hospitals. LBJ experienced marked performance improvements, and many goals were achieved as a result of the big data and analytic initiatives that were employed. However, these outcomes represented only the beginning of the improvement journey.

Although volume increased by 10 percent, LBJ was able to lower expenses by over $3.1 million, reduce expenses per patient day (total, labor, and supply) by 16 percent, and reduce the benchmarked opportunity by 21.5 FTEs and $1.7 million. Supply chain improvements and cost reductions also solidified LBJ's place as a GHX "Best 50" Healthcare Provider for Supply Chain Excellence. A portion of the labor expense reductions were from the replacement of premium labor (contract, agency, and so on) with regular full-time staff. This shift to more permanent staff is also posited to have supported quality of care improvements. Finally, systemwide revenue cycle initiatives aimed at ensuring the timely management of invoices, receivables, rebates, and discounts assisted in the resulting 28 percent revenue increases.

Intent on ensuring that quality would not be compromised during major efforts to improve financial performance and close deficits, the LBJ team proactively monitored clinical outcomes via system, hospital, quality, case management, and nursing indicator scorecards (see exhibit 13.3). Consistent monitoring, auditing, and sound action plans for fallouts ensured LBJ's very successful DNV, College of American Pathologist (CAP), and trauma surveys, as well as the American Nurses Credentialing Center's Pathway to Excellence designation. Additionally, the hospital had low or nonexistent CLABSI, methicillin-resistant Staphylococcus aureus (MRSA), and vancomycin-resistant Enterococcus (VRE) rates; consistently outperformed case mix index–adjusted length of stay, readmission, and surgical site infection benchmarks; and obtained patient satisfaction scores in the 91st percentile for the first time in the hospital's history. As a final achievement for the year, Harris Health / LBJ was named a *Houston Chronicle* "Top Workplace."

Conclusion

Big data analytics initiatives are increasingly important tools in the Harris Health and LBJ arsenal. In light of the challenges of securing data while ensuring functionality, significant effort has been, and will continue to be, invested in sustaining high quality, managing costs, and improving efficiency through the use of evidence-based management. The future will undoubtedly provide further opportunities to leverage the benefits of big data in decision making. For instance, using the International Statistical Classification of Diseases and Related Health Problems (ICD-10) code for patient noncompliance could provide evidence to support a business case initiative around more proactive patient management. Additionally, traditional demographic, socioeconomic, utilization, and diagnosis-related group predictive models can be enhanced by big data to increase their predictive power and the cost-effectiveness of decisions. Epic's STARS and Honor Roll programs provide

EXHIBIT 13.3
Executive
Summary
Scorecard

LBJ EXECUTIVE SUMMARY SCORECARD

Indicator	Data Source	Frequency	Outcomes	Jun	Jul	Aug	Sep	Oct	Nov	Dec
Cost effectiveness compared to peer group (FTE/$ opportunity)	Action OI	Quarterly	Actual	53.8/$3.9M		58.5/$4M			32.3/$2.2M	
			Target	0 FTEs/$0s		0 FTEs/$0s			0 FTEs/$0s	
Hospital total expenses per patient	Financials	Bimonthly	Actual	$3,455			$3,260		$3,279	$3,324
			Target	$3,515			$3,515		$3,515	$3,515
ED boarder hours	EC Timings Workbook	Monthly	Actual	10,023	10,762	9,938	10,424	7,369	3,572	2,997
			Target	8,529	8,529	8,529	8,529	8,529	8,529	8,529
ED LWBS for ESI 1s, 2s, & 3s	EC Timings Workbook	Monthly	Actual	12.3%	11.2%	8.8%	8.7%	5.1%	4.9%	5.2%
			Target	8.0%	8.0%	8.0%	8.0%	8.0%	8.0%	8.0%
Hospital 1-day admissions	Epic	Monthly	Actual	66	43	57	52	69	62	64
			Target	65	65	65	65	65	65	65
ED door-to-provider for ESI 3s, 4s, & 5s	EC Timings Workbook	Monthly	Actual	2:52	2:37	2:32	2:16	1:21	1:17	1:13
			Target	2:15	2:15	2:15	2:15	2:15	2:15	2:15
ED provider-to-disposition for discharged patients	EC Timings Workbook	Monthly	Actual	4:56	4:59	4:43	4:17	4:21	4:55	4:34
			Target	4:30	4:30	4:30	4:30	4:30	4:30	4:30
ED screen-out of nonemergent ESI 4s & 5s (ages 18–64)	EC Timings Workbook	Monthly	Actual	32.1%	26.4%	25.4%	28.6%	37.0%	35.8%	28.9%
			Target	30.0%	30.0%	30.0%	30.0%	30.0%	30.0%	30.0%
Quality scorecard fallout rate	System Scorecard	Monthly	Actual	17.2%	0.0%	6.9%	3.4%	3.4%	0.0%	3.4%
			Target	5.0%	5.0%	5.0%	5.0%	5.0%	5.0%	5.0%
Medical necessity physician-clinical case management discordance rate	Epic	Monthly	Actual	42.4%	43.4%	24.3%	19.2%	17.0%	19.7%	19.9%
			Target	<45%	<45%	<25%	<25%	<25%	<25%	<25%
Overall patient satisfaction	NRC Picker	Monthly	Actual	73.8	82.2	79.3	80.8	80.9	82.8	78.1
			Target	73.5	73.5	73.5	73.5	73.5	73.5	73.5

Source: Data from LBJ General Hospital.

electronic patient record functionality and analytics best practices derived from clinical and financial evidence from the field of Epic users. Hamad and colleagues' (2015) big data–based DxCG Intelligence patient risk stratification tool can assist in the development of interventions to move high- and rising-risk patients to lower-risk strata and produce significantly improved clinical and financial outcomes.

References

Bottles, K., E. Begoli, and B. Worley. 2014. "Understanding the Pros and Cons of Big Data Analytics." *Physician Executive* 40 (4): 6–12.

Davenport, T. H., P. Barth, and R. Bean. 2012. "How Big Data Is Different." *MIT Sloan Management Review* 54 (1): 43–46.

Ferguson, R. 2014. "Crafting Health Care's Future at Kaiser Permanente." *MIT Sloan Management Review* 56 (1): 1–5.

Fogarty, D., and P. C. Bell. 2014. "Should You Outsource Analytics?" *MIT Sloan Management Review* 55 (2): 41–45.

Gandomi, A., and M. Haider. 2015. "Beyond the Hype: Big Data Concepts, Methods, and Analytics." *International Journal of Information Management* 35 (2): 137–44.

Hamad, R., S. Modrek, J. Kubo, B. Goldstein, and M. Cullen. 2015. "Using 'Big Data' to Capture Overall Health Status: Properties and Predictive Value of a Claims-Based Health Risk Score." *PLoS One* 10 (5): 1–14.

Harris Health System. 2016. "Lyndon B. Johnson Hospital." Accessed November 15. www.harrishealth.org/en/services/locations/pages/lbj.aspx.

Harrison, J. P., and L. R. Lambiase. 2007. "The Improving Efficiency of University Health Consortium Hospitals." *Journal of Public Budgeting, Accounting & Financial Management* 19 (3): 385–99.

Hogarth, R. M., and E. Soyer. 2015. "Using Simulated Experience to Make Sense of Big Data." *MIT Sloan Management Review* 56 (2): 49–54.

Hood, L., J. Lovejoy, and N. Price. 2015. "Integrating Big Data and Actionable Health Coaching to Optimize Wellness." *BMC Medicine* 13 (4): 1–4.

Institute for Healthcare Improvement (IHI). 2016. "The IHI Triple Aim." Accessed July 25. www.ihi.org/engage/initiatives/tripleaim/Pages/default.aspx.

Postel, M., P. Frank, T. Barry, N. Satou, and R. Shemin. 2014. "The Cost of Preventing Readmissions: Why Surgeons Should Lead the Effort." *American Surgeon* 80 (10): 1003–6.

Rabin, E., K. Kocher, M. McClelland, J. Pines, U. Hwang, N. Rathlev, B. Asplin, N. S. Trueger, and E. Weber. 2012. "Solutions to Emergency Department 'Boarding' and Crowding Are Underused and May Need to Be Legislated." *Health Affairs* 31 (8): 1757–66.

Robert Wood Johnson Foundation. 2016. "Our Approach." *County Health Rankings & Roadmaps*. Accessed October 6. www.countyhealthrankings.org/our-approach.

Roski, J., G. Bo-Linn, and T. A. Andrews. 2014. "Creating Value in Health Care Through Big Data: Opportunities and Policy Implications." *Health Affairs* 33 (7): 1115–22.

Sharma, R., S. Mithas, and A. Kankanhalli. 2014. "Transforming Decision-Making Processes: A Research Agenda for Understanding the Impact of Business Analytics on Organisations." *European Journal of Information Systems* 23 (4): 433–41.

Shulan, M., K. Gao, M. Kelly, and D. Crystal. 2013. "Predicting 30-Day All-Cause Hospital Readmissions." *Health Care Management Science* 16 (2): 167–75.

US Census Bureau. 2011. "Small Area Health Insurance Estimates: One-Year Estimates, 2011." Accessed February 2014. www. census.gov/did/www/sahie/data/interactive.

Wyber, R., S. Vaillancourt, W. Perry, P. Mannava, T. Folaranmi, and L. A. Celi. 2015. "Big Data in Global Health: Improving Health in Low- and Middle-Income Countries." *Bulletin of the World Health Organization* 93 (3): 203–8.

AN ACADEMIC PRACTICE PARTNERSHIP TO SUPPORT EVIDENCE-BASED MANAGEMENT AT RUSH UNIVERSITY MEDICAL CENTER

by Andrew N. Garman, Tricia J. Johnson, Shital C. Shah,
W. Jeffrey Canar, Peter W. Butler, and Chien-Ching Li

Introduction

The purpose of this chapter is to provide a generalizable case example of how the principles of evidence-based management (EBMgmt) can be taught at the graduate level, using a hands-on approach involving real-world problems in healthcare management. Beyond the education of future graduates, the approach can also be used to increase working managers' exposure to EBMgmt principles through their involvement in the student project teams. Our hope in sharing our experiences is to enable others to adopt the approach for their own uses and to help spread the use and application of evidence-based management as a cornerstone of learning health systems.

Within the US healthcare sector, recognition of the role and importance of evidence-based management has moved beyond early efforts to build awareness (Hewison 1997; Walshe and Rundall 2001) and toward a clear mandate for action (Institute of Medicine Committee on the Learning Health Care System in America 2012). At the same time, the availability of data of all kinds has been expanding at an unprecedented pace—bringing with it an increased risk of data misuse and illusory or politically driven interpretations resulting from chance patterns or weak research designs (Boyd and Crawford 2012). For a health system to fully benefit from the value data can provide, users must develop not only an appreciation for data-driven decision making, but also an understanding of such concepts as statistical power, generalizability, and sampling error. These and related concepts might be collectively referred to as "evidence literacy," and a thorough understanding and appreciation of the concepts may require substantial applied experience.

At Rush University Medical Center (RUMC), we provide opportunities for practitioners and graduate students to gain this experience through the Masters Project Program (MPP), which operates within the university's Master of Science in Health Systems Management (MS-HSM) degree program. MPP students benefit from hands-on experience applying evidence to real-world management questions and also generating new evidence to support decisions where prior knowledge is lacking. In the sections that follow, we describe the context in which the program operates and discuss the program itself.

Rush University Medical Center

Originally founded in 1837 as Rush Medical College, Rush University Medical Center originally had an academic mission: It trained people to become doctors (which in that era took just 16 weeks), and the actual provision of healthcare was a side concern necessary to support this mission (Bowman 1990). Its flagship affiliate hospital, the Presbyterian Hospital of Chicago, opened in 1884. During World War II, Rush Medical College ceased admissions; however, the affiliated Presbyterian Hospital continued operations, eventually merging with another hospital to become Presbyterian-St. Luke's. Some 20 years later, responding to a shortage of medical personnel, the leadership of Presbyterian-St. Luke's began to investigate reopening the Rush Medical College charter. After weighing the costs and benefits of pursuing another university affiliation, the leaders asked a bold question: Might we be able to launch the college within the hospital itself?

Accrediting bodies were unable to provide any specific reason that this approach could not be taken, so Rush took the unprecedented step of launching the medical college as a fully integrated component of the hospital. The college's leadership comprised the current leaders of the hospital in broadened roles. The model proved successful enough that the charter was eventually expanded to turn Rush into a full health sciences university, one that would eventually include a full complement of programs to address healthcare workforce needs (Goldsmith 1980; Montgomery, Enzbrenner, and Lerner 1991; Williams et al. 1987).

Toward the end of the 1970s, a graduate-level healthcare management program was also launched, the Master of Science in Health Systems Management (Flanagan 2005). Designed to be a generalist management program for preparing future hospital executives, the MS-HSM program entered its first cohort of students in 1979. In keeping with the practitioner-teacher model, a vice president in the medical center was appointed the program's first chair, and course faculty members were selected from among the leadership of the medical center and its affiliated organizations. From its inception, the program also included a graduate research project, which over time evolved into the current Master's Project Program.

Today, RUMC has more than 9,500 employees (RUMC 2016). Its HSM department includes more than 100 part-time, professionally qualified faculty members who work as managers, directors, or senior leaders within the medical center or other healthcare organizations. Strategic leadership is provided by the department chair, a practitioner faculty member with a dual role as RUMC's president. The MS-HSM program accepts up to 27 students per year—23 to 25 full-time students and 2 to 4 part-time students. Full-time students in their first year spend half their time in internship positions at the medical center or other healthcare organizations. Both the internships and the curriculum itself are organized around the interdisciplinary leadership competency model maintained by the National Center for Healthcare Leadership (Calhoun et al. 2008).

Like all US hospitals, RUMC is evolving in response to the Affordable Care Act of 2010, the most significant legislation to influence healthcare delivery in the past generation (Federal Register 2016). Additionally, the field has placed increasing emphasis on the effective leveraging of care process and outcomes data to continuously improve care models, as described by the Institute of Medicine's "learning health system" concept (Institute of Medicine Roundtable on Evidence-Based Medicine 2007; Institute of Medicine Committee on the Learning Health Care System in America 2012). This expanded focus on meaningful use of data has enhanced the visibility of the MPP and heightened the medical center's expectations for the program's role in supporting practice improvements.

Description of the Masters Project Program

The MPP is designed to provide participants with hands-on experience in the practice of all aspects of evidence-based management, up to and including the processes involved in the creation and dissemination of new scientific evidence (Barends, Rousseau, and Briner 2014). The formal MPP coursework involves a two-course sequence, with an optional third course if the student and practitioner faculty want to pursue publication. However, the EBMgmt education and acculturation process itself unfolds throughout the student's two years in the master's program. The concept of evidence-based management is first introduced during new student orientation, and it is described at that time as foundational to the curriculum. First-year students (known as HSM-1s) attend three events that provide them with additional exposure to the masters project (MP) and EBMgmt processes. The first two of these events are the proposals and final project presentations by the second-year students (HSM-2s), which occur in the fall and winter quarters, respectively.

The third event, a "meet and greet" kickoff to the HSM-1s' own MPs, occurs in late spring.

Exhibit 14.1 provides a summary of the MPP as it currently operates. In the sections that follow, we describe the steps in the MPP in greater detail. We organize this description around an eight-step model, adapted from the model provided by Kovner and Rundall (2006). We have expanded upon the model to incorporate an emphasis on evidence creation as well as application.

Step 1: Formulating Research Questions

During the spring prior to the start of the MPP sequence, the teaching team (i.e., the four PhD faculty members with primary responsibility for the MPP) actively solicits practitioners for management questions that might benefit from an evidence-based approach. Initially, the teaching team would attend senior leadership meetings at RUMC and affiliated organizations to build awareness about the MPP. Today, most of these requests are gathered via an online survey, which is distributed to practitioner faculty members, prior MPP participants, and other key stakeholders. This data collection is supplemented by some direct outreach on the part of the teaching team to help managers formulate their questions as "testable," and to ensure that data will be available to address these questions. The teaching team's goal is to collect more management research questions than there are students to pursue them, so that demand favors the students, and project sponsors need to actively promote their questions as important opportunities to the prospective student leads. The approach better ensures a high level of intrinsic interest on the part of practitioners as well as students, balancing autonomy with relatedness.

Step 2: Setting Priorities for Research Questions

Around the same time, the teaching team schedules a "meet and greet" session to connect students with prospective project sponsors. The session is held during a lunch hour and lasts 75 minutes. It begins with a brief (15-minute) introduction to the MPP, including a description of the characteristics of a successful project. Successful projects are characterized as "sitting on a three-legged stool," or simultaneously meeting three criteria: (1) a high-value management question, (2) a committed project champion, and (3) a feasible set of project requirements.

A management question is considered high value to the extent that it possesses two key characteristics. The characteristic of utmost importance is *salience*: The results of the project should guide a specific decision that managers will make at some future point. A second important characteristic is *generalizability*: All else equal, decisions that have relevance beyond the

EBMgmt Step	Program Step	Time Frame	Actions	Participants
1. Formulating research questions	Faculty survey	Spring, Year 1	Structured survey is sent to practitioner faculty and other key contacts, requesting project topics.	• MP teaching team • Practitioner faculty
2. Setting priorities for research questions	MP "meet and greet"	Spring/ summer, Year 1	MP teaching team provides introduction to the process; faculty "pitch" their topic ideas; students follow up as interested and assemble project committees.	• Teaching team • Practitioner faculty • Students
3. Searching for evidence	MP Course 1	Fall, Year 2	Students conduct scan of peer-reviewed and gray literature.	• Students • Faculty mentor
4. Clarifying where more evidence is needed	MP Course 1	Fall, Year 2	Students identify gaps in existing knowledge base that a project could address.	• Students • Faculty mentor
5. Defining the approach to new evidence creation	MP Course 1	Fall, Year 2	Students work with faculty mentor and project committee to define research question and present proposed approach to an open forum.	• Students • Faculty mentor • Project committee • MP community
6. Developing new evidence	MP Course 2	Winter, Year 2	Students collect/ obtain data, run analyses, and develop findings.	• Students • Faculty mentor
7. Communicating results	MP Course 2	Winter, Year 2	Students present findings to an open forum.	• Students • MP community
8. Contributing to the evidence base	MP Course 3 (optional)	Spring, Year 3	MP faculty work with students to develop publishable works.	• MP faculty • Interested students

EXHIBIT 14.1
Evidence-Based Decision Making and the Masters Project Curriculum

specific context in which the question is being asked stand to make more valuable contributions overall.

The project champion for a given management question is typically the person who generated that question. To be capable in this role, a champion needs to possess five qualities. First, the champion must be committed to supporting the student in seeing the project through to its completion. Typically, this quality is closely related to the second critical quality: influence over the people, processes, and sources of information that the project will require. Evidence-based management frequently involves challenging established ways of working (Speicher-Bocija and Adams 2012). For example, prior projects have involved testing the potential impact of significant changes in how staffing decisions are made, how specific populations of patients are managed, and how surgical cases are prioritized and scheduled. In such projects, students often encounter problems accessing necessary resources, such as data or input from key people. The project champion needs to be in a position to help the student navigate these barriers and step in as necessary. For the third critical quality, a champion needs sufficient expertise to provide guidance about the context of the management question, the availability and limitations of data needed to answer that question, and the gap between previous findings and the local context in which these findings will be applied. Fourth, the champion needs to be able to hold the student and the project committee accountable for timely completion of tasks for which they are responsible. Fifth, the project champion should be someone whom a given student can view as a professional role model, thus maximizing the relatedness component of intrinsic motivation.

Once the student has selected a topic and a project champion, she assembles a project committee including at least two other members. The committee meets with the student periodically throughout the course of the project and also provides competency-based feedback at the conclusion of each of the two main courses. The committee is required to include a member of the academic faculty, who is assigned from the MP teaching team. This requirement ensures that each committee includes both practitioner and academic perspectives that are relevant to the research question at hand. The remaining committee members are selected by the student. Often these additional members are selected based on their familiarity with the area of practice under study, though frequently they are selected based on the student's interest in working with specific individuals.

With respect to project feasibility, the program takes great care to ensure that pursuit of the project will reinforce a student's sense of confidence. In particular, the scope needs to fit within the limited resources that a student and his committee will have to bring to bear on the research question. Constraints exist in terms of both total hours available (the typical HSM-2 student is taking a full-time course load and working 20 hours per week) and project duration (the project does not formally commence until September, the proposal must be completed by November, and the project findings must be finalized by early March). Therefore, a general rule of thumb is that the student should spend about 12 hours per week during the core seven months of the project, supported by 2 to 4 hours per month from the other committee members.

Step 3: Searching for Evidence

The formal coursework supporting the MPP begins during the fall quarter of the student's second year. During this quarter, students enroll in Masters Project 1, the first of two required courses to support the MPP. Many elements of both Masters Project 1 and Masters Project 2, taken in the following quarter, were designed with a recognition of self-efficacy as a driver of students' intrinsic motivation. In particular, throughout both quarters, the project has weekly deliverables. The deliverables are graded primarily on a pass/fail basis, and students typically receive full credit if the assignments are completed and turned in on time. This approach affords students the opportunity to receive feedback along the way without an expectation that they must get everything right the first time.

In terms of searching for evidence, students are encouraged to recognize the importance of all four major sources of evidence (Briner, Denyer, and Rousseau 2009). However, the course work places special emphasis on developing skill in accessing best available research evidence. The early weeks of the Masters Project 1 course focus on developing students' skills in searching peer-reviewed sources as well as gray literature (i.e., non-peer-reviewed research, such as white papers from associations and consulting firms); assessing the quality of the evidence they are identifying; and understanding the importance of data security and privacy rights in the EBMgmt process. The approach reflects two design elements that we believe are highly relevant to how practitioners actually use evidence. First, recommended sources of evidence include practitioner-focused (e.g., consultant white papers, research reports from private services) as well as academic-focused (peer-reviewed) publications. Second, recommended search strategies are designed to be highly efficient and targeted, rather than highly systematic and exhaustive. In support of both elements, the course discusses the concept of a hierarchy of evidence quality. Though students are encouraged to find the strongest evidence they can, the value of best available evidence is also reinforced. In addition, students are often coached to be mindful of the time–cost trade-off associated with continuing a search for evidence, especially in light of the value of the decision at hand.

Step 4: Clarifying Where More Evidence Is Needed

An important goal of the literature scan is to ensure that the team is designing an approach that will meaningfully contribute to the confidence with which a given management question can be answered. Almost without exception, the literature scan not only identifies some evidence that can inform the management research question but also surfaces many other unanswered questions that would be helpful to address. The student assembles the evidence, as well as gaps in evidence, into a conceptual model to visually communicate the contribution the MP will make to existing knowledge. As the quarter progresses, the student vets both the findings of the literature scan and the conceptual model with her project committee, and typically the model evolves iteratively through these ongoing discussions. This step has an important side benefit of exposing the participating committee members to research they would not be likely to see if not for their participation in the MPP (Rynes, Giluk, and Brown 2007).

Step 5: Defining the Approach to New Evidence Creation

The first course culminates in a presentation to the broader healthcare community. Structured in alignment with the goal of creating "sticky" evidence (Bartunek, Rynes, and Ireland 2006; Leung and Bartunek 2012; Rousseau and Boudreau 2011), the MP presentations are designed more as "pitches" than as traditional academic proposal defenses. Each student is provided ten minutes to convey his project concept, why it is important, and how it will be studied. The presentation is followed by five minutes of open questions and answers with the audience. Once feedback has been received, students finalize their proposals, and the first quarter concludes.

Step 6: Developing New Evidence

To help provide participants with exposure to the various aspects of the EBMgmt process, all projects are considered to be research studies, and as such they are submitted to the medical center's institutional review board (IRB) for approval. Student investigators submit their IRB applications by the end of the first quarter, so they can begin any necessary data collection by the start of the second quarter. The second quarter then focuses on executing the project. Class sessions in the second quarter are primarily focused on hands-on data management and analysis. Each class session starts with a discussion of the quarter timeline and expectations for upcoming deliverables. Sessions are held in a computer lab so that course instructors can work hands-on with students individually or in small groups. Cross-exposure of students to one another's projects also helps broaden their experience in applying evidence to a range of management applications and fosters a sense of relatedness across students.

Step 7: Communicating Results

The student communicates results of her MP in two formats: a presentation and a final paper. The final presentation is similar in format to the proposal, and it is intended as much to enhance persuasive impact as to rigorously defend the approach taken. A series of practice presentation sessions takes place, in which student investigators do "dry runs" of their oral presentations, with a small number of practitioner faculty members in the audience to provide feedback. For the presentation itself, each student has ten minutes to convey the importance of the management question being addressed, the approach taken to applying evidence, what was learned, and the implications for management practice. All presentations are given on the same day to an audience that primarily consists of healthcare managers but also includes academic faculty. All audience members are asked to complete a structured evaluation for each of the presenters, on dimensions including clarity, engagement, confidence, and overall quality.

Final papers are designed to follow the style of modern evidence-based medicine articles—that is, "significantly shorter, written in easy-to-read English, and the theoretical underpinning of the research outcomes is of secondary importance to the practical relevance and applicability" (Barends, ten Have, and Huisman 2012, 33). Students are provided a white paper template that guides formatting to ensure completeness and uniformity of presentation, as well as an emphasis on practical implications over theory.

Step 8: Contributing to the Evidence Base

By the end of the second quarter of the MP, students are required to either communicate their intent to pursue external publication of their project or release the opportunity to do so to their other committee members. Students interested in pursuing publication are provided the option to complete a third MP course in the spring quarter, focusing on preparing their results for peer-reviewed publication. This third course is taught as an independent study; the goal at the end of the ten weeks is to have a manuscript ready for submission—although frequently the process extends into the summer and occasionally beyond. Typically, between six and eight MPP teams have pursued this elective option each year, and from any given year as many as five will eventually see their manuscripts accepted for publication. Exhibit 14.2 provides a listing of publications from 2012 through 2015.

Evaluating Results

The MPP as a course sequence is evaluated annually by its student participants. Student feedback on the MPP is collected most directly via course

EXHIBIT 14.2

Published
Master's
Projects,
2012–2015

- An Evaluation of International Patient Length of Stay, *International Journal of Healthcare Management*
- Cost and Quality Implications of Discrepancies Between Admitting and Discharge Diagnoses, *Quality Management in Healthcare*
- Empirical Analysis of Domestic Medical Travel for Elective Cardiovascular Procedures, *American Journal of Managed Care*
- Factors Influencing Medical Travel into the United States, *International Journal of Pharmaceutical and Healthcare Marketing*
- Impact of a Combined Pharmacist and Social Worker Program to Reduce Hospital Readmissions, *Journal of Managed Care Pharmacy*
- Impact of an Education Intervention on Red Blood Cell Transfusion Rates in an Academic Medical Center, *American Journal of Managed Care*
- The Impact of Electronic Health Records as an Enabler of Hospital Quality and Patient Satisfaction, *Academic Medicine*
- The Impact of Hospital and Surgeon Volume on In-Hospital Mortality of Ventricular Assist Device Recipients, *Journal of Cardiac Failure*
- Impact of a Centralized Inpatient Hospice Unit in an Academic Medical Center, *American Journal of Hospice and Palliative Medicine*
- Impact of the Unit-Based Patient Safety Officer, *Journal of Nursing Administration*
- The Impact of the Resident Duty Hour Regulations on Surgical Patients' Perceptions of Care, *Patient Experience Journal*
- Kidney Stone Protocols to Reduce Emergency Department Overcrowding, *Medical Research Archives*
- Managing Patient Expectations at Emergency Department Triage, *Patient Experience Journal*
- The Relationships Between HCAHPS Communication and Discharge Satisfaction Items and Hospital Readmissions, *Patient Experience Journal*
- Strategic Human Resource Management and Health System Adaptability, *Advances in Health Care Management*
- Case Volume and Outcomes in Neonates Undergoing Repair of Congenital Diaphragmatic Hernia in Academic Medical Centers, *Journal of Perinatology*
- Using Administrative Data for Mortality Risk Adjustment in Pediatric Congenital Cardiac Surgery, *Pediatric Critical Care Medicine*
- Single-Level Anterior Cervical Discectomy and Fusion Versus Minimally Invasive Posterior Cervical Foraminotomy for Patients with Cervical Radiculopathy: A Cost Analysis, *Neurosurgical Focus*
- The Relationship Between Hospital Value-Based Purchasing Program Scores and Hospital Bond Ratings, *Journal of Healthcare Management*

evaluations. Evaluations have been consistently favorable, with perceived quality of the course and its teaching team scoring above the 70th percentile for both peer programs and other courses in the university. Qualitative feedback also reflects a favorable reception of the course, with most of the critical feedback focusing not on the value of the program but rather on the difficulties students can experience completing deliverables within the program's strictly enforced timeline. The most frequently cited specific challenge involves access to and preparation of the necessary data, tasks that are frequently outside the committee's control.

As students graduate and begin their first postgraduate positions, favorable perceptions of the MPP tend to carry forward and strengthen. Immediately prior to graduation, students complete an exit survey that asks them to reflect on the perceived importance of each of the program's core competencies for their career success, providing a programmatic assessment of affective outcomes (Sitzmann et al. 2010). In 2015, 96 to 100 percent of respondents rated each of the components of the "information-seeking" competency—the competency most directly relevant to evidence-based management—as "very important" or higher.

The impact of the MPP on Rush's culture can be seen in changes in the composition of practitioners participating. Although the ratio of total participating practitioners to student projects has remained steady at roughly 2:1, the percentage of practitioners outside the HSM faculty has grown, from 44 percent in the 2008–2009 academic year to 67 percent in the 2012–2013 year. Having received feedback from participants, we attribute this change to the greater visibility of the program across the medical center and greater recognition of the value in participating. In terms of ongoing impact, the results of MPs continue to inform everything from the redesign of care processes to Rush's most recent philanthropic report.

Although the MPP is well received, its influence on subsequent EBMgmt attitudes and implementation has not been systematically evaluated. In particular, we have not yet assessed the extent to which practitioners apply EBMgmt practices to other management decisions beyond the MPs they are involved with, or how effectively the core EBMgmt principles are applied. To address this gap, we have begun collecting additional survey data from practitioners and alumni about their perceptions of the importance of evidence-based management, their self-confidence with regard to the EBMgmt skill components, and the application of evidence-based management in the workplace. This work is itself being guided by reviews of the literature on self-efficacy and self-determination theories, as shown in exhibit 14.3.

EXHIBIT 14.3
Conceptual
Model for
Evaluating the
Impact of the
Masters Project
Program on
Management
Practices

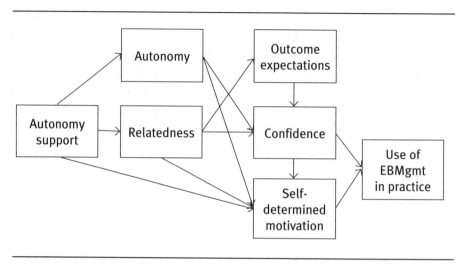

Source: Adapted from Sweet et al. (2012).

Conclusion

Over the years, the MPP has become embedded in Rush's culture in a way that has helped advance the role of EBMgmt principles in management decision making. The MPP strives not only to provide its participants with hands-on experience with evidence-based management but also to promote an appreciation for the importance of rigorous evaluation in management. Furthermore, external dissemination of EBMgmt results helps others who are facing management challenges similar to the ones investigated. Through these activities, our goal is to support a learning health system in the broadest sense of the term, as well as to disseminate a collaborative and user-friendly approach to the evidence creation process itself.

References

Barends, E., D. M. Rousseau, and R. B. Briner. 2014. *Evidence-Based Management: The Basic Principles.* Center for Evidence-Based Management. Accessed June 9, 2016. www.cebma.org/wp-content/uploads/Evidence-Based-Practice-The -Basic-Principles.pdf.

Barends, E., S. ten Have, and F. Huisman. 2012. "Learning from Other Evidence-Based Practices: The Case of Medicine." In *The Oxford Handbook of Evidence-Based Management,* edited by D. M. Rousseau, 25–42. New York: Oxford University Press.

Bartunek, J. M., S. L. Rynes, and R. D. Ireland. 2006. "What Makes Research Interesting, and Why Does It Matter?" *Academy of Management Journal* 49 (1): 9–15.

Bowman, J. 1990. *Good Medicine: The First 150 Years of Rush-Presbyterian-St. Luke's Medical Center.* Chicago: Chicago Review Press.

Boyd, D., and K. Crawford. 2012. "Critical Questions for Big Data: Provocations for a Cultural, Technological, and Scholarly Phenomenon." *Information, Communication & Society* 15 (2): 662–79.

Briner, R. B., D. Denyer, and D. M. Rousseau. 2009. "Evidence-Based Management: Concept Cleanup Time?" *Academy of Management Perspectives* 23 (4): 19–32.

Calhoun, J. G., L. Dollet, M. E. Sinioris, J. A. Wainio, P. W. Butler, J. R. Griffith, and G. L. Warden. 2008. "Development of an Interprofessional Competency Model for Healthcare Leadership." *Journal of Healthcare Management* 53 (6): 375–89.

Federal Register. 2016. "Health Care Reform." Accessed July 26. www.federalregister .gov/health-care-reform.

Flanagan, M. J. 2005. *To the Glory of God and the Service of Man: The Life of James A. Campbell, M.D.* Winnetka, IL: FHC Press.

Goldsmith, J. C. 1980. "The Health Care Market: Can Hospitals Survive?" *Harvard Business Review* 58 (5): 100–112.

Hewison, A. 1997. "Evidence-Based Medicine: What About Evidence-Based Management?" *Journal of Nursing Management* 5 (4): 195–98.

Institute of Medicine Committee on the Learning Health Care System in America. 2012. *Best Care at Lower Cost: The Path to Continuously Learning Health Care in America.* Washington, DC: National Academies Press.

Institute of Medicine Roundtable on Evidence-Based Medicine. 2007. *The Learning Healthcare System: Workshop Summary.* Accessed July 26, 2016. www.nap .edu/openbook.php?record_id=11903.

Kovner, A. R., and T. G. Rundall. 2006. "Evidence-Based Management Reconsidered." *Frontiers of Health Services Management* 22 (3): 3–22.

Leung, O., and J. M. Bartunek. 2012. "Enabling Evidence-Based Management: Bridging the Gap Between Academics and Practitioners." In *The Oxford Handbook of Evidence-Based Management*, edited by D. M. Rousseau, 165–80. New York: Oxford University Press.

Montgomery, L. D., L. R. Enzbrenner, and W. M. Lerner. 1991. "The Practitioner-Teacher Model Revisited." *Journal of Health Administration Education* 9 (1): 9–24.

Rousseau, D. M., and J. W. Boudreau. 2011. "Sticky Findings: Research Evidence Practitioners Find Useful." In *Useful Research: Advancing Theory and Practice*, edited by S. A. Mohrman and E. E. Lawler, 269–88. San Francisco: Berrett-Koehler.

Rush University Medical Center (RUMC). 2016. "Rush Facts: FY2015." Accessed July 26. http://annualreport.rush.edu/rush-facts.

Rynes, A. M., T. L. Giluk, and K. G. Brown. 2007. "The Very Separate Worlds of Academic and Practitioner Periodicals in Human Resource Management: Implications for Evidence-Based Management." *Academy of Management Journal* 50 (5): 987–1008.

Sitzmann, T., K. Ely, K. G. Brown, and K. N. Bauer. 2010. "Self-Assessment of Knowledge: A Cognitive Learning or Affective Measure?" *Academy of Management Learning & Education* 9 (2): 169–91.

Speicher-Bocija, J., and R. Adams. 2012. "Designing Strategies for the Implementation of EBMgt Among Senior Management, Middle Management, and Supervisors." In *The Oxford Handbook of Evidence-Based Management*, edited by D. M. Rousseau, 293–306. New York: Oxford University Press.

Sweet, S. N., M. S. Fortier, S. M. Strachan, and C. M. Blanchard. 2012. "Testing and Integrating Self-Determination Theory and Self-Efficacy Theory in a Physical Activity Context." *Canadian Psychology* 53 (4): 319–27.

Walshe, K., and T. G. Rundall. 2001. "Evidence-Based Management: From Theory to Practice in Health Care." *Milbank Quarterly* 79 (3): 429–57.

Williams, A. P., G. M. Carter, G. T. Hammons, and D. Pointer. 1987. *Managing for Survival: How Successful Academic Medical Centers Cope with Harsh Environments*. Santa Monica, CA: RAND.

15

TEACHING CAPSTONE AT NYU WAGNER: DEMONSTRATING COMPETENCY AND APPLYING THE PRINCIPLES OF EVIDENCE-BASED MANAGEMENT

by John Donnellan

Introduction

Over the course of my 40 years of federal service, my 20 years as a senior executive at a veterans' hospital, and my graduate study in healthcare management, I learned a great deal about the management of public and health services organizations. One of the key things I learned about problem solving and decision making is that it is important to know what you don't know. Another is that "ready-aim-fire" is generally a more effective decision-making strategy than "ready-fire-aim." Regardless of how much or how little time you may have to make a decision, the odds of making a better decision improve if you invest time and effort in learning what strategies are more likely to result in your objective.

At a relatively early stage in my career in healthcare administration, I realized that I lacked management discipline and technique, so I enrolled in the graduate program in healthcare management at New York University (NYU). The formal education I received was outstanding, although at that time the emphasis was much more on imparting knowledge than on the practical application of that knowledge. Fortunately, I attended graduate school while working full-time as a midlevel healthcare manager, so I had a personal laboratory at which I could begin to apply what I was learning. I also had the benefit of university faculty with whom I remained connected long beyond graduation. Most significant among them was Professor Anthony Kovner, who kept me abreast of his evolving vision to train healthcare managers and leaders on techniques for systematically gathering and appraising evidence in an effort to make better decisions—what came to be known as evidence-based management (EBMgmt) in healthcare.

As I neared the end of a career in healthcare management, I found myself drawn to teaching—a passion I had always harbored. I began teaching the Capstone course at NYU's Robert F. Wagner Graduate School of Public Service in 2006. In 2009, upon retiring from my position as CEO of a US Department of Veterans Affairs healthcare facility, I expanded my teaching role at NYU Wagner.

The purpose of this chapter is to describe how the principles of evidence-based management are applied in the Capstone course specifically designed for students in an executive master of public administration (EMPA) program for nurse leaders at NYU Wagner. I will also reflect on lessons learned and implications for graduate education in healthcare management.

Capstone at NYU Wagner

In 1995, NYU Wagner incorporated a Capstone experience into the curriculum for a degree of master of public administration (Schachter and Schwartz 2009). At NYU Wagner, Capstone is a two-term course in which students, working in teams of four or five, perform a project for a client healthcare, nonprofit, or public agency. The course is intended to guide students as they define a problem currently facing the client and develop solutions for the client in real time (NYU Wagner 2016a). Students design the approach, conduct the data collection and analysis, and present findings, both orally and in writing, to the client. The goal of Capstone is to determine the degree to which students can apply the knowledge imparted to them in a "real-life" setting.

Since the course's inception at NYU Wagner, some 5,300 students have conducted more than 1,100 Capstone projects. Approximately 800 organizations have sponsored an NYU Wagner Capstone project and benefited from the work of a Capstone team.

The EMPA Program for Nurse Leaders

In 2006, in conjunction with Wilhelmina Manzano, the senior vice president and chief nurse executive at New York-Presbyterian Hospital (NY-P), Professor Kovner initiated a new executive master degree program, EMPA Nurse Leader, at NYU Wagner. The program was specifically intended for registered nurses (RNs) who, having earned bachelor's degrees and already in leadership and management roles, aspire to further their careers (NYU Wagner 2016b). It was designed to be completed part-time over the course of two academic years while the students continued to work full-time (Kovner 2010).

Professor Kovner, Ms. Manzano, and other senior leaders at NY-P shared a common goal: to identify nurses working in frontline managerial positions and provide them with a rigorous course of study that emphasized both management theory and practice. The results would be better-trained nurse managers, more effective management decisions by the nursing department, and a more satisfied and organizationally committed cadre of nurse leaders.

The EMPA Nurse Leader program curriculum consists of four required courses on healthcare policy, health systems management, healthcare financial management, and quality measurement and improvement; graduate elective courses tailored to the student's individual interests, which can be selected from such options as public health, public policy and management, international health, and business administration; and a two-semester Capstone course. The syllabus for the EMPA Nurse Leader Capstone and the process for carrying out client-directed projects were modeled on Professor Kovner's experiences in evidence-based management (Kovner 2012).

Senior leadership at NY-P invested considerable resources and talent to assist in this effort. It committed money, in the form of full tuition support for RNs employed by NY-P who enrolled in the program. It committed space and logistical support: Three of the four core courses, as well as the Capstone course, meet in classroom space at NY-P. It also committed executive talent: The director of nursing external affairs and affiliations, Rosemary Sullivan, was charged with coordinating NY-P's sustained efforts for student recruitment, curriculum development, and reevaluation; assisting in teaching the Capstone course; and serving as a liaison to the NY-P community for students and faculty. In addition, NY-P committed a culture of inquiry based on the principles of evidence-based management to support Capstone. Ten years after the start of the program, more than 85 percent of the Capstone project proposals offered to EMPA Nurse Leader students are put forward by clinical managers at NY-P. These managers look to the program for evidence-based recommendations to address management problems and strategic decisions—a testament to the continued enthusiasm for and perceived value of the program by NY-P leadership.

The Capstone Experience

As previously stated, the NYU Wagner Capstone takes place over two academic terms, and students, working in teams of four or five, examine a "real-life"/"real-time" management problem for a client healthcare organization and provide evidence-based recommendations. The phases and timeline for the two-term Capstone engagement are displayed in exhibit 15.1 and summarized in the next sections of this chapter. An EMPA Nurse Leader participant's particular experience in Capstone is described by Bryce Clark in chapter 18 of this book.

EXHIBIT 15.1
A Year of
Capstone at
NYU Wagner

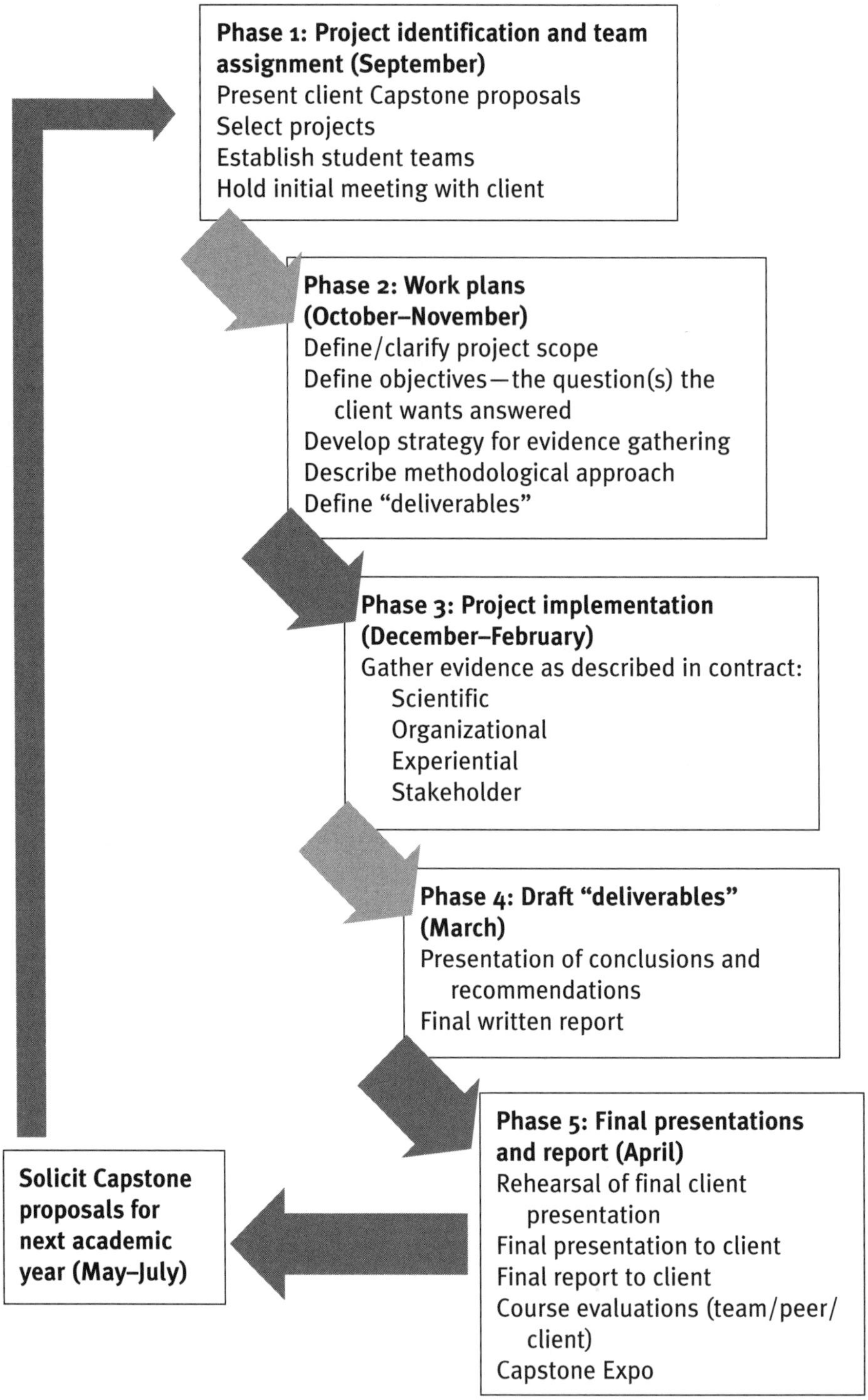

Phase 1: Project identification and team assignment (September)
Present client Capstone proposals
Select projects
Establish student teams
Hold initial meeting with client

Phase 2: Work plans (October–November)
Define/clarify project scope
Define objectives—the question(s) the
    client wants answered
Develop strategy for evidence gathering
Describe methodological approach
Define "deliverables"

Phase 3: Project implementation (December–February)
Gather evidence as described in contract:
    Scientific
    Organizational
    Experiential
    Stakeholder

Phase 4: Draft "deliverables" (March)
Presentation of conclusions and
    recommendations
Final written report

Phase 5: Final presentations and report (April)
Rehearsal of final client
    presentation
Final presentation to client
Final report to client
Course evaluations (team/peer/
    client)
Capstone Expo

Solicit Capstone proposals for next academic year (May–July)

Phase 1: Project Identification and Team Assignment

Client Organization Proposals

Several months in advance of the Capstone academic year, faculty and administration at NYU Wagner actively solicit proposals from prospective client agencies. For the EMPA Nurse Leader program, Capstone proposals are sought from the nursing departments at several large academic medical centers in New York City. At NY-P in particular, Ms. Manzano and Ms. Sullivan challenge senior nursing leaders to consider management problems that they currently face and that might benefit from more in-depth data gathering and analysis. A list of NYU Wagner EMPA Nurse Leader Capstone engagements is shown in exhibit 15.2.

The best proposals are those that describe important problems the organization faces and for which an in-depth analysis over a two-semester, nine-month academic period is acceptable. Successful proposals articulate one or more problems the organization wishes to examine in greater depth, but with an understanding that a more precise description of the scope of the problem, the specific questions to be addressed, and the analysis methodology will be developed by the Capstone team, in consultation with the client.

EXHIBIT 15.2
NYU Wagner EMPA Nurse Leader Capstone Projects, 2009–2015

Client Organization	Project Title
Hospital for Special Surgery	Assessment of Nursing Professional Development
Hospital for Special Surgery	Evidence-Based Practices Supporting Clinical Nurse Ladder
Hospital for Special Surgery	Evidence-Based Practices for RN-Driven Community Outreach Education
Hospital for Special Surgery	Assessment of RN Manager Development Program
NY-Presbyterian Hospital	Improving RN Time at the Bedside
NY-Presbyterian Hospital	Optimizing Health Information Technology Tools for Nurse Managers
NY-Presbyterian Hospital	Improving RN Retention
NY-Presbyterian Hospital	Hearing the Virtual Voice of the Patient
NY-Presbyterian Hospital	Identifying Discharge Barriers and Improving Discharge Processes

(continued)

EXHIBIT 15.2
NYU Wagner
EMPA Nurse
Leader
Capstone
Projects,
2009–2015
(Continued)

NY-Presbyterian Hospital	Optimizing RN Satisfaction with Bedside Technology
NY-Presbyterian Hospital	Improving Pre-Admission Processes for Bariatric Surgery
NY-Presbyterian Hospital	Assessment of Operational Efficiency of Hemodialysis & Apheresis Unit
NY-Presbyterian Hospital	Assessment of RN Hourly Rounding Processes
NY-Presbyterian Hospital	Improving Early Mobilization of ICU Patients
NY-Presbyterian Hospital	Assessment of Staff Beliefs and Attitudes re: Organ Donation
NY-Presbyterian Hospital	Improving the Discharge Process for Short-Stay Urology Patients
NY-Presbyterian Hospital	Improving Communication and Collaboration for the Allen Hospital and Its Community
NY-Presbyterian Hospital	Improving Interdisciplinary Communication
NY-Presbyterian Hospital	Case Management at NY Presbyterian: An Opportunity for Change
NY-Presbyterian Hospital	Improving the Dissemination of Nursing Practice at NY Presbyterian
NY-Presbyterian Hospital	Empowering Nurses in the Capital Equipment Procurement Process at NY Presbyterian
NY-Presbyterian Hospital	Introducing RNs at the Allen Hospital to Community Outreach
NY-Presbyterian Hospital	Improving Supply Procurement on Nursing Units at Columbia Presbyterian Hospital
NY-Presbyterian Hospital	Improving Supply Procurement on Nursing Units at the Weill-Cornell Hospital
NY-Presbyterian Hospital	Streamlining Restraint Data Monitoring at NY Presbyterian Hospital
NY-Presbyterian Hospital	Assessment of Patient Acuity Systems at the Morgan Stanley Children's Hospital

Capstone proposals submitted for consideration are carefully vetted by course faculty. The vetting process seeks to ensure that the problems and client organizations are appropriate to the academic and competency-based objectives of the particular Capstone section, and also that the client understands the Capstone process and timeline. The client must be agreeable to further refinement of problem definition and scope as necessary and must commit to designate specific personnel to serve as project liaisons to students and faculty throughout the academic year. Client Capstone proposals determined to be appropriate to the course are presented to students by the client in the first Capstone session of the academic year.

Student Teams

After the client presentations, students rank the projects, one through four, based on their preference for the client/project, and they justify their rankings based on academic interest, professional experience, and personal preference (e.g., team partners). Student rankings and justifications serve as the basis from which faculty then selects the client organizations best suited to the student cohort and most closely matched with student preferences.

Initial Client Conference

Immediately after the Capstone teams are formed, meetings are arranged with each of the project sponsors. The initial meeting formally brings together student team members and faculty with the client liaisons and seeks to clarify the project's scope and the client's expectations. During this meeting, the team members strive to better understand what internal or external factors make the project important at the time, what key questions the client wants answered, how the client will determine project success, what obstacles the team can expect to encounter, and who the key organizational stakeholders in the outcome of the project are. The team members and client should reach agreement about the process for and frequency of ongoing team–client communication; the persons/parties inside and outside the organization that the team might need to engage; how the client wishes to facilitate that communication; and how access to organizational data, reports, records, and other materials will be managed.

Phase 2: The Contract and the Work Plan

The Capstone process now enters Phase 2: the development of a team–client contract. This phase is generally accomplished within four to six weeks, during which time the team works with the client to better define and clarify the project scope and objectives and to design a methodological approach to gathering evidence from a variety of sources to answer the client's questions.

Objectives and Methodological Approach

The agreed-upon methodology takes the form of a written and signed agreement—the contract—between the team and the client. The contract defines the elements of a working partnership, and it describes mutual expectations, deliverables, and what constitutes a successful and completed project.

The contract includes the following components:

- *Background description and summary*—the problem the client organization wishes the team to address
- *Project objectives*—an articulation by the team of the specific and "researchable" questions to be probed and answered
- *Methodology*—the process the team will follow to gather scientific, organizational, experiential, and stakeholder evidence to reach credible conclusions and rational recommendations to remedy the situation identified by the client
- *Assumptions*—individual and shared responsibilities of the client and the team
- *Communication*—expectations for the methods and frequency of team–client communication
- *Deliverables*—a description of the reports, surveys, presentations, and other items that the team will provide to the client at the conclusion of the engagement
- *Phases*—a description of the project phases, with a timeline and milestones

The Researchable Question(s)

At this point in the process, considerable emphasis is placed on asking the right questions in the right way. People who have taught Capstone at NYU Wagner have generally found that clients submitting proposals are able to recognize, and can to some degree articulate, the managerial problems or decision challenges they face. They are less good, however, at framing a problem as a question (or questions) for which evidence can be systematically gathered and actionable and measurable recommendations put forward.

Consider the following example: A 2014 proposal from NY-P's director of nursing informatics wanted a Capstone team to examine what prevents RNs from devoting an additional 15 minutes each day to uninterrupted, face-to-face conversation with hospitalized patients. The problem was stated by the client in this manner:

> Registered nurses in the inpatient, acute care setting are faced with a myriad of tasks and responsibilities, many of which do not directly involve the patient.

Research shows that increased time by the nurse at the patient bedside results in better quality outcomes and increased satisfaction (both patient and nurse). This Capstone will analyze how nurses spend time on a shift and identify opportunities for increasing time at the patient bedside.

The client identified an important problem: Nurses are burdened with a multitude of tasks that are essential but that appear to take them away from spending time at the bedside with patients. In addressing this problem, the Capstone team carefully considered the precise questions the client sought to answer and the ways the team might gather evidence to provide effective answers and actionable recommendations. The Capstone team reframed the problem in the written contract as follows (NYU Wagner 2014):

Project goals:
- Assess the current state of . . . lack of uninterrupted time spent [by RNs] at the bedside through surveys, focus groups, and interviews.
- Refine data collected to determine the top three commonly reported limitations.
- Present research-based recommendations, strategies, best practices, processes, and models for increasing uninterrupted nurse time at the patient's bedside.

Questions to be answered:
- What do RNs . . . believe limits their uninterrupted time spent with patients at the bedside? (surveys and focus groups)
- What does literature show to be the common barriers preventing uninterrupted time spent with patients at the bedside?

Tasks to be accomplished:
- Analyze the current limitations to uninterrupted nursing time spent with patients at the bedside.
- Analyze nurse perceptions regarding limitations to uninterrupted time spent with patients at the bedside.
- Analyze perceptions of patient care directors regarding nurses' uninterrupted time at the bedside.
- Analyze current evidence-based best practices regarding uninterrupted time spent with patients at the bedside.

In addition to the contract, the team developed an internal work plan that further described the following:

- A detailed timeline and list of project milestones
- Assignment of team member responsibilities for each component of the project
- A critical path diagram that specified and sequenced activities

Phase 3: Project Implementation

The teams now begin the real work of Capstone—Phase 3, devoted to executing the contract. To convince the client that the final recommendations have a high likelihood of attaining the desired outcomes, Capstone teams follow a structured evidence-gathering and decision-making process. The process, as described by Barends, Rousseau, and Briner (2014), emphasizes the systematic gathering of the "best available" evidence, drawn from multiple sources. The sources include findings from published and peer-reviewed scientific research; findings from non-peer-reviewed reports of successful organizational practice; facts, figures, and other data gathered from within the organization; the professional experience and judgment of internal and external practitioners; and the values and concerns of people who will be affected by the recommended action. Capstone teams follow Barends' six-step process (Barends, Rousseau, and Briner 2014):

- *Ask.* Translate the issue or problem into an answerable question.
- *Acquire.* Systematically search for and retrieve relevant evidence.
- *Appraise.* Critically judge the trustworthiness and relevance of the evidence gathered.
- *Aggregate.* Assemble and weigh the evidence.
- *Apply.* Incorporate the evidence into recommendations for action.
- *Assess.* Propose measures for evaluating the outcome of recommended action.

During the *ask* and *acquire* steps, students are provided in-depth instruction from guest faculty who have expertise in focused and evidence-based literature searches. Students also receive training in methods by which the quality of evidence gathered can be appraised, assembled, and weighed. Details of the instruction are provided by Susan Kaplan Jacobs in chapter 5 of this book.

The training emphasizes the importance of gathering evidence from multiple sources: scientifically acquired and validated facts, best practices at comparable organizations, opinions, surveys, and internal reports and data sources. It makes clear that effective management decision making most often requires that decisions be made based on incomplete evidence; however, it also stresses that adhering to a process based on a systematic evidence-based evaluation of management choices increases the likelihood of selecting options with high probability of a favorable outcome.

Because acquiring evidence often takes the form of gathering important knowledge from less quantitative sources, students also learn from guest faculty with expertise in gathering qualitative data. Students receive instruction and ongoing consultation on methods to design and carry out interviews, surveys, and focus groups and to evaluate the quality, relevance, and applicability of information obtained from such sources. The sources of this information may be internal to the client organization (e.g., staff, managers, patients) or external (e.g., thought leaders, community stakeholders, staff at comparable organizations).

The implementation stage requires great commitment by students and faculty outside the classroom setting. Though Capstone teams meet weekly with course faculty during the fall and spring semesters, they also meet at least one additional time each week, sometimes face to face and often using virtual media. They discuss work plan progress; distribute individual and group task assignments; and try to reach agreement on findings, conclusions, and recommendations. The teams are strongly encouraged to keep their client engaged throughout the process; a formal report of team progress is provided to the client no less than two times each month.

Phases 4 and 5: Project Deliverables

Capstone teams now enter the final phases, which focus on the preparation and presentation of findings, conclusions, and recommendations. Success in this effort requires that the teams carefully examine the evidence that has been acquired (appraise) and assemble and present it in a manner that reflects the source, validity, reliability, and organizational applicability of each finding (aggregate). Conclusions and recommendations then follow from the findings (apply, assess). How do the findings serve to answer the agreed-upon question(s)? What actions, supported by the evidence and examples provided, should the organization undertake, and what metrics should be enacted to measure the degree to which organizational objectives are achieved?

The Capstone team delivers an in-person oral presentation of the work to the client, covering the team's most important findings, conclusions, and recommendations. A formal, written report discusses findings, conclusions, and recommendations more extensively and provides a full description of the methodological steps taken to acquire the evidence to support the recommendations. Final Capstone reports generally adhere to the following outline:

- Table of contents
- Executive summary
- Introduction

- Methodology
- Findings
- Conclusions
- Recommendations
- Acknowledgments
- References
- Appendixes

In this phase, students receive formal instruction in making an effective business presentation and writing a management consulting report. In advance of delivering the final presentation, teams rehearse their presentation in class with faculty and student peers, who provide critical but constructive feedback. The final written report that is given to the client must also be submitted for multiple reviews and critique by faculty.

The final grade assigned to each student in Capstone is based on the degree to which the presentation and final report meet the requirements of the agreed-upon deliverables. Grading criteria include the extent to which evidence has been gathered and used to persuasively support findings, conclusions, and recommendations. Feedback from the client is incorporated, and students have the opportunity to provide input about their own contributions to the final product, as well as the contributions of their peers. The Capstone team receives an overall grade based on the degree to which the final work represents a professional management consultant document clearly delineating the problem faced by the organization, the steps taken by the team to address the problem, and recommendations. Findings and recommendations must be comprehensively stated and supported by relevant evidence. The grade of any individual student may be adjusted downward from the overall team grade if sufficient evidence indicates a lack of commitment, engagement, and contribution to the team.

Lessons Learned / Next Steps

Feedback from EMPA Nurse Leader students who have completed Capstone has been consistently and remarkably positive throughout the program's ten-year history. Students have especially appreciated the up-front commitment of clients, as demonstrated by the in-person meetings to discuss proposals/problems; the time and effort devoted in Phase 2 to carefully defining the project scope, objectives, and questions; and the instruction provided in Phase 3 and Phase 4 about effectively conducting literature searches and collecting, assembling, and interpreting data (quantitative and qualitative).

Students comment favorably about faculty's availability for consultation throughout the process, coaching on presentation skills, and guidance in the preparation of business-style consulting reports (as opposed to academic analyses). Finally, students speak positively about the experience of working in teams and the skills they acquire through sequencing tasks to be completed, reaching consensus, identifying and resolving conflict, and becoming more effective team members.

Students also mention elements of Capstone that can be improved. Some have found that clients do not always remain consistently engaged in the process from beginning to end. Client engagement thus needs to be more vigorously emphasized by course faculty and project sponsors. Also lacking is a comprehensive approach to following up on completed Capstone projects. To what extent are the recommendations from Capstone teams implemented? Are there measurable improvements in performance as a result of Capstone? Can faculty and NY-P leadership do a better job of educating prospective clients (both at NY-P and at other healthcare institutions) about the benefits of Capstone, describing the elements of a successful Capstone engagement, and encouraging managers to submit prospective projects well in advance of the start of the academic year?

Opportunities for strategic program expansion must also be considered. Should the EMPA Nurse Leader program be expanded to include physicians, allied health professionals, and experienced nonclinical middle managers? Should an online component of the program be integrated into the curriculum? How would each of these ideas affect the current structure of Capstone?

Acknowledgments

I would like to acknowledge with gratitude the contributions to this chapter from two of my colleagues, Professor Anthony Kovner and Professor Sarah Gurwitz.

Tony has inspired me and challenged me throughout my career—as my professor, my mentor, and more recently my colleague. His enormous knowledge of and insight about management and the US healthcare system have made me a better executive. His passion for sharing knowledge inspired me to teach and makes me a better teacher.

Sarah is always willing to share ideas, insights, and knowledge about what makes a successful Capstone engagement—knowledge she acquired over the course of an extensive career as a human resources manager, healthcare consultant, and teacher of the Capstone course at NYU Wagner. Sarah also designed the framework for depicting "A Year of Capstone" in exhibit 15.1.

References

Barends, E., D. M. Rousseau, and R. B. Briner. 2014. *Evidence-Based Management: The Basic Principles.* Center for Evidence-Based Management. Accessed June 9, 2016. www.cebma.org/wp-content/uploads/Evidence-Based-Practice-The-Basic-Principles.pdf.

Kovner, A. R. 2012. "Adventures in the Evidence-Based Management Trade." In *The Oxford Handbook of Evidence-Based Management,* edited by D. M. Rousseau, 183–90. New York: Oxford University Press.

———. 2010. "Teaching a Capstone Course: Using Evidence-Based Management." *Journal of Health Administration Education* 27 (1): 55–62.

New York University Robert F. Wagner Graduate School of Public Service (NYU Wagner). 2016a. "Capstone Program." Accessed May 3. http://wagner.nyu.edu/capstone.

———. 2016b. "EMPA for Nurse Leaders." Accessed May 3. http://wagner.nyu.edu/executivempa/nurseleaders.

———. 2014. "Improving Registered Nurse Time at the Bedside." Capstone team–client contract, November.

Schachter, D. R., and D. Schwartz. 2009. "The Value of Capstone Projects to Participating Clients." *Journal of Public Affairs Education* 15 (4): 445–61.

16

THE CONSULTING APPROACH AS AN APPLICATION OF EVIDENCE-BASED MANAGEMENT: ONE FIRM'S EXPERIENCE

by Kim Carlin

What does evidence-based management (EBMgmt) have to do with management consulting services in healthcare? The answer lies in the similarities between the two approaches in improving performance. Evidence-based management is a process of making decisions about management interventions using the best evidence available. Management consulting is based on assisting healthcare organizations to improve the performance of their assets using the best information available to them. The goals are similar: to improve performance and thus generate positive results. In addition, both evidence-based management and management consulting use a similar process of idea generation and outcome implementation. Both start by asking a research question, obtaining and weighing evidence, deciding on interventions, and sustaining the improved results.

The purpose of this chapter will be to provide background about the role of management consultants in healthcare and how their process and methodology align with evidence-based management. For the purpose of illustration, I will outline work we have done at Carpedia Healthcare Ltd., a division of Carpedia International Ltd., a tactical consulting resource based in Oakville, Ontario, and New York City. I will review the ways consultants contribute to the healthcare field and the value they provide for the generation of evidence and use of evidence-based practice. The chapter will review the steps of a typical consulting engagement and explore the common issues identified through engagements. It will also examine the approach we have taken at Carpedia to address these issues and create sustainable value for healthcare clients.

Why Healthcare Clients Use Consultants

Clients can use consultants for a variety of purposes: to fix a known operating problem; to address a business challenge resulting from an unknown problem; to provide unique skills as an extension of the management team; or to act as a trusted adviser, with knowledge built from experience tackling a variety of issues with other clients.

In our experience, our client partners have no shortage of good ideas. However, synthesizing these ideas, generating the evidence to evaluate these ideas, and getting people to work across functions to implement these ideas are time-consuming and difficult. Managers who are extremely busy running their departments often lack the time and resources to carry out these tasks in an efficient manner. Management consultants can help by harnessing good ideas and organizing them through a continuous improvement methodology, ultimately implementing method changes to create sustainable value. We are often asked in our sales process, "Why should I use a consultant when I have a series of highly paid managers here?" We have a number of answers to that question.

First, in most cases, our client's managers are extremely busy running their business. Operating problems may be known to exist, but the organization's leaders simply do not have the time and human capital bandwidth to address the problems in a timely and efficient manner. An outside consulting resource, on the other hand, can devote 100 percent of its attention to addressing the operating problems. We are free from the business distractions that tend to preoccupy managers and take them away from continuous improvement processes. As a result, we can help accelerate time lines and maximize benefits. A typical consulting engagement requires approximately 2,500 hours to identify, quantify, communicate, train, install, and sustain change. Our clients' managers simply do not have these additional hours available in their schedules. Consultants allow clients to engage in continuous improvement while continuing to operate their departments, providing them with the information, tools, and training to move their business forward.

A second advantage to using consultants is that outside advisers bring with them a sense of objectivity. Clients may perceive that they have operating problems, but an impartial external viewpoint can point out the specific root causes. As external parties, we are free from bias and the "sacred cows" that persist in most organizations. Consultants bring a perspective of objectivity because they are not driven by the organizational politics, promotions, and internal personal relationships that so often influence decision making.

Client resources today are stretched more than ever before. With labor budgets under constant pressure, many clients are unable to finance the ongoing skill set of continuous improvement. As such, a third advantage of using consultants is that we bring a short-term infusion of a particular skill set or expertise to address a particular issue at a lower long-term investment. Consultants tend to be formally educated, often with master of business administration degrees or experience in industrial engineering. Such individuals provide a balance of theoretical and experiential knowledge that can work in tandem with the functional expertise of the client management team to maximize benefits.

Finally, the very nature of consulting work means that we have considerable experience with a broad range of clients. This experience with numerous leaders across industries provides consultants with a wealth of evidence and research. When presented with a challenge, consultants are able to capitalize on insights and solutions from other clients because they have likely "seen it before." Though no two clients are alike, often experiences and problems that confront leaders in one organization can be cross-utilized in another business. In this way, a consultant can provide another organization with a fresh perspective and a new way of looking at recurring problems.

The type of management consulting done at Carpedia International Ltd. is general in nature, meaning we have experience across a variety of industries including healthcare, hospitality, financial services, and manufacturing. We do not claim to be experts in any one particular industry; however, through our operating divisions, such as Carpedia Healthcare Ltd., we have expertise in dealing with similar operating problems in specific industry concentrations. Our consultants have a wealth of common leadership practice knowledge that they bring to each engagement, and they can and do have their fingers on the pulse of current best-demonstrated practice. Multiple clients, cross-industry experience, and significant theoretical research all strengthen our capacity for scientific and practical evidence application.

Stages of a Carpedia Engagement

Carpedia International Ltd. is a mid-sized international consulting company that serves customers in various industries and sectors. A key differentiator of the Carpedia methodology is the implementation nature of the work that is done. We do not write reports for our clients to self-implement in our absence; instead, we physically work with clients to implement changes while on-site. The benefits of these implemented changes are measured directly on our client's financial statements and calculated against a required return on investment. Carpedia has done a number of large projects in healthcare, including work at the Yale New Haven Hospital, the Hospital for Special Surgery in New York City, and New York-Presbyterian Hospital, to name a few.

Establishing a new consulting partnership is a lengthy and complex process, often encompassing many years. Most Carpedia consulting projects go through four stages: (1) needs identification, (2) opportunity analysis, (3) project delivery, and (4) sustaining of results (Carpedia 2013).

Needs Identification

The first step in the process is to meet directly with the organization's top executives. The purpose is for the consultants to better understand the client's business, including key priorities and issues, and for the client and the consultants to determine whether they have a good organizational fit in terms of methodology, experience, and approach. The consultants look to develop an early hypothesis and a working research question that will guide how the consultants approach the client's issue. If a mutual fit seems to exist, Carpedia will provide more detailed information about how the consultants can help in the next stage—a comprehensive, two-week "opportunity analysis."

Opportunity Analysis

Carpedia conducts the on-site opportunity analysis to determine whether our methodology will provide tangible financial, quality, and service improvements to the client's operation. During this phase, we acquire the evidence to determine the nature and magnitude of the opportunity, as well as the opportunity's financial impact. We then develop a business case for working together with the client to recover a portion of that opportunity. During the analysis phase, we invest more than 400 hours interviewing, observing, and analyzing the business process, the management tools currently in place, and management's mind-set and behavior. We are able to provide a full operational assessment of the organization, which allows us to build a case for change and show the magnitude of the opportunity. Based on the evidence collected, we prepare a detailed proposal and financial business case for the client.

The financial business case for any one of our projects is based on a detailed evaluation of the client's own data—in particular, their historical financial and operating information. Following the analysis process, we define a percentage of "recapturable" opportunity based on our observations and analysis, which is then correlated to a financial indicator (e.g., cost recapture, revenue improvements, capital improvements). This percentage is then applied to the financial statements to determine the financial benefit of the engagement.

The project approach or project plan is built up independently, with a detailed summary of tasks and a defined schedule. This information allows us to determine the magnitude of work effort and the time required on-site, along with the associated consulting and travel costs. The client receives a summary of the project's financial requirements and investments, along with a detailed project cash flow based on a pro forma income statement. The client is then in a position to make a decision about whether to move forward with the project. Exhibit 16.1 presents a sample projection for a typical project.

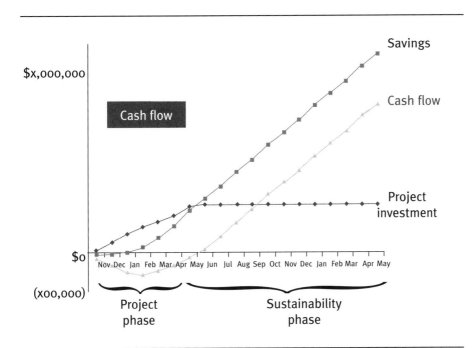

EXHIBIT 16.1
A Typical Carpedia Project Cash Flow Projection

Project Delivery

The delivery phase generally occurs over a four- to six-month time horizon and begins by working with our clients to refine the current state and identify recurring operating problems and the resulting performance gaps. From this baseline, we help develop new processes, management tools, and methods that result in the desired improvements that we defined in the analysis. We prototype and simulate these changes to test how effective they will be, and we physically work with client managers to get all the changes installed and working. Together, we make any alignments or revisions necessary and then lock in the new way of doing things. The changes are understood and agreed upon by operating managers, and they become embedded in the DNA of the organization.

The key outputs from this phase are better methods, better tools, and stronger and more effective managers. Program outcomes contribute to a new set of metrics that managers understand and are held accountable to. These metrics inherently link to the financial requirements of the organization, and managers learn to understand how controlling variances in these metrics can produce positive financial outcomes.

Sustaining of Results

The sustainability phase can last from 12 to 24 months, depending on the extent of the changes and the stability of the workforce. This phase recognizes that familiar patterns of behavior are difficult to change and that people have a natural tendency to want to revert back to the way things used to work. Only through compliance to the new way of doing things and confidence gained from the resulting success will the new behaviors eventually become habits. Periodic reviews help ensure that the changes stick and provide guidance to managers as they move from pure compliance to understanding to, eventually, full ownership of the changes.

Why We Need Evidence-Based Management in Business—A Consultant's Experience

Organizations are complex, and the leaders who manage them sometimes face extreme demands. Over the course of our more than 600 successful engagements, we have found that most businesses—despite variances in products, markets, and processes—face similar operating problems, most often tied to breakdowns in operating processes, planning mechanisms, and management behaviors (Follows 2005). Under most improvement initiatives, managers tend to address only one of these three problem categories, failing to recognize the interconnectivity and mutual dependence among them. Sustainable performance improvement requires a methodology that integrates process, a management operating system, and organizational behavior to change the way managers act and think (Follows 2005).

Before beginning to harness this opportunity in the current operating world, leaders must first recognize their present performance levels in relation to maximum achievable performance. To demonstrate opportunity to our clients, we believe fundamentally in the process of observation (Carpedia 2002c). This method of data collection is a critical component of our consultants' evidence research. Not only does observing a process in real time allow us to collect fundamental data related to productivity, quality outcomes, and service levels; it also enables us to collect evidence regarding constraints or process impediments. We are able to correlate these findings with past observations and experiential learning to see trends and similarities. In this way, the observation process resembles the methods used in the collection of scientific research for evidence-based management.

The process of observation isn't about walking by and quickly checking in on an employee's day. Instead, consultants engaged in observation will closely job-shadow employees for half or full shifts. The exercise is not about individual performance but rather about how the employees being observed react within their processes. During this exercise, we take detailed notes about the activities individuals perform and categorize their time into one of two color codes, red or green. Green time is the productive part of a process; red time is the nonproductive time. The rough litmus test we use for red time is whether the time is devoted to "something a customer of a client's business is unwilling to pay for."

Green time typically takes up 50 to 60 percent of a process, and red time takes up 40 to 50 percent. Over the course of 500,000 hours of real-time observations at more than 600 businesses throughout North America, we have found this average of 50 percent utilization to be quite consistent regardless of business health, industry, or market segment (Follows 2005). In our evaluation of reasons for the lost time, we found that employees are busy reworking errors, searching for missing information, and trying to fix recurring problems.

Most managers are surprised to learn how much time falls into the red category. One of the reasons for this surprise is that people often equate productive time with effort, when in fact the two are not necessarily related (Follows 2005). Nonproductive time can take as much effort as productive time, or even more. Nonproductive time rarely means the person is not busy; often the employee is working incredibly hard, just not in the most effective or efficient manner.

That said, we are not suggesting that an employee's day should be 100 percent green, because recapturing all lost time is impossible. Some nonproductive time is actually required to allow flexibility in operations. Other factors can have an impact on the amount of nonproductive time—for instance, the degree to which processes are machine- versus people-driven, or differences between union or nonunion environments. Even so-called world-class processes generally have 10 to 15 percent red time related to real-life variability, which is natural in every process.

The Application of Evidence-Based Management Theory in the Carpedia Approach

Though our consultative method is not rooted directly in evidence-based management per se, tenets of the approach are woven within our consulting concepts and method. The key stages will be reviewed in this section.

The very nature of what we do in helping clients achieve sustainable financial improvement is based on harnessing good evidence. In most cases, evidence is developed through an introspective look at the organization. As mentioned previously, we have found that the issues our clients face typically fall into three broad categories: process-related problems, planning problems, and gaps in management mind-set and behavior. The following sections will describe common problems we see associated with each category, as well as the changes we typically put into place to solve those problems and improve productivity, service, or quality.

Process-Related Problems

A process, by definition, relates to the method or steps one employs to move an input, and then add value to it, to create some kind of output (Carpedia 2002d). Problems, breakdowns, and constraints will impede a process from optimal performance, meaning that efficiency is hampered by less-than-ideal and systemic handoffs throughout the process. In the most general terms, process problems can become apparent through observation of the process and through variability in the pace of outputs. Typical process-related problems that we encounter include the following:

- Too many touches, handoffs, and nonrequired steps
- Reworking of the process, whereby something is touched multiple times to fix an error or mistake
- Process variability, whereby different points or different people within the process do not follow the steps as defined, creating anomalies
- Workload imbalances, when work volume is assigned to employees in an uneven distribution (meaning some people or work areas are busier than others, or one process step is waiting on another, causing constraints and idle time)

Process Changes

To address a process problem, we introduce a process or method change. A process change refers to a modification or augmentation in how work is performed between the input and output (Carpedia 2002b). This change could involve fixing a piece of equipment that has created a work-around or eliminating a step that is deemed unnecessary. At times, a change may address a combination of work functions through the modification and restructuring of layouts or the adjustment of equipment speeds. Generally, the more concrete the changes are, the more sustainable the changes can become—reducing the likelihood of reverting back to the old methods (Follows 2014a).

Planning-Related Problems

The key to improved operating and financial performance and long-term sustainability is to address planning problems. In general, planning mechanisms tend to be complicated, often with gaps in standards and scheduling tools. These gaps create challenges for leaders aiming to evaluate performance in a proactive way. The planning mechanisms of any business are embedded in a management operating system, which we deem to be the most critical tool to provide visibility for leaders into area performance. The management operating system is an integrated control tool that translates the strategic plans of an organization into the specific activities and accountabilities required (Carpedia 2002a). It links operating activities to financial systems and allows management to proactively manage against the business plan. Typical planning-related problems include the following:

- Often, the financial and operating worlds tend to be poorly linked. In such cases, the financial requirements of the business are not translated into well-defined key performance indicators (KPIs) that are well understood throughout the organization.
- In many cases, volume forecasts lack accuracy, which prevents the operations groups from understanding what volume is required and what timing is expected to plan effectively.
- Performance planning tends to be inaccurate and outdated. Resource requirement plans (e.g., plans for people, equipment, material, capital) often have inaccurate work-to-time standards that are embedded with inherent lost time, making the effective scheduling of resources impossible.
- Scheduling tools are prone to inaccuracy. Schedules often include little more than work start and stop times, and they often lack volume and output requirements.
- At the point of execution, managers often lack the tools necessary for assigning work in a volume-to-time relationship. Furthermore, tools may fail to provide real-time performance information to leaders, which would provide leaders with insights into variances against plan.
- Many organizations are data rich and have access to information through a variety of queries and reports. However, we often find that we are measuring too many things, on too macro a scale. Most businesses are not focused on the "universal values" to the organization: cost, quality, and service.

Management System Changes

A carefully designed management system is the cornerstone of sustained process planning, control, and management variance resolution. Management system changes generally require tightening up the mechanisms that are used to plan, measure, and monitor the organization (Carpedia 2002a). Generally observable work-to-time standards are aligned with accurate volume forecasting to better schedule the business. Managers are then provided the tools to plan, monitor, and report on the attainment of the plan at the point of execution. The reporting elements of the management operating system provide a direct link between the short-interval operational metrics and the financial statements, and KPIs directly align to the universal values of cost, quality, and service. The management system is only as good as the numbers put into it, so the effectiveness of any system relies on the accuracy and integrity of the numbers (Carpedia 2002a). The management system is arguably the most important tool for leaders to use in measuring performance, holding onto improvement gains, and building upon them in the future.

Management Mind-Set and Behavior Problems

Sustained continuous improvement requires a change in leadership mind-set and behavior at all levels of the organization. Changes in management behavior represent the most critical aspect of ensuring long-term sustainability. Managers, like all of us, tend to repeat the same behaviors over and over again. Behaviors help form individual management styles and are the basis of familiar, comfortable work routines (Follows 2014b). These behaviors are developed over long periods of time, and they tend to become entrenched and difficult to change. Common problems in management behavior include the following:

- Most managers' time is spent troubleshooting and firefighting, rather than proactively gauging performance at the front line.
- Too little time is dedicated to resolving the root cause of problems; as a result, the problems continue to perpetuate.
- Based on our observations, managers spend very little time actively managing employees at the point of execution, even though they perceive that they spend upwards of 30 percent of their time actively managing their staff. A disconnect exists between management perception and reality.
- Managers generally do not have a good handle on the day-to-day variances that take them off schedule. Discussions regarding variances tend to be "high level" and generic, rather than focused on specific examples of operating issues at the point of execution.
- Without point-of-execution problem solving and variance resolution, problems become all-consuming and unmanageable.
- Operating problems persist because management time is consumed in reactionary mode (i.e., "putting out fires").

Management Mind-Set and Behavior Changes

Changing management behavior requires getting managers to actually act differently from the way they have acted in the past. It could involve setting clear daily expectations for staff, following up on planned work, actively listening to others, or giving useful feedback. Though these behaviors may seem basic, they are not always common practice (Follows 2014b). If managers do not perform such behaviors currently, they will have difficulty doing them in the future. Not only do such managers not know how to perform the behaviors; employees do not know how to respond to them (Follows 2014b).

Another aspect of changing management behavior is to modify the style of management that people use. We are strong believers in an active management style that is controlled, collaborative, and focused on results (Follows 2014b). We believe fundamentally that the role of manager is to remove the performance barriers that impede individual employee performance. Without actively following up with one's staff, a leader cannot possibly have visibility into lost time and work proactively to resolve it. An important distinction must be made, however, between active management and micromanagement. In active management, the intent is not to aggressively manage output but rather to understand variances and then work with the employee to resolve the root cause of the issue.

Modifying specific behaviors is easier to accomplish than modifying a person's management style. Behaviors usually develop as a person repeats an action over and over, and they can often be tweaked or adjusted. Management styles are more complicated, in that they tend to reflect both the social style of the individual and the culture of the organization (Follows 2014b). When a performance improvement project is under way, a heightened intensity surrounds the project, and managers are expected to change their patterns of behavior. When the project ends, however, a feeling of relief at all levels emerges, and some of the intensity naturally dissipates (Follows 2014b).

The simple truth is that operating at a higher level of performance is more difficult, and it requires more planning and more active management. The real responsibility for sustainability always falls on executive leadership, because the improvement effort needs continual reinforcement. Although most system and process changes directly affect frontline levels, frontline managers simply do not have sufficient authority to sustain the integrity of the changes.

The Process of Implementing Change Based on Evidence

The process of implementing change in an organization is highly structured to provide managers with the best available evidence related to process changes, management system changes, and behavior changes. Consultants by their very nature cannot implement anything in an organization themselves, so a project's success depends on the empowerment of leaders with the right evidence and information to make decisions. The five phases of the typical Carpedia project delivery, as interpreted from Follows (2005), are (1) target, (2) develop, (3) focus, (4) install, and (5) sustain. The phases align with the steps of an EBMgmt approach as described by Barends, Rousseau, and Briner (2014): (1) asking, (2) acquiring, (3) appraising, (4) aggregating, (5) applying, and (6) assessing.

Phase 1: Target

In the target phase, we begin to formulate the management problem into a research question. This phase starts with discovery and looks to frame the business problem as a tangible issue. The target phase aligns with the EBMgmt step of asking, whereby a practical issue is translated into an answerable research question (Barends, Rousseau, and Briner 2014).

We begin this phase by understanding the cost and revenue drivers affecting the business, and we visually depict these drivers in a simple financial model, called a profit driver model (PDM). The PDM helps us align revenue with the drivers of cost and their associated volumes, called *operational levers.* This exercise helps us see what key financial metrics drive operational performance, and it enables us to demonstrate to managers how operational levers can affect the cost base. At this point, we start determining what levers we need to affect in what quantities to improve performance.

The output of the PDM exercise is a measurement and evaluation system through which we will evaluate the project. The operational evaluation allows us to track results on a weekly basis that aligns to the client's financial statements. The key output in this phase is a document we call the *results strategy.* This document articulates the research question, states where specifically the results are going to come from, and explains how the results will be measured. The presentation and review of the results strategy allow both the client team and the consulting team to ensure that they are fully aligned toward the strategy of the project and the measurement methodology moving forward.

Phase 2: Develop

The second phase of any engagement is the period of method change development, and we begin the phase by acquiring evidence and analyzing the current state of the business. This segment of our project aligns with the second and third EBMgmt steps, acquiring and appraising (Barends, Rousseau, and Briner 2014).

Through interviews, data analysis, focus group process critique sessions, and observations, we identify recurring problems and determine the magnitude of opportunity. During this phase, process, system, and behavior changes are developed and evaluated by managers for validity and feasibility. The quality of the evidence presented is critically evaluated as method changes are proposed. The evidence generated can be organizational evidence, including financial and operating information from the client; experiential evidence, based on the professional experiences of our client managers, staff, and consultants; or stakeholder evidence, which takes into account the values and concerns of people affected by the decisions (Barends, Rousseau, and Briner 2014). At times, we may also draw upon evidence from published scientific research about a specific business issue, but most of our scientific research is self-generated through our observation and analysis processes. The outcomes of these studies are used as a research tool and compared with our past research from similar environments.

Phase 3: Focus

In the third phase, local area managers—not the consultants—present findings back to the top client decision makers in a *focus meeting*. They describe the current-state issues; the opportunity; and the process, system, and behavior changes they would implement to achieve the required financial benefits and to address the research question formulated in Phase 1. At this aggregating phase (Barends, Rousseau, and Briner 2014), the client managers and consultants have weighed and pulled together the available evidence to develop method changes and to present implementation plans. The focus meeting often serves as a turning point for a project: The managers take ownership of the results, and specific roles and requirements of employees and managers in the change process are defined.

Phase 4: Install

The evidence that has been gathered, assessed, and presented is now applied during the fourth phase, the installation stage—the point at which process, system, and behavior changes are physically put into practice. This phase most closely matches with EBMgmt's applying phase, in which evidence is incorporated to make decisions (Barends, Rousseau, and Briner 2014).

The install phase generally consists of a number of key steps and stages over many weeks. The early stages include a significant amount of testing, or *prototyping*, to mitigate risk. Trial runs of method changes allow us to test the feasibility of the changes in a safe and controlled manner to gauge how the management team will react. Following the testing, managers will begin the process of actually implementing new methods, processes, procedures, tools, and behaviors. Effective implementation requires careful attention to the coaching and training of new tools and techniques. Changes in each area must reinforce the financial benefits that have been defined. The outcome of the implementation phase corresponds with EBMgmt's assessing phase, whereby the results of the decision outcomes are measured (Barends, Rousseau, and Briner 2014). This activity will continue in perpetuity through the sustain phase.

Phase 5: Sustain

Sustainability is the most critical phase of any engagement, and it challenges the stability of the method changes as the business moves forward from the routine of the project. The phase can last for 6 to 12 months and often beyond, depending on the organization. During this phase, we recognize people's natural tendency to want to revert back to the old way of doing things; however, we must continue to support the behavior changes and use of the management system to tackle business variances. This phase is the most volatile period of the project, because familiar patterns and bad habits threaten to creep back into processes. During this phase, the consulting team supports formalized reviews, and longer-term auditing ensures that the changes are solidified and that managers are compliant to the new tools and behaviors.

We help our client organizations incorporate continuous improvement and the control of process variances as key elements of their routine business operations. Through the steps outlined here, we ensure that the concepts of evidence-based practice become embedded within the organization to support further improvement.

Case Example

Perioperative Services, Nursing Productivity, and Patient Flow at a Canadian-Based Academic Medical Center

The Challenge

As a Canadian-based academic medical center, our client is accountable to provincial taxpayers who expect their tax dollars to be spent appropriately. In recent years, perioperative expenditure at the center has grown exponentially, as case volumes and patient acuity have increased. Approximately 30,000 surgical cases are performed per year. With decreasing budgets and capacity constraints, our client needed solutions quickly to manage the cost of surgical care.

The medical center engaged Carpedia to assist with improvements to nursing and support staff productivity, patient flow, and patient service. The project scope included two hospital sites within close proximity, comprising 31 operating room (OR) theaters, 12 tertiary surgical service suites, and 4 litho rooms. Both hospital sites have preadmission clinics, sterile processing departments, postanesthetic care units (PACUs), and sterile supply departments.

Applying Evidence-Based Management

Formulating the Research Question

Within the confines of the current operating model, capacity was constrained. Sixty-five percent of patients were past their recommended date for surgery, and leadership was concerned that the health of the population would suffer if the center did not find a way to deliver services more efficiently. A working research question was developed: *What is the current level of operating room utilization, how well are surgical blocks utilized, how standard is case duration, and what is affecting patient throughput?*

Acquiring the Evidence

Carpedia was invited to conduct a two-week opportunity analysis, during which we generated a preliminary overview of the opportunity and developed a project plan and financial cash flow objectives. Based on the outcome of that exercise, Carpedia was further engaged to conduct a consulting project over 20 calendar weeks. To acquire the evidence and make a case for change, a number of key activities took place over the life of the project.

First, we set up interviews with the chief operating officer (COO), the director of perioperative services, OR managers, and physician stakeholders who formed part of an OR executive committee. Management and employees showed strong support for continuous improvement; however, current benchmarking reporting and performance KPIs were hiding some opportunities to improve, and many people felt they were operating at high performance levels already. We quickly realized that the tools were not adequate to provide real-time, accurate reporting and that considerable variability existed in the definitions of key terms (e.g., *start time, procedure duration*). As a result, not all parties were measuring performance in the same way.

Hundreds of hours of point-of-execution observation in the operating rooms demonstrated that nursing and staff labor productivity varied between 45 and 60 percent. Staffing levels did not align with operational and procedural requirements, and schedules did not take current OR procedural times into account. Virtually no cases ever started on time, and 10 percent of cases were being cancelled or rescheduled because of end-of-day constraints.

Assessing the surgical block schedules, we found that planning standards and case durations were largely outdated and were not relied upon for scheduling decisions. Scheduling was based on gut feel and historical past practice. Case duration standards were measured differently by different employees and did not consider the unique variances between cases. Simple benchmarking was used, but it was largely ineffective, with no complexity indexing by case or between surgeons.

Observations with OR supervisors identified an absence of active management. Managers lacked the tools necessary to follow up on the schedule within the day at the point of execution. Leadership behaviors were highly reactionary.

Assessing the Validity, Quality, and Applicability of the Evidence

The academic medical center has a long history of collaboration between administrators and medical staff, and it had a highly engaged OR executive committee that consisted of the COO, the director of perioperative services, surgical chiefs, and a representative from corporate procurement. This group came together to form a steering committee for the consulting project.

As part of the method change development process, each change was assessed for validity, quality, and applicability using evidence collected through data analysis or observation. We developed method changes in tandem with the OR supervisory and management team, and the OR executive committee reviewed and signed off on them. Prior to finalization, each method change was prototype-tested to ensure that all risk mitigation strategies had been dealt with in a safe environment. The OR executive committee then reviewed the output off all prototyped method changes and verified all final implementation plans to ensure that stakeholder concerns were addressed.

Presenting the Evidence

The final method changes were presented over a three-hour focus meeting. At the meeting, the director of perioperative services and various department supervisors reviewed the changes, their impact, and their value and worked to achieve consensus from the entire OR executive steering committee. Following the focus meeting, all parties agreed that the changes represented the "go forward" plan for the implementation portion of the project.

Applying the Evidence

The following are some of the key changes implemented based on the evidence collected:

- Streamlined and redesigned intershift reporting
- Adjustment to staffing levels and hours of operation for admissions to reduce morning bottlenecks
- Electronic transfer of chart documentation from physicians' offices
- A new process for clinical review of chart readiness
- Elimination of staff rotations and the chart prep desk to create consistency
- Defined time and performance standards for room turnover cleaning
- Creation of the room turnover facilitator role to expedite the entry of patients into the OR
- Standardization of the PACU handoff by the anesthetist to reduce wait times
- Updated preference cards to minimize material and equipment shortages
- Improved scheduling rules and controls to reduce volatility in surgical blocks
- Daily operating reports and weekly management reports with key metrics and a formal variance review process

Evaluating the Results

After implementing more than 60 unique process changes and providing hands-on support to managers and charge nurses for several months, all key operational indicators improved from their baseline values. Targeted improvements included the following:

- 75 percent reduction in OR/PACU holds
- 75 percent reduction in controllable case cancellation (i.e., cancellations from hospital resource issues, such as instrumentation, staffing, bed availability, and so on)
- 50 percent improvement in OR turnaround times, resulting in improved access to care and effective use of resources
- 72 percent improvement in OR start-up times
- Modifications to the staffing and organizational structure to optimize the skills of the staff, ensuring that the right care providers are performing the right tasks
- Standardization of instrumentation across sites and procedures
- Identification of data sets (metrics) to manage the perioperative environment

- Improved surgical experience for the patient, as noted in patient satisfaction scores and reduced wait times

The project focus was designed to balance the diverse aspirations of the key stakeholders in a perioperative environment, including the administrative, clinical, and medical staff. Significant initiatives satisfied each of these groups' collective objectives. A key win for the surgical staff was the alleviation of bottlenecks in the PACU, which had delayed surgical cases and often led to cancellations. In a win for the nursing staff, case turnovers were compressed, which contributed favorably to timely case starts.

A variety of factors go into a successful engagement, and this case shares many positive characteristics that can apply broadly to any academic medical center. Such factors include the following:

- *Broad engagement and participation at all levels of the organization.* For positive changes to occur, buy-in must occur throughout the organization, from the front line to the executive offices. Managers internalized the improvement potential and promoted the changes in their work areas. The OR executive steering committee remained engaged, supported the results, and advanced the interests of a complex group of stakeholders.
- *A focus on quality, patient satisfaction, employee engagement, and profitability.* Key metrics were developed to tie real-time reporting to the KPIs that capture improvements, to aid with focus and accountability.
- *Attention to implementation.* Recommendations alone do little to help the organization; changes must be implemented, not just talked about. The engagement started and continued with an implementation mind-set and accountability.
- *Sustained results.* The organization must be able to sustain the results and continue to improvement. By developing and empowering management skill and by providing access to integrated tools, the engagement helped frontline leaders drive sustainable results and continue to track favorably to the project requirements.

Conclusion

Though no two consulting engagements are alike, many organizations possess distinct similarities. These similarities have allowed us to develop a structured and systematic methodology aimed at harnessing the best available evidence to empower leaders to address issues of process, system, and management behavior in a constructive way. Through the training received during our engagement and the ongoing proliferation of new tools, leaders are better positioned to tackle operating challenges and ultimately continue the cycle of continuous improvement.

But if evidence-based management and Carpedia's application of it are so good, then why aren't prospective clients buying more of it? And why isn't this methodology revolutionizing business school teachings? The simple answer is that, even with solid returns and sustainable value, misconceptions continue to create objections to our service offerings and barriers to the sales process. These barriers closely correlate with the ones noted by Barends, Rousseau, and Briner (2014) regarding the universal uptake of evidence-based management.

The first objection is that consulting based on evidence-based management ignores the practitioner's own experience (Barends, Rousseau, and Briner 2014). This misconception directly contradicts the definition of evidence-based management, which incorporates a combination of evidence types, including experiential. Similarly, the fear that consultants will somehow disregard managers' expertise is completely unfounded. The role of consultants is to harness the best ideas from both the organization and their own experience. These ideas are vetted, challenged, and, eventually, fully agreed to by the client management team. The experiential knowledge of the leadership team is the most valuable asset we use in an engagement.

Another common objection is based on the misconception that evidence-based management is only about the numbers (Barends, Rousseau, and Briner 2014). In reality, neither evidence-based management nor a consulting engagement requires a manager to become a statistician. Though we enforce accountability through the use of metrics, we work with our clients to ensure that leaders have thorough training and full understanding of the key metrics and analytics being used. For us, the emphasis is not so much on the generation and manipulation of the numbers; it is on the need for decisions to be made in relation to what the numbers are telling you.

A third common misconception is based on the idea that managers must make decisions quickly and therefore don't have time for evidence-based practice (Barends, Rousseau, and Briner 2014). We acknowledge that managers make many decisions, some in quick succession and others over longer time horizons; however, the magnitude of this decision making is precisely the reason that managers should step back, evaluate available evidence, and weigh alternatives. With a solid continuous improvement methodology in place, supported by the key metrics and performance indicators of the management operating system, managers now more than ever can use good and trustworthy evidence to make decisions.

A final objection involves the idea that the uniqueness of each organization limits the usefulness of evidence from other organizations (Barends, Rousseau, and Briner 2014). One of the most common things we hear from our clients is how unique their business is and how difficult it will be for us to comprehend it. And while, yes, many businesses are unique, the problems they face share marked similarities, and the businesses can benefit from consultants' experience in having seen similar issues before. Consultants by their very nature provide this kind of "been there, seen that" experience, which managers often lack when embedded within their own organization. Evidence-based management is flexible enough to take similar yet different qualities into account (Barends, Rousseau, and Briner 2014).

Future research and application should continue to address these misconceptions and promote the benefits of critical appraisal—particularly the use of the best available evidence to make the most informed and scientifically advanced decisions possible. Though little academic literature has been written on the topic, the consulting industry will continue to benefit from a deeper understanding and a broader acceptance of EBMgmt principles and their applications for continuous improvement.

References

Barends, E., D. M. Rousseau, and R. B. Briner. 2014. *Evidence-Based Management: The Basic Principles.* Center for Evidence-Based Management. Accessed June 9, 2016. www.cebma.org/wp-content/uploads/Evidence-Based-Practice -The-Basic-Principles.pdf.

Carpedia. 2013. *Carpedia Overview.* Oakville, Canada: Carpedia International Ltd.

———. 2002a. *Management Action Plan: Management System and Critique.* Oakville, Canada: Carpedia International Ltd.

———. 2002b. *Management Action Plan: Method Changes.* Oakville, Canada: Carpedia International Ltd.

———. 2002c. *Management Action Plan: Observations.* Oakville, Canada: Carpedia International Ltd.

———. 2002d. *Management Action Plan: Process Flow and Critique.* Oakville, Canada: Carpedia International Ltd.

Follows, P. 2014a. "The Red Flags of Process Changes." Carpedia International Ltd. Published September. http://blog.carpedia.com/bid/90966/The -red-flags-of-process-changes.

————. 2014b. "What Does Changing Management Behavior Really Mean?" Carpedia International Ltd. Published December. http://blog.carpedia.com /bid/90978/What-does-changing-management-behavior-really-mean.

————. 2005. *Managing Profits at the Front Line.* Oakville, Canada: Carpedia International Ltd.

V

EXPERIENTIAL EVIDENCE

17

EXPERIENCE OF A HOSPITAL MANAGER

by Lynn McVey and Eric Slotsve

Introduction

I (Lynn) was a 26-year-old radiographer with a new baccalaureate degree when a large inner-city medical center in New Jersey hired me as a radiology quality manager. My introduction into management began rather blindly. I received no job description, training, orientation, or mentoring of any sort, and I had no idea where to start or what to do. All I had was advice from my father, telling me to start counting everything that could be counted—unbeknownst to me at the time, that is exactly how I started developing evidence-based management (EBMgmt) practices.

I captured all the metrics in the radiology department every month, looking for anything that I could analyze and spot as a trend. At the end of the year, I would find the median of the prior 12 months and calculate a 10 percent improvement benchmark for my upcoming year. Like a marathon runner, my goal was to always best myself. This humble early model was so incredibly powerful that I followed it for the next 20 years at nine radiology departments. I also worked for consulting firms, where I would compare my benchmarks to other radiology department metrics to quickly locate their weak points.

After I entered graduate school, I learned that my management style had a name—*evidence-based management*—and a body of literature supporting its theory. I devoured the works of Eric Barends, Denise Rousseau, Anthony Kovner, Rob Briner, Jeffrey Pfeffer, and Robert Sutton, just to name a few. These scholars furthered my passion for evidence-based management, and I was fortunate to be able to teach and implement these theories as chief operating officer at my hospital. At this point, I accept nothing less.

Moving from Old to New Management

Under traditional management, decisions are based on professional experience, personal education (no matter how outdated), and the emotions and biases carried by managers. This management style was adequate in an "assured payment" industry, which is what Medicare originally created in 1965 by reimbursing charges at 80 percent. For many years, every hospital claimed to be "unique," healthcare claimed to be "local," and healthcare standards were evaded. "Silos" were everywhere. Hospitals, clinics, and doctor's offices all kept close tabs on their information, as did departments within a hospital or health network (Wicklund 2014).

This secrecy of information has proved to be trivial, because Medicare-certified institutional providers are required to submit annual cost reports to a Medicare administrative contractor. The cost reports contain such information as facility characteristics, utilization data, cost and charges by cost centers (in total and for Medicare specifically), Medicare settlement data, staffing information, and financial statement data (CMS 2016). But as one might expect, the data that Medicare publishes are excessive and unwieldy; the data have therefore failed to provide a simple, macrocosmic set of expense, revenue, and productivity standards.

When I was a radiology manager, my expenses were $50 per exam, which I tracked monthly, and my revenues always exceeded $50. In addition, I publicly trended individual staff productivity data as a means of keeping an equitable workload. My goal each month was to exceed my prior month's performance. However, because I was trapped in my own silo, I had no idea whether $50 per exam was good or bad. Years later while conducting research, I captured similar data from hundreds of radiology managers, only to find extreme variations: The median cost of a radiology exam was $70, with highs and lows ranging from $30 to $130. Suddenly, my $50 seemed quite reasonable!

Hospital executives have used some of the metrics from the Centers for Medicare & Medicaid Services (CMS) data sets as their own management metrics. But with only this high-level set of comparative benchmarks, the metrics can only trigger across-the-board staffing adjustments—meaning that staffing reductions would be uniformly applied to all hospital departments, regardless of whether the departments are managed efficiently or inefficiently. For the efficiently managed departments, the cuts would have a negative impact on patient care.

When every hospital department manager uses a common set of measurements, we can make apples-to-apples comparisons. For example, salary expense per unit of service, nonsalary expense per unit of service, revenue per unit of service, and full-time equivalent (FTE) per unit of service can provide comparative benchmarks across all hospital departments. I captured these internal key performance indicators (KPIs) monthly for 30 years at multiple hospitals. Unfortunately, no other hospital managers were capturing the same data. To break out of our silos, hospital managers need to input this data into a national data warehouse to develop external comparative benchmarks for all departments in all hospitals.

Putting It All Together

In 2008, I had the great fortune of serving as the national president of the Professional Association of Medical Imaging Leaders (AHRA). In that role, I had the opportunity to test my internal KPIs against data submitted by hundreds of medical imaging managers. After I discovered extreme variations in imaging spending, I further compared my newly expanded data collection to Medicare's imaging spending data, accessed via the CMS website (www.cms.gov).

CMS has developed a collection of data that enables researchers and policymakers to evaluate geographic variation in the utilization and quality of healthcare services for the Medicare fee-for-service population. The data are aggregated into a geographic variation public-use file that has demographic, spending, utilization, and quality indicators at the state level (including the District of Columbia, Puerto Rico, and the Virgin Islands), the hospital referral region (HRR) level, and the county level.

In my research, the geographic variations revealed that the highest costs per beneficiary are in the ten states that also have the highest imaging costs per exam. Because the utilization of imaging for both the highest and lowest utilizers is less than 20 percent, one might suspect that these ten states are using high-tech imaging (e.g., magnetic resonance imaging, computed tomography, positron emission tomography) at a higher rate than less expensive, low-tech imaging. To the hospitals in question, this overutilization of services would seem surprising. Without access to metrics from comparable hospitals, how were they to know that they themselves were outliers? Fortunately, the Affordable Care Act includes provisions for transforming clinical practices—reflected in CMS's Transforming Clinical Practice Initiative (TCPI)—that will decrease unnecessary testing and treatments, reduce costs, and eventually create standards of care. The TCPI is Medicare's pathway to reach the Triple Aim of better care, better health, and lower costs (CMS 2015).

I was able to witness and address these kinds of variations first-hand at a newly purchased hospital within my health system. The failing hospital, which used traditional management, was losing $12 million per year, received a Leapfrog grade of C, and had a Hospital Consumer Assessment of Healthcare Providers and Systems (HCAHPS) overall ranking of 61.8. The sustainability of this hospital was certainly in question. The new ownership moved to replace traditional management with evidence-based management. After a year of evidence-based practices in all 40 hospital departments, the hospital posted an $8.4 million profit, received an A rating from Leapfrog, and saw a 4.1 percent increase in its HCAHPS ranking score. This exercise revealed practice variations similar to those found in the overutilization of medical imaging across the 50 states. Across 40 hospital departments, we found some expensive outliers, which we swiftly eliminated by standardizing the KPIs. We were able to compare apples to apples when we took these individual departments out of their silos.

We rolled out a rudimentary evidence-based program at the hospital, but its implementation was far from simple. For 30 years, traditional managers in this facility relied on making decisions based on their personal opinion, experience, education, and bias. Now they were being told that their personal opinion and professional experience were no longer the focus; instead, we would be measuring their management skills using internal and external benchmarks. One does not need to be a manager to appreciate how frightening this might be to people who have never used metrics in their operations. Without any prior baseline measurements for comparison, hospitals have not been able to analyze or rank their managers' performance; therefore, existing hospital managers have not been aware of whether they are high or low performers.

Under our system, all managers were required to capture ten data sets each month and input them into a data warehouse. A standard departmental dashboard is shown in exhibit 17.1. This practice created internal, dynamic operational KPI benchmarks. The data provided senior leadership with the ability to locate exactly where expensive variations existed, enabling leaders to eliminate or correct them.

Now, imagine that process on a national level. All 5,000 US hospitals would capture the same monthly data and input them into a data warehouse. Every hospital would have the information it needed to identify department outliers. Evidence-based management could give us the ability to find efficiencies that could potentially preserve failing hospitals. And who knows where the possibilities could go after that?

Standardized KPI data provide a means of comparing managers from all hospital departments. For example, when KPI data are transparent, the manager with the highest overtime is revealed. The ER manager whose expenses are increasing while volume is decreasing is revealed. The nurse manager using more FTEs than last year, despite lower admissions, is revealed. Merely identifying the metric that needs to be tracked can lead to vast improvements, described in a phenomenon called the Hawthorne effect. The Hawthorne effect refers to improvements that occur as a result of subjects' awareness of what is being watched, counted, or measured. Some of the low-hanging fruits for evidence-based management include departmental absenteeism and overtime rates. Every department manages absenteeism and overtime, so they are easy points to illustrate at management meetings.

The peer pressure that comes from transparent rankings is also an effective tool when dealing with group dynamics. After all, nobody wants to

	Year 1	Year 2
Salary expenses	$997,348	$677,908
Nonsalary expenses	$194,652	$150,565
Total expenses/costs	$1,192,008	**$803,379**
Gross charges	$25,758,108	$19,058,895
Collections (15%)	$2,574,827	$2,858,834
Profit/loss	$1,382,820	**$2,037,037**
Volume inpatient	37,320	27,478
Volume outpatient	4,688	4,129
Volume total	42,008	**31,607**
Supply per unit	$58.92	$58.40
Salary per unit	$286.68	$268.29
Cost per unit	$345.60	$316.96
Revenue per unit	$735.84	$755.59
Profit/loss per unit	$403.92	$438.63
Average overtime %	0.94%	0.7%

EXHIBIT 17.1
Standard Departmental Dashboard for the Respiratory Department

Note: The bolded numbers in Year 2 reflect improved efficiency: Even when volume decreased, profit increased.

look at a presentation on the big screen and discover that his department has the highest absenteeism or overtime rates. In most cases, immediate improvements are made after implementing evidence-based practices; exhibit 17.2 provides a sampling of such improvements. In one example, after reducing overtime from 18 percent to 9 percent in one payroll, a manager was congratulated and asked why she did not reduce this earlier. "Nobody ever asked me," she replied. This kind of statement—that the manager was unaware or never asked—is common in instances where major improvements are made quickly. This particular manager reduced her overtime to 4 percent by the second post-EBMgmt payroll.

Results Achieved

The most impressive results occur during the first year of converting from traditional management to standardized, evidence-based management. During this period, expensive variations are revealed and adjusted, and a standard dashboard is established and used throughout all hospital departments.

EXHIBIT 17.2
Examples of
Annual Expense
Variations
Before and After
Implementation
of Evidence-
Based
Management

Department	Before EBMgmt	After EBMgmt	% Change
Respiratory	$1,450,139	$761,435	47.5
Emergency	$2,314,560	$1,935,912	16.4
Laboratory	$2,911,790	$2,267,706	22.1
Facilities	$1,235,210	$1,067,881	13.5
Surgery	$11,838,833	$10,197,393	13.9
Radiology	$4,141,410	$3,048,924	26.4
Total	$23,891,942	$19,279,252	19.3

Looking at exhibits 17.1 and 17.2, we can see the significant results gained in the respiratory department from a single year of evidence-based management. The original respiratory manager was in his role for more than 20 years at the time the switch was introduced. When asked for improved efficiencies, he had repeatedly reported that none were available. The excessive layers of management and failure to charge inpatients for respiratory services were identified as potential dampers on the department's performance, but the traditional manager's reply was simply, "That's how it's always been." After we eliminated his position, the new manager quickly discovered several other expensive variations throughout, which resulted in a 47 percent annual increase to the bottom line after the appropriate adjustments were made—our highest improvement.

The Persisting Problem

Research literature has identified a gap in knowledge between clinical expertise and business skills. Douglas (2010) says that the call for deeper understanding of finance among clinical leaders has been long and loud and for good reason. Historically, hospitals have relied on the finance office to handle the business end, while the department managers handle the clinical end. Clearly this gap needs to be bridged.

We need to establish a process crosswalk between clinical and financial departments. When we only rely on finance employees to manage patient accounts, we assume that all appropriate tests and treatments have been properly charged. This approach is imperfect. For instance, it does not capture any missing or inaccurate charges because we have excluded the only person who knows what actual tests and treatments were done. One recommendation is to have the clinical manager review a daily activity report while the activity is still a fresh memory.

Hospitals have had a less-than-optimal approach to patient billing for many years, and the area needs attention, especially considering today's tough markets. And who would know their department's activity better than the manager who manages it on a daily basis? When we train clinical managers to use evidence-based management, we close the gap between the business and clinical domains.

Conclusion

Looking back on my 30-year career, I realize the tremendous impact of evidence-based management. I have worked for more than one COO or CEO who believed that his job was to hire "great" managers and to "not micromanage." This line of thinking is still common today. The problem is that the COO or CEO cannot reliably know which of the managers is "great" without operational metrics. Many declarations are perceptions based on emotions, biases, and anecdotal experiences—not hard facts.

Because we have only one Medicare "piggy bank," we must identify which hospitals are overspending in order to reduce the risk that such practices put on other hospitals. A study by former CMS administrator Donald M. Berwick and RAND Corporation analyst Andrew D. Hackbarth estimated that waste consumed $476 billion to $992 billion, or 18 to 37 percent, of the approximately $2.6 trillion of total health spending in 2011 (Advisory Board 2012). Spending in Medicare and Medicaid, including state and federal costs, was estimated to contribute about one-third of this waste (*Health Affairs* 2012). My passion and belief is that if we standardize operations in all 5,000 hospitals using evidence-based practices, we can locate inefficiencies, reduce waste, and preserve those hospitals that want to survive.

When traditional managers are asked how their department is running, they may reply with a canned answer: "We're busy, patients are satisfied, and staff morale is high." Unfortunately, they answer with anecdotal, observational information because they do not manage with metrics. An evidence-based manager would likely answer with a more factual statement: "Volume is 5 percent higher than last year, expenses are 10 percent lower, and our HCAHPS scores are forecast to be 6 points higher." Lord William Kelvin, British mathematical physicist, said an important adage for all future evidence-based managers: "If you cannot measure it, you cannot improve it."

References

Advisory Board. 2012. "Berwick: Cut These Six Forms of Waste to Rein in Costs." Published April 10. www.advisory.com/daily-briefing/2012/04/11/berwick -cut-these-six-forms-of-waste.

Centers for Medicare & Medicaid Services (CMS). 2016. "Cost Reports." Updated July 27. www.cms.gov/Research-Statistics-Data-and-Systems /Downloadable-Public-Use-Files/Cost-Reports.

———. 2015. "Transforming Clinical Practice Initiative Awards." Published September 29. www.cms.gov/Newsroom/MediaReleaseDatabase/Fact-sheets/2015 -Fact-sheets-items/2015-09-29.html.

Douglas, K. 2010. "Taking Action to Close the Nursing–Finance Gap: Learning from Success." *Nursing Economic$* 28 (4): 270–72.

Health Affairs. 2012. "Health Policy Briefs: Reducing Waste in Healthcare." Published December 13. www.healthaffairs.org/healthpolicybriefs/brief.php ?brief_id=82.

Wicklund, E. 2014. "Healthcare's Four-Letter Word? It's 'Silo.'" *mHealthNews.* Published April 9. http://mobihealthnews.com/news/healthcares-four-letter-word -its-silo.

18

HOW TO DO EVIDENCE-BASED MANAGEMENT: A DEMONSTRATION

by Bryce Clark

I n the fall of 2012, I began a team-based Capstone project as part of a graduate program in healthcare management. This project was based on the success of a prior intervention in an orthopedic clinic at an urban academic medical center, in which a preadmission patient educator was able to reduce the length of stay for elective surgical admissions by helping patients form realistic expectations about surgery. Our project sponsor initially charged my team with transferring this intervention to a new patient population; however, by following an evidence-based management (EBMgmt) approach, we quickly learned that our sponsor had jumped to a conclusion about how to solve a problem without first evaluating the evidence for the intervention. In this chapter, I discuss how my team applied EBMgmt methodologies to make an informed decision to better address our client's management problem.

Framing the Question Behind the Decision

Without a thoroughly developed management question, locating the necessary evidence is nearly impossible. My team faced this challenge when our client originally proposed the purpose of our Capstone project, which was to take the success of an intervention done for one specific group of patients and apply it to a different patient population. From our client's perspective, the management question was, *How do you take a successful preadmission patient education program from one clinic and make it work in a different clinic?* The issue, however, was that no one had first asked whether compelling evidence existed to suggest that this intervention would be translatable to a different setting.

We therefore worked with our client to reframe the management question as, *Can a preadmission patient education program be successful at reducing the length of stay for another elective surgery population at the hospital?* From this management question, we developed a research question:

Note: This chapter describes the author's experience in the Capstone program at NYU Wagner. Please see chapter 15, by John Donnellan, for in-depth information about the program's development and approach.

Does preadmission patient education reduce the length of stay for elective surgical patients? With this reframed question, we could now better evaluate the literature for preadmission patient education programs to determine whether sufficient evidence supported use of the intervention.

When we formed our research question, we purposely wrote it as a closed-ended question, because we specifically needed to know whether evidence supported use of a preadmission education intervention in another population. In addition, when we developed the management question with our client, we did not consider a time frame. In hindsight, a time frame might have been useful, because it would prevent us from recommending an intervention that would take an unreasonable amount of time to implement. A more complete management question, therefore, might have been, *Can a preadmission patient education program be implemented within one year and be successful at reducing the length of stay for another elective surgery population at the hospital?*

Finding Sources of Information

My team used both key informant interviews and scholarly literature searches to locate our evidence. Because the original orthopedic project was conducted at our client's hospital, we had the opportunity to interview the patient educator who developed and maintained that program. From this interview, we were able to ascertain the key factors that led to the program's success, which were not entirely evident from a published article on the program.

To specifically answer our research question of whether preadmission patient education reduces the length of stay for elective surgical patients, we spent the majority of our time querying articles in the MEDLINE database (accessed via PubMed) and the Cochrane Database of Systematic Reviews. Prior to initiating our literature search, we completed a "literature search strategy worksheet" with guidance from a university librarian (see the example provided in exhibit 18.1). This worksheet helped us clearly define our research question, decide which databases to search, determine our search terms (e.g., Medical Subject Headings, or MeSH, terms; synonyms), map out search strategies with Boolean connectors, and set search limits and filters (e.g., publication types, year of publication, age groups). We then used the worksheet to systematically enter search criteria into the MEDLINE and Cochrane databases. We saved electronic copies of all of the articles we located.

In reflecting on this literature search process, two key factors helped our team efficiently find our evidence (or lack thereof). The first was the use of our literature search strategy worksheet, which made our search more

EXHIBIT 18.1
Literature
Search Strategy
Worksheet

1.   Develop the research question.

Problem:	Increased length of stay
Patient population:	Elective surgical patients
Intervention:	Preadmission patient education

Research question: Does preadmission patient education reduce the length of stay for elective surgical patients?

2.   Decide which databases to use.

Name of Database	Yes/No/Maybe	Why?
PubMed/MEDLINE	Yes	Biomedical literature
CINAHL Plus	Yes	Nursing/allied health
PsycINFO	No	Not relevant to surgical populations
ProQuest (includes Joanna Briggs evidence summaries)	Maybe	Evidence-based reviews
Cochrane Database of Systematic Reviews	Yes	Systematic reviews/ metadata on human healthcare

3.   Determine terms/concepts, synonyms, MeSH terms, and so on, to use.

Term/Concept	Synonyms	MeSH terms
Decreased length of stay	Hospital days, hospitalization, hospital stay, LOS	Length of stay, patient discharge, LOS
Preoperative teaching	Presurgical education, preop teaching, preadmission education	Teaching, preoperative period
Elective surgery patients	Elective procedures, surgery, surgery patients, preop patients, planned surgeries	Elective surgical procedures

(continued)

EXHIBIT 18.1
Literature
Search Strategy
Worksheet
(Continued)

4.   Determine the search strategy.

Strategy Number	Database	Strategy (Terms with Boolean Connectors)	Number of Hits
Strategy 1	MEDLINE	(Length of stay OR LOS OR decreased length of stay) AND (preoperative OR presurgical OR elective surgical procedure) AND (teaching OR education)	49

5.   Specify limits and filters.

Publication types:	Systematic reviews / critically appraised
Year(s) of publication:	2002–2012
Age group, if appropriate:	Adults (18 years and older)
Research methodology limits:	None
Other limits:	None

systematic. Instead of randomly typing search terms into a database, we let the worksheet guide every step of our search process. The worksheet also served as documentation of our search strategy, which was useful whenever our client or advisers had questions about our process. The second helpful factor was the guidance of a librarian. Because some members of the team were inexperienced in conducting literature searches, we asked a librarian for feedback on our research question and search strategy before we began.

Because this project was part of an academic program, we had the luxury of spending time and resources on our evidence search. If we were to do this project as managers, however, we likely could have obtained similar evidence in a shorter amount of time by focusing primarily on research syntheses as opposed to individual research studies.

Evaluating the Evidence (Assessing the Accuracy, Applicability, and Actionability of the Information)

Our initial literature review from the MEDLINE and Cochrane databases yielded 49 articles. To organize these articles, we listed each article in a row of a spreadsheet and labeled columns for study type, population type, main findings/conclusions, and other notes. By keeping all the high-level findings in one spreadsheet, we were able to more efficiently evaluate the articles and sort through those that were most appropriate. Similar to our search strategy worksheet, this spreadsheet was an invaluable tool for documentation of our literature review. We updated and referenced it throughout the duration of the Capstone project

When assessing accuracy, we examined how true the articles were to the study type; we placed greater emphasis on systematic reviews and meta-analyses than on retrospective case studies. Next, to determine the applicability of the evidence, we looked specifically at the patient populations studied (e.g., surgery type, type of hospital, location of hospital) and considered whether the evidence was able to correlate preadmission patient education with an outcome, such as length of stay. Finally, we prioritized the articles based on the quality of their designs and their applicability to elective surgery populations. We used a systematic process to evaluate scholarly evidence; however, we did not apply the same rigor to the colloquial evidence that we obtained from the orthopedic patient educator.

We did not specifically measure the actionability of the evidence, because we did not find a sufficient volume of high-quality evidence supporting a relationship between preadmission patient education and length of stay. If stronger evidence had existed, however, we likely would have examined the costs of the orthopedic patient educator and the resources needed to implement such a program.

Determining If the Information Is Adequate

Overall, we did not find conclusive evidence to support implementing a new preadmission patient education program to reduce length of stay. Our evaluation of the evidence obtained by interviewing the orthopedic patient educator led us to conclude that the educator was able to decrease the length of stay in her particular setting by helping patients clearly set realistic expectations about the surgical procedure, the hospital admission process, and postdischarge follow-up care. The key elements of this program were the educator's motivation and her ability to form close relationships with patients—both of which were individual, person-based elements that may not have been easy to replicate in a new system or population.

During our literature review, we found no meta-analyses or systematic reviews that conclusively showed a significant relationship between preadmission education and length of stay. Two individual studies reported a significant decrease in length of stay after implementing preadmission educational interventions, and both hypothesized that the success of the interventions resulted from the format of the education. Neither study, however, was designed as a randomized controlled trial, and in both cases the authors acknowledged that more research would be needed to determine which elements of the education would most likely reduce length of stay. We therefore concluded that we did not have adequate evidence to support implementation of a similar preadmission patient education program for another elective surgery population.

Instead, we proposed a new management question: *What can be done preadmission to decrease the length of stay for elective surgical patients?* By making this new question broader and more open-ended, we hoped to find evidence for other interventions, besides patient education, that might decrease the length of stay for an elective surgery patient population. Of course, we could have chosen the more open-ended management question from the beginning. However, our team benefited from the experience of evaluating the evidence for our initial management question and demonstrating to our client the need to modify the purpose of the project.

Lessons Learned

Overall, by using an EBMgmt approach, our team was able to reframe the objectives of our Capstone project so that a successful outcome would be more achievable. Had we not used this approach, we may have proposed interventions that were not based on evidence and therefore would have had a greater potential for failure. By changing our management question to focus on any preadmission practices that might reduce length of stay, we were able to identify evidence-based interventions that went beyond patient education, and we were able to make recommendations to our client that had a greater likelihood of success. In addition, by using this systematic process to make an informed decision, we were able to streamline the work of collecting, reviewing, and analyzing the evidence, which made the overall process more efficient—something any full-time manager should appreciate.

19

PERSPECTIVE ON HOSPITAL PERFORMANCE

INTERVIEW WITH DAVID FINE, PRESIDENT AND CEO, CATHOLIC HEALTH INITIATIVES INSTITUTE FOR RESEARCH AND INNOVATION, ENGLEWOOD, COLORADO

This interview was conducted in June 2015.

What is your understanding of evidence-based management?
The most elegant definition is (Denise M.) Rousseau's from the first edition: using the best available research combined with practitioner experience and customer preference. This is pragmatic and not geeky. We are talking about using a body of research knowledge as tempered by the practical experience of those who have traveled the same path, whose experience is subjective but bona fide. This collaboration between best research evidence and best practitioner experience produces much better decision making.

What has been your experience implementing evidence-based decision making?
This has been the centerpiece of my career. Early on, I was viewed based on my track record as a turnaround CEO. My niche was delivering results to a troubled environment where a great deal of change was necessary, focusing on clinical processes and outcomes and finance. I have been concerned with patient satisfaction and financial variables. My approach was to compare outcomes and processes at a new employer with those of comparably situated hospitals that perform better on the same metrics. When demonstrated objectively, this reveals opportunities for improvement. Executives can get useful "a-ha" moments and hopefully enthusiastic buy-in.

For example, consider a nationally ranked clinical service, positioned in *US News and World Report* as one of the ten best of its kind nationally. Upon closer examination, I saw that a number of embedded metrics were no better than median performance in its class. At the time, national rankings were heavily weighted toward "reputation," which had been built upon historical performance many years earlier. This was reputation among clinical specialists doing the same work. But when we looked at certain specialty-specific performance data, including morbidity and mortality, performance was no better than the 50th percentile. There was incredible denial when I shared these findings. We were looking at data that had not been manufactured by the management team but rather taken from performance norms developed by professional societies and government. The local physicians argued that their organization was different, treating "sicker patients." I have found this to be a common defense that seldom holds up to careful scrutiny or reasonable statistical adjustments based on comorbidities or other objective factors.

At the same organization, the hospital had been supporting research at a rate of $6 million per year. Performance of the clinical service was examined at the board level, where it was decided to offer the opportunity for staff to earn $1 million on each of ten quality performance variables. The targets were national professional society performance at the 50th percentile. We selected the criteria carefully and in concert with the affected medical staff. For several years, less than a quarter of the pay-for-performance was earned. In one year, none was earned. Needless to say, this became a material, if controversial and painful, wake-up call for the involved physicians, board members, and management.

Describe the work of your current employer, the Catholic Health Initiatives (CHI) Institute for Research and Innovation (CIRI). How is its work influenced by evidence-based management?
There are three components to the CIRI operation: (1) clinical trials of experimental devices and drugs, (2) translational research, and (3) a Center for Healthcare Innovation. Several current innovation projects illustrate our activities. The first is in a Lincoln, Nebraska, hospital and concerns registered nurse (RN) staffing in medical-surgical units, which is typically in a ratio of four patients to one RN on day shifts. The CHI corporate chief nursing officer has asked the question, "What happens if we transform the labor combination by reducing RN hours on the unit, adding lower-cost support personnel, and using 'virtual' nurses to answer clinical questions and give advice electronically?" We have demonstrated results on 1 bed and on 12 beds, and we are about to launch on a 40-60-bed trial. Scale is everything. If you are implementing in over 100 hospitals, the virtual backup could include multiple nursing subspecialists, clinical pharmacists, and potentially physician hospitalists as well. Our working hypothesis is that aggregate costs will be lower, patient/nurse/physician satisfaction will improve, and clinical outcomes will be enhanced or held constant.

In Washington state, we piloted a program for 20 intractable diabetics in a primary care practice. What kinds of interventions make sense? From actions already taken, we see a 20 percent improvement in patient outcomes, as measured by hemoglobin A1C levels. Now, how do we get the payers to support the costs of such improvements? The Institute for Research and Innovation receives block grants from the national CHI budget to run such pilots. We started modestly with overall funding of $2 million but will expand. CIRI also competes for federal and private funding to support specific projects and receives philanthropic support.

What kind of uptake has evidence-based management and decision making been getting in the hospital and healthcare industry?

Things are happening as a result of pay-for-performance and shared risk arrangements, which encourage long-embedded processes to be reexamined. This is the motivation needed at CHI and other providers to experiment with new pathways. The CHI corporate CEO takes pride in the work we are doing in research and innovation. Our institute was recently budgeted to hire an epidemiologist and a health economist. I am thinking about approaching other large systems for a joint venture in evidence-based decision making. This is scalable.

To sum up, we must act based on the popular song "Let the Sunshine In" (from the 1967 musical *Hair*). Health systems must shine a light in dark corners and make the not-for-profit sector more transparent. Comparisons raise the performance bar and stimulate improved effectiveness and efficiency in a sector that has not performed to the levels achieved in other industries.

PERSPECTIVE ON HOSPITAL PERFORMANCE

INTERVIEW WITH RICHARD D'AQUILA, PRESIDENT, YALE NEW HAVEN HOSPITAL

The first part of this interview was conducted in July 2014.

You were interviewed in 2008 for the first edition of this book. What have you accomplished since the first edition?
We have made significant progress advancing our academic medical center in the face of a very unforgiving financial and regulatory environment. Our major accomplishments include the successful acquisition and integration of the Hospital of St. Raphael, a 511-bed hospital in New Haven that became part of Yale New Haven in 2012. We accomplished a very successful integration of these two hospitals, which rationalized services and created significant long-term cost savings. As a 1,541-bed hospital with two campuses and over 50 ambulatory sites, it is one of the largest in the United States. This integration is especially noteworthy since it fully integrated a Catholic and non-Catholic hospital, a large academic medical center and a community teaching hospital, and two institutions with different labor unions.

By way of background, I have been at Yale New Haven since 2006. My focus has been to build a team and lead the transition of our institution to a regionally prominent destination hospital. Our accomplishments have included a period of unprecedented growth and successful implementation of major clinical service lines in areas such as cancer, heart and vascular disease, neurosciences, solid organ transplantation, and our children's hospital. We have also made great strides in an innovative approach to enhancing the value of care we provide through clinical redesign and a high-reliability patient safety environment, which has reduced costs, eliminated waste, and improved clinical outcomes. Despite several years of successful operating margins in a fee-for-service environment, we are preparing for the next wave of payment shifts from episodic care to risk-based models which will tie our reimbursement to population health and performance-based targets. This is definitely a transition time for our hospital as we build on past progress but prepare ourselves for the next level of sustained success.

How has your philosophy of management changed since 2008?

I don't think my philosophy of management has changed as much as I have tried to continuously refine my skill set, particularly in selecting, motivating, and developing members of my team. I continue to believe the people equation is the most critical single factor in organizational success, and getting it right has to be a career-long learning experience. I'm still amazed at how much I don't know and what new techniques can be applied to finding great talent, building high-performance teams, developing leadership skills, and managing conflict. It's the most challenging and rewarding aspect of my work.

Have your thoughts about evidence-based management changed over the years?

We use evidence-based management mostly in the way we empower and engage our physicians in clinical redesign. It's a very structured process which is grounded in sophisticated analytics and Lean-based methodologies to reduce variation and restructure the care process aimed at reducing waste and improving outcomes. We have as many as 20 physician-led teams working on clinical redesign at one time, and our physicians are enthused because the focus is on improving outcomes and patient satisfaction, not just lowering costs.

What keeps other managers from managing as you do?

I spend only a limited time interfacing with colleagues from around the country, but I get a very real sense that there is still great reluctance to embrace innovation and to continuously work at improving your skillset. Many hospitals are struggling financially right now, so they can't take the long view on work like clinical redesign and high reliability that takes a long time to pay off. I also think there is still great reluctance to engage and embrace physicians at the highest leadership levels, like service line management and clinical strategies. These are all things we have tried to do better, with great success.

Do you see any increased uptake in your kind of management practice?

As I mentioned earlier, my national experience is limited. I do see a great deal of relevance in the work done by the University HealthSystem Consortium (now Vizient) in their research series led by Tom Robertson. Vizient regularly spotlights and encourages the sharing of best practices in transforming academic medical centers, patient safety and high reliability, and adaptive strategies for coping with payment system changes.

How do you train your managers to use an evidence-based approach?

We have a corporate college at Yale New Haven Health System called the Institute for Excellence. It offers courses and leadership development programs for our managers across the health system. We also collaborate with the Yale School of Medicine and Yale School of Management to offer training and skill enhancement programs for our physician leaders, especially those who are emerging talent.

How do you use consultants?

As a consultant in a previous life, I view them as a valuable asset under the right circumstances. The benefits of using consultants include having specialized expertise and efficiency supporting time-limited projects where the resources they bring to bear can be concentrated in a short period of time to get the job done. They can also be extraordinarily useful in bringing parties together and constructively managing conflict. But their work has to be clearly scoped and closely managed, with clear boundaries defined.

What have you learned in getting good results?

I still think the most important requirements are the people. Having the right people on the team, fostering an environment where they can grow and support each other, and being intolerant of behaviors that undermine the team are critical. It's also essential to have a very clear plan and strategy, continuously challenge it, and hold both individuals and the team accountable for staying on track and fostering frequent and meaningful communication. We are in an unforgiving environment with very little margin for error, which requires this kind of leadership precision and attention to team dynamics.

What has been your greatest failure?

As I think back over the years, I can trace every failure in some way to a bad hiring decision. In leadership roles, we often see shortcomings or blind spots in the interview process but feel it is something that can be addressed or remedied. It's always a mistake to think that way rather than to hold out for the best possible candidate who has thoroughly demonstrated both the technical and personal qualifications to thrive. It's a tough lesson to learn the hard way.

What does the future hold for Yale New Haven and your management skills?

At the risk of oversimplifying a very complicated question, there are common themes here. Both as institutions and individuals, we have to adapt and thrive in a complicated and rapidly changing environment.

At Yale New Haven, our focus is on what we call the "value equation." This includes a relentless focus on high reliability, better outcomes, a better patient experience, and lower cost. We are building scale through clinical service lines, partnerships, and integration success like the Hospital of St. Raphael. And all of this has to be done in a manner that does not lose sight of engaging our physicians and employees as they adapt to the new healthcare environment.

As individuals and executive leaders, you have to be energized by these challenges. These are demanding roles that require intellectual curiosity and adaptive skills. You have to be exceptionally organized and comfortable with multiple priorities and complex situations. You have to be excited by lifelong learning and embracing innovation. And you have to keep it all in perspective with a work–life balance and a sense of humor. We owe it to our healthcare system, our patients, and our staff to lead this transition to greater value.

The second part of this interview was conducted in 2015.

How did you decide to integrate with the Hospital of St. Raphael?
The Hospital of St. Raphael is located six blocks from Yale New Haven Hospital, and like a number of community hospitals, it had been in significant financial distress due to declining patient volume and growing debt obligations for a number of years. Hospital of St. Raphael leadership was looking to partner with another Catholic hospital / health system in the region but, due to its precarious financial situation, was unable to find a suitable partner. At the same time, Yale New Haven Hospital was experiencing rapid outpatient and inpatient growth, and we were exploring the addition of a new inpatient bed tower to address our growing clinical needs. There was a change in Hospital of St. Raphael leadership in 2011, and the stars aligned for us to become one organization.

From an economic standpoint, there was no need for two separate hospitals within such close geographic proximity of each other. Coming together allowed us to provide the region with more coordinated care, to reduce duplicative clinical and administrative services, and to become more efficient. It also provided us with much-needed bed relief and allowed us to avoid an estimated $650 million investment in a new patient tower. Proceeds from the transaction allowed the Hospital of St. Raphael to pay off its debt and address its pension liabilities. Finally, integrating helped prepare us for the transition to risk-based payment reform, as we are now the primary care provider in the region and have implemented one standard of care across all our inpatient and outpatient sites, along with a single electronic medical record.

How did you decide which clinical services to focus on?
From the onset, we decided that it was very important that each inpatient campus have its own identity, in addition to a common core of medicine, surgery, behavioral health, and emergency medicine services. This was an important guiding principle for us, as we did not want employees or physicians to

feel that we were minimizing the clinical expertise of the St. Raphael campus to fulfill our bed needs.

The Hospital of St. Raphael had a number of high-quality clinical programs and strong outcomes in areas such as orthopedics and geriatric services that we wanted to make sure we continued to develop. Additionally, we had made a number of investments in high-technology destination services at the York Street campus in areas such as solid organ transplantation that we did not want to duplicate.

In collaboration with our consulting team from Kurt Salmon and Associates, and based on recent investments and volume and outcomes data, we developed a clinical vision that leveraged the unique strengths of each campus. We were also mindful to respect the Ethical and Religious Directives for Catholic health facilities, which we continue to abide by on the St. Raphael campus. The St. Raphael campus is the primary site for musculoskeletal, specialty geriatrics, and low-risk high-amenities OB services. The York Street campus houses children's services, oncology, solid organ transplantation, trauma, and cardiac surgery programs.

We were mindful to get input and buy-in for the vision from our physician and other clinical leaders, as their support is a prerequisite to implementation success. Physician engagement in clinical services planning should not be minimized, and we have found it to be invaluable in all the planning projects we accomplished.

Over the last four years, we have made over $80 million in investments on the St. Raphael campus, consistent with the aforementioned vision, including the creation of a new inpatient musculoskeletal unit, state-of-the-art musculoskeletal operating rooms designed by the physicians, and a specialty restorative care / geriatric unit designed by renowned architect Michael Graves, with innovative features for fall prevention and cognitive support.

In addition to investing in our inpatient services, we have also made a number of investments on the ambulatory front. We have decommissioned a number of duplicative ambulatory practices and instead created multispecialty ambulatory satellites in surrounding suburbs and across the Connecticut shoreline. This allows us to grow our geographic footprint and make it easier for our patients to access our services by bringing the Yale New Haven Hospital services and standards of care directly to local communities.

How did you track integration progress?
In order to get the integration approved by the Federal Trade Commission and Connecticut Office of Healthcare Access (CON authority), we had to develop out a robust plan to integrate services and commit to synergies. This was challenging to do, since we were competitors up until the date of closing and were legally not allowed to see each other's financials and operating

reports. To this end, we, Yale New Haven Hospital and the Hospital of St. Raphael, jointly retained Alvarez and Marsal as our independent third-party consultant to help us develop an integration plan and validate synergies.

Alvarez and Marsal helped us establish a project management office, which was responsible for defining and tracking progress against a set of metrics and implementation timetables. We tracked implementation progress through a set of dashboards. We put in place a designated site leadership team, which included members of the senior leadership team who were based at the St. Raphael campus and could ensure timely resolution of issues. This included a chief integration officer overseeing all aspects of the integration, a dedicated vice president of nursing, a vice president of human resources, a vice president of finance, and an executive director, Catholic heritage. The site leadership team reviewed issues and progress on a weekly basis.

The site leadership team was instrumental in helping us develop a new culture at the St. Raphael campus and reinforcing the message that we are truly one medical center with two inpatient campuses. We achieved our integration milestones ahead of schedule and have now moved to an integrated leadership structure with responsibilities for activities across both campuses.

What are some of the lessons learned from the integration?
Although we are seeing an increase in hospital acquisitions and integrations across the country, the reality is that each transaction is unique. It is truly a balance of art and science. There are common success factors, such as identifying demonstrable synergies, engaging medical staff, ensuring that there is a robust vision endorsed by all stakeholders, appointing a dedicated project leader, and having an appropriate mix of internal and external resources working on the project. Those are all part of the mechanics / technical skills required for successful integration.

But above all, there is the intangible and probably most challenging component, which is engaging employees in creating a new culture. Yale New Haven Hospital is a very different hospital today than it was four years ago, before we integrated with the Hospital of St. Raphael. Yet it is very hard for us to remember what it was like before. This has become our new normal—our new Yale New Haven Hospital.

One item I think is important to do very early on is recognizing and emphasizing the common values shared by both organizations that are coming together and embracing each organization's rich history. When I was talking with employees on both campuses before integration, the one item that stood out to me was the fear in people's eyes. Although they were committed to the vision and looking forward to the future, the fear of the unknown and where they would fit into the vision was palpable. As leaders, we sometimes take for granted how important the daily relationships and activities are for our employees and how discombobulating a change is for employees.

Creating a new culture is not without its challenges, and I liken it to adding a new child to a family. There is always that transition period where the existing children question why there is a new addition and why things can't go back to "the good old days" when things were simpler. We experienced something very similar in the first few months after integration, and we were able to work through it by engaging our employees in coming up with communications, activities, and celebrations that would allow everyone to come together and truly foster that sense of team. Although it may feel a little uncomfortable at first, we found it to be instrumental in helping us define the new normal. It has truly been a positive transformational journey for our medical center and helped us further our destination hospital aspirations.

PERSPECTIVE ON HOSPITAL PERFORMANCE

INTERVIEW WITH MICHAEL DOWLING, CEO, NORTHWELL HEALTH

This interview was conducted in March 2015.

Please explain your philosophy of management and how it incorporates evidence-based practice.
Managers can do what needs to be done today—effectively and efficiently. Our focus is on implementation. We are looking for leaders who can take a longer view and take us where we want to be five years from now. These leaders have to evaluate the overall context and trends, understand key demographics, be familiar with government policy and regulation, and—especially important—think outside the box to help create the future. Individuals who can both *manage* in the short term and *lead* in the long term are unique.

An example of our approach to management involves our decision to start our own medical school (in partnership with Hofstra). We recognized that medical education had not kept pace with the demands of a changed environment. New doctors need preparation to practice effectively in the world of 2030, where transparency, quality outcome measurement, teamwork, interdisciplinary practice, prevention, wellness, and the impact of the social environment will be extremely important. We knew we had to create something different.

The same set of dynamics affected our initiative to begin our own nursing school. Nurses need to be at the forefront (with physicians and other team members) of primary care. They can be leaders in administration as well as clinical care delivery. But to get improved outcomes in the future, we need to train differently today. Many schools are constrained by history, tradition, and long-standing bureaucracies. Even if they want to pursue innovation, they have difficulty achieving it. Seeing a need for change, we developed a new curriculum—a new approach—focused on how to *do*, not just to *know*. It's a move away from just teaching facts toward teaching students how to analyze and apply. After all, facts can be accessed from your iPhone.

Note: See chapter 9, by Sofia Agoritsas, Steven Fishbane, and Candice Halinski, for an in-depth look at one specific program implemented at Northwell Health.

How do you train and hold your management team accountable for using an evidence-based process?

We created, in 2001, the equivalent of an in-house corporate university. We called it the Center for Learning and Innovation (CLI). The inclusion of the word *innovation* was not an accident—it represents a core part of our culture. CLI is the epicenter of our educational enterprise. We provide comprehensive training in leadership development, process improvement methodologies, performance management, evidence-based care, and so on. We create, build, and adapt program offerings based on the needs of individuals and of the organization as a whole. Our leaders, at the various levels, are responsible for holding their teams accountable for both doing things right and doing the right things.

We also expose employees to best practices both in the US and abroad, both by researching results and making in-person visits. Many of our team members hold leadership positions in regional and national organizations.

One other important point: We like to give responsibility to individuals who "haven't done it before." We want new blood, new thought processes, new curiosity. For example, I recently promoted an operating manager to head of human resources (HR) for the whole organization, even though he has never had HR experience. He provides a new perspective.

How have Northwell's philosophy and practice adjusted in the face of a fast-changing environment?

Balancing consistency of purpose and strategy with continuous tactical change is an ever-present component of leadership. Years ago, we were very hospital inpatient focused. More recently, we have placed much more of an emphasis on outpatient and ambulatory expansion. The shift has been pronounced and requires a refocus on talent and leadership selection. Consistent with that shift is our emphasis on customer service—looking at the business from the outside in, not just from the inside out. Customer service and the overall customer experience must become a distinguishing characteristic. Organizations that fall short in these areas will fail.

What keeps managers of other large healthcare organizations from adopting the management practices that Northwell follows?

I believe most are attempting to move in a similar direction and build the necessary infrastructure. Our history—being the first integrated health system in the region—and the way we are organized give us an advantage. The move also requires a philosophic and cultural shift in how you look at the business, envision the future, and prepare your staff. Some organizations are "hostage to precedent," can't successfully let go of tradition, and view current reform efforts incorrectly as temporary. One other point: We see the commitment to learning and training as an investment, not an expense. We want to promote a continuous culture of learning.

For a management decision made recently, discuss how an evidence-based process was followed at Northwell.
There are many examples I could discuss, but I will briefly mention two. One was our breakthrough effort on sepsis reduction. We brought the best experts from around the world together, analyzed best practices, and then created a comprehensive program that has been extraordinarily successful and led to government regulatory changes. It is, of course, a continuous work in progress.

The other was our decision two decades ago to create our corporate university (CLI). In this case, we looked at the best such organizations in nonhealthcare companies—IBM, General Electric (GE), Motorola, and so on. We engaged experts from GE to help us initially, and once we created the competence, we moved ahead independently. Later on, when we decided to build a Patient Safety Institute, we engaged with the aviation industry to help design our innovative simulation training center—currently a national model.

All decisions, in my view, are the combination of expert input, internal debate, evidence-based research, and a large dose of vision, risk taking, and good old-fashioned common sense.

What have been Northwell's greatest achievements in implementing evidence-based decision making? How have they been accomplished?
We define ourselves as an entrepreneurial organization. As we approach decision making on any issue, we research the literature, we search for best practices, and we visit other organizations (both healthcare and nonhealthcare). We collect as much relevant information as we can, and we allow open, constructive internal discussion. There are times, however, when decisions have to be made in the absence of clear evidence or historical perspective. In these cases, you apply the old-fashioned method—the combination of common sense and gut reaction. Our decision on moving into Manhattan to assume Lenox Hill Hospital was, for the most part, in this category. And it was one of the best decisions we have made. It meant taking a risk—an essential part of leadership.

Can you provide an example of a decision where evidence-based processes were faulty or lacking? Please explain what caused these situations.
A willingness to fail is essential if progress is to be attained. Every failure is a learning experience, so we should always look at its positive aspects and its optimistic potential. About 15 years ago, for example, we entered into a total risk capitation payment program with Oxford Insurance Company

for Medicare. We made many assumptions, and it turned out to be a major failure. We had to terminate the relationship, but we learned many valuable lessons that served us very well recently as we engaged in starting our own insurance company, CareConnect. Was the original idea a failure? The answer has two parts—yes and no.

Please discuss any future plans you have for implementing and improving evidence-based decision making at Northwell.
We plan to keep doing what we have been doing and continuously attempting to get better. We use evidence-based methodologies when possible, but healthcare is going through such transformation that decisions have to be made in a dynamic environment and through a forward-looking lens. For many decisions, "evidence" (as we traditionally define it) may not be available, but that should not lead to fear or inaction. As Samuel Beckett once said, "No matter, try again, fail again, fail better."

STAKEHOLDER CONCERNS

PERSPECTIVE ON MEDICINE

INTERVIEW WITH ETHAN BASCH, MD, UNIVERSITY OF NORTH CAROLINA

This interview was conducted in June 2015.

What do you consider evidence-based medicine in cancer care, and to what extent do you think it is practiced?

The practice of evidence-based medicine aligns medical decision making for individual patients with scientific evidence to optimize outcomes at the population level. Oncology is a highly evidence-based clinical discipline, and it generally uses the best evidence that is available. Clinical practice guidelines based on rigorous research are widely used. Nonetheless, a number of limitations are beginning to be acknowledged: First, people in clinical trials don't always resemble people in real life. Clinical trial participants are often healthier, younger, and whiter than the general population with cancer, and follow-up time in trials is usually not long enough to understand long-term effects of treatments. Second, most medical decisions don't have supporting evidence to inform them. Decisions are multifaceted, and we don't have evidence for all the facets. For example, with an advanced cancer, say a patient unfortunately has metastases in three or four areas of his body. We may have evidence for what works if the patient has one small metastasis, or if he has metastases in many areas. But what about the people in between? Should we recommend a highly toxic therapy in this situation? Although rigorous evidence exists for treatment in this cancer type, that evidence leaves a gray area for his particular scenario.

In fact, we lack evidence for many facets of care—how many scans to do, how often to see patients in clinic, how often to check the toxicity of treatment at home. We lack evidence for how much psychosocial support is needed and what outcomes it can be expected to achieve. With major evidentiary gaps, we lean on the evidence we have and on personal experiences and anecdotes. Doctors are culturally committed to evidence-based medicine. But often the evidence doesn't match the patient's situation, so evidence is lacking for appropriate care. Is there any special evidence-based medicine movement within cancer care?

Yes. The main oncology specialty society, the American Society of Clinical Oncology, runs a large guidelines program and offers a quality-of-care symposium. The National Comprehensive Cancer Network also provides clinical guidelines that are widely used. There are numerous drivers of guideline use: Treatment is often very complicated for the provider, and guidelines are useful. Following guidelines is also perceived to protect the doctor from malpractice exposure. In addition, guideline-compliant care can serve as a basis for reimbursement authorization.

There are also local-level processes to encourage applications of evidence and guidelines. "Tumor boards" are multidisciplinary meetings where practitioners discuss patients and how best to apply existing evidence.

How do you use an evidence-based process in your own practice of diagnosis and treatment of cancer?

I use the approaches mentioned previously, including guidelines and tumor board discussions. I follow the scientific literature and attend national conferences to understand the evidence landscape. I discuss evidence with my patients when making shared decisions, recognizing that this is only a part of decision making. Patient preferences and values, logistics, and other patient-level characteristics also must be considered and balanced with the science piece.

Have you had any experience with evidence-based processes being used in management? What generally happens when doctors ask managers, "What is your evidence?" or say, "I don't see that there is sufficient evidence to adopt what you as a manager are suggesting"?

I haven't had much experience with this. I have had some experience at the institutional level looking at the evidence for integrating nurse navigators and lay navigators in cancer care delivery. Evidence was used to make the case that nurse navigators lead to better outcomes. The program would not have existed without a review of the evidence to convince administrator stakeholders that it was worth the investment. One of the clinical departments at my institution has adopted Lean management. There is evidence for this approach, and the result has been more efficient operations and greater net revenue—although some practitioners have felt strained by increased workload.

What is your understanding of the evidence base available for coordinating cancer care? Why isn't there more funding for interventions so we can know more about what works and doesn't work and why?

Care is highly fragmented. As providers, we often are unable to effectively communicate with other providers or with caregivers due to infrastructure and time limitations. Innovations such as medical homes and more integrated accountable care models promise a better future. I am impressed by the recent emphasis by the Centers for Medicare & Medicaid Services and other federal agencies on managing the whole patient, as well as on the interoperability of electronic systems, which is essential. Funding is available from the Patient-Centered Outcomes Research Institute and the Agency for Healthcare Research and Quality (AHRQ) related to care coordination.

To what extent is your own work increasingly evidence based, and how would you see what it takes to increase production of better evidence for diagnosis and treatment of cancer?
More providers and administrators are focused on quality and evidence these days, which culturally makes it easier to be an evidence-based physician. Quality and value are at the forefront of discussions in oncology now—for example, reducing overuse and underuse and eliminating low-value treatments. There is also a substantial promise of harnessing big data—linked data sets including cancer registries, electronic health record information, and insurance claims—to generate evidence tailored to individual patient characteristics. However, there are also persistent limitations. Some people in the country resist the generation and use of evidence, as seen in proposed legislation to defund AHRQ. There is also a persistent problem related to health disparities and low health literacy in some populations; we will need to address such issues with research, education, and outreach moving forward.

PERSPECTIVE ON NURSING

INTERVIEW WITH MAJA DJUKIC, ASSISTANT PROFESSOR, RORY MEYERS COLLEGE OF NURSING, NEW YORK UNIVERSITY

This interview was conducted in February 2016.

Please explain your philosophy of management and how it includes evidence-based practice (EBP).

I don't have experience being a manager, but since I left bedside nursing, my interest has been in nursing management. I left bedside nursing because of bad management, and ten years of research have led me to the conclusion that many nurses leave hospitals for the same reason. I have been devoting my career to ensuring that nurses get enough support in their work environment to deliver the best care to the patient.

The job of the manager is to ensure a good work environment for nurses, so that nurses can provide a high quality of care. One thing I believe is not happening is tying patient outcomes to staff outcomes such as job satisfaction and turnover. The focus now is on patient outcomes such as pressure sores, falls, and infections—not on the management of staff as an independent outcome. We must marry clinical evidence-based practice to best management practice.

Management practice is broad. I'm not familiar with research in areas such as budgeting and mergers. I focus on decision making to improve the nurses' working environment. A lot of hospitals have to collect data from nurses evaluating the working environment in these areas:

- Involvement in organizational decision making
- Staffing
- Support from managers—for example, giving praise and recognition for a job well done or backing up decisions made by nurses on the spot, even if the decisions are criticized
- The degree to which doctors and nurses collaborate
- Professional development—for example, having assignments that foster continuity of care or working with a champion for quality improvement

The nurse manager should review data and ratings for the above work environment factors, look for gaps in performance, and search for evidence for best practice in improving nurses' work environments. The nurse manager can look at teamwork as a work environment factor to improve (e.g., search the literature, learn from consultants, draw from personal work experience). She should examine existing evidence. If evidence on how to improve teamwork is not available or sufficient to inform improvement at the unit level, the nurse manager can conduct research in her local units. Nurse managers do innovate, but they don't usually write up and disseminate the interventions and resulting outcomes. Note: The Agency for Healthcare Research and Quality has a website where innovations are discussed outside of the formal publishing process (https://innovations.ahrq.gov).

How is evidence-based practice currently used in nursing management?
EBP is occurring, but it is focused on clinical care. Nurse managers are accustomed to using EBP to improve falls but not to improve teamwork, although the process of applying EBP is the same. One significant barrier is perhaps that EBP for improving nurses' work environments is not required for accreditation or reimbursement, even though the problem of patient falls may result from poor teamwork among nurses or between nurses and other clinicians.

How is evidence-based practice used in graduate nurse teaching and in nursing research?
EBP focused on clinical issues is well integrated into graduate nurse teaching, but EBP focused on management of the work environment or other management topics is not. Only 12 percent of nurses in management positions have master's degrees, and those degrees are not necessarily in nursing administration but in clinical areas. Lack of graduate education is likely to hinder nurse managers' use of EBP in their management practice.

There is a push nationally to teach EBP content so that more nurses will be ready to implement it. QSEN—Quality and Safety Education for Nurses—is a national effort funded by a foundation to teach six competencies to undergraduate and graduate nurses: teamwork, quality improvement, patient-centered care, patient safety, evidence-based practice, and informatics. This can change the way nurses think, going beyond individual care to systems of care.

How do you use evidence-based practice in your own work?
I am interested in obtaining the best available evidence for the problem at hand. The first step is producing evidence as a researcher. For example, my research has shown that procedural justice, or involving staff nurses in organizational decision making, is an important predictor of staff nurses' job satisfaction. The second is to use an implementation science framework to move

research evidence into practice. Implementation science identifies personal and organizational factors and strategies that promote the use of research and other evidence in everyday practice.

The Magnet movement is a strategy facilitating implementation of management-focused EBP. It provides resources and develops infrastructure for EBP. Magnet also creates many outlets to involve nurses in organizational decision making. However, only 7 to 8 percent of hospitals are Magnet-accredited, so we must research other ways to facilitate implementation of EBP at non-Magnet organizations.

What are the barriers to further adoption of EBP by nurse managers in the field? How, if at all, can these barriers be overcome?
I'm trying to study this right now. One barrier is nurse managers not having a master's-level education. I found that nurse managers with a master's-level education are more likely to implement evidence focused on improving the work environment.

Managers are extremely busy, so we must routinize EBP focused on improving nurses' work environments and other domains of management practice. Clinicians have tools to implement EBP through protocols that are part of electronic health records so that they don't have to search for evidence themselves. Having someone in charge of management-focused EBP would be huge, as it is in clinical decision making. EBP needs to have organizational support and a supporting culture. We need resources and leadership, with CEOs who believe in EBP and the importance of support for nurse managers in translating management research into management practice.

How can nurse managers work with other clinician and nonclinician managers to improve EBP in healthcare organizations?
We must extend discussions of gaps in clinical care, such as treating pressure sores and preventing falls, to include discussions on how to best improve teamwork or staff involvement in organizational decision making across professions and departments. This hasn't yet penetrated, by and large, the DNA of healthcare organizations. We must marry clinical and systems issues.

Please share any additional thoughts you have about implementing and improving evidence-based decision making in nursing management.
Decision-making support for nurse managers remains in the background. We must discuss patient outcomes affected by nurse outcomes and areas of improvement. Nurse managers are inundated with data, but data are cheap and information is expensive. We must make an investment into building better decision-making tools for managers to support them in using management research in their everyday practice to improve staff outcomes and patient outcomes.

PERSPECTIVE ON BIG DATA

INTERVIEW WITH JOHN BILLINGS, PROFESSOR, NYU WAGNER

This interview was conducted in October 2015.

Everyone is talking about the increasing use of big data to respond to management challenges; to address uneven quality, poor care coordination, and bad customer service; and to decrease waste and contain healthcare costs. Define *big data* and explain why its use is becoming more important.

I don't think there is a single definition. The way I think about it is "lots of data." A big data set often contains many millions of records. The data are often gathered for one purpose and used for another. For example, Medicaid or Medicare claims data that were generated for payment are also used for research and evaluation. With these data, we can identify patients in the Medicaid database who are at risk for future hospitalization. Managers are coming to realize that large data sets exist and that analysts can use them to improve operations. A lot of government agencies have huge amounts of data and don't know what questions to ask or don't have the resources to mine the data effectively.

A big data set might contain millions of records that can be examined for risk of hospitalization. A small data set might involve surveys of several hundred patients with a focus on other information, such as why patients have poor access to care or what their social circumstances are—information that is not available in the claims data. A third data set could be qualitative. Such a data set could include interviews with providers carrying out an intervention, explaining how or why something has occurred—for example, why some patients order prescription drugs but do not take them. Mixed-method approaches make sense, and they have varying costs to get different kinds of information.

What are the answerable questions for which big data can help the manager and the researcher?

Managers can try out new interventions for specific groups—for example, diabetes patients—and explore different ways to reach out to patients and use community health workers. We can identify the people at risk and watch for any change in utilization rates (hospital admissions) or adherence to medications after an intervention is implemented. For example, we can analyze filled prescriptions by patient each month. There are, of course, limits to the use of big data, and many questions cannot be answered with a particular big data set. We can identify some people who are at risk for future hospital admissions (based on whether they have chronic disease, abuse substances, see a regular provider of care, and so on). However, the Medicaid administrative data set does not say if the patient is socially isolated, has no family or friends, lives in a shelter, or is homeless. Therefore, a design intervention may have to deal with social, housing, and transportation factors.

How does big data facilitate or limit evidence-based management as you understand it?

With regard to treating diabetes, for example, hospitals are doing all kinds of things without knowing what works. We haven't had the same evidence standard in management as we've had in medicine. Predictions of changes in outcomes based on low-quality data often get fanfare. We don't know if we can design the right intervention but then go ahead with large interventions based on low-quality evidence. For example, Obamacare launched programs targeted at high-cost/high-risk patients without evidence about what interventions did or didn't work. In a similar way, the calorie labeling that was legislated for New York City restaurants was also included in Obamacare, although the available data at the time of Obamacare's passage showed no effect on consumer calorie intake.

How do you respond to the criticism that use of big data and evidence-based management often costs more than it is worth and often doesn't definitively answer questions of what interventions work and do not work?

Big data sets may not always work to definitively answer specific questions, and new questions often arise from analysis of the data. But the promise that big data shows in answering many questions definitively is enormous.

Our new big data collaborative involving Medicaid claims and encounter data at New York University (NYU) will provide answers to many questions cheaply and quickly. That way, managers can find out whether interventions are working, then recalibrate the interventions or stop the interventions altogether if they are not working. We are creating a data set closer to real time, and we are talking with potential clients and collaborators about questions they might like answers to. For example, with the New York State Delivery System Reform Incentive Payment program—a major Medicaid initiative with a $9 billion federal waiver—we can provide information about what works and what doesn't work in achieving program utilization goals. Similarly, the New York State Office of Mental Health is interested in learning what impact its initiative to integrate mental health and primary care has on utilization patterns.

There are two costs for our work. The first is that we must create the analytical database that is updated monthly and can be used by many users, not just one. This costs about $10,000 to $15,000 per project. The other cost is for analysts of the data, which amounts to $40,000 to $50,000 per project. Three months after we get the data, we plan to provide analysis to the participant that can be immediately put to use.

We are moving from theory-based or faith-based rationales to evidence-based decision making. The response to our NYU cooperative has been promising—we've had 15 to 20 positive inquiries.

What is it like to work with managers or clients who want quick answers and validation for interventions that they already want to do?

We've always been successful in "speaking truth to power." When we provide the data, show how we gathered the evidence, and how we analyzed the data, managers are willing to change their minds. We say some things don't work and provide the evidence, and managers usually respond appropriately.

Intermountain, Kaiser Permanente, and Geisinger are all examples of large health systems using big data and evidence-based management to improve their operations. Kaiser Permanente, for instance, "blew the whistle" on the drug Vioxx after it found that cardiac risk associated with the drug had not been identified in trial use because the size of the sample was not large enough to track related complications.

How should graduate programs in healthcare management be organized to teach students to use big data and evidence-based management?

All management and policy students at the graduate level should be shown examples with lessons learned about the use of big data to answer questions that impact decision making. At NYU, we show students variations in utilization presented in the *Dartmouth Atlas* and ask them to consider why the variations exist and to pose alternative responses to reducing high variation. We teach them that big data sets are unlikely to answer every question; some questions can best be answered through the use of smaller data sets or qualitative surveys. But it may be cheaper to analyze millions of records to determine the risk of hospitalization for different categories of patients than to use small surveys or qualitative methods.

PERSPECTIVE ON EVIDENCE-BASED PRACTICE

INTERVIEW WITH ERIC BARENDS, CENTER FOR EVIDENCE-BASED MANAGEMENT, AMSTERDAM, THE NETHERLANDS

This interview was conducted in June 2015.

What do you consider the chief benefits of implementing evidence-based practice?
The bottom line of evidence-based practice is that it provides people with trustworthy evidence to inform their decisions. If it is done in a conscientious, explicit, and judicious way, people will increase the likelihood of a desired outcome, which in the case of healthcare management means better patient and business outcomes. But there is more at stake here. Whether it's in the realm of medicine, education, public policy, or daily life, people are bombarded with unreliable or even misleading information. As a result, they believe weird stuff and take wild claims for granted. I believe that the world would be a better place if we taught evidence-based practice to young kids starting in primary school.

How exactly does evidence-based practice produce better outcomes?
Evidence-based practice produces better outcomes in two different ways. The first is by asking questions. This creates moments of contemplation: If someone claims that A will lead to B (or that A causes B), how do we know whether that is likely to be true? What is the evidence for this claim? Asking questions is a powerful way to create awareness. For what problem is this the solution? How do you know there is a problem? Why is this a problem, and what are its organizational consequences? Do experienced professionals agree there is a problem? How trustworthy are the data? It is important that people question themselves, check their assumptions, and consider options. After all, scientific literature suggests that considering multiple options tends to lead to better outcomes than fixating on "yes/no" or "either/or" choices.

The second way evidence-based practice leads to better outcomes is through critical appraisal. How trustworthy is the evidence? Could there be confirmation bias? Groupthink? Evidence-based practice is a good way to differentiate trustworthy from untrustworthy evidence. But again, it goes further than that. Critical appraisal applies to claims made in daily life. How do you know whether the claims for an advertised product are valid? Or whether a claim made by a politician is based on trustworthy evidence?

What do you see as the chief obstacles to implementing evidence-based practice, and how may these obstacles be overcome? In large firms? In academia?

I think our greatest obstacle is ourselves. As human beings, we are overconfident. We think we know what the problem is and how to solve the problem. Managers and business leaders with an MBA do this in a split second. The three hardest words in management and leadership are "I don't know." Daniel Kahneman and Amos Tversky demonstrated with their research that this is how our brains are wired. People often say that evidence-based practice is nothing more than common sense, but taking an evidence-based approach can be very counterintuitive to the way human beings usually make decisions.

Another barrier is that, in the corporate environment, managers and leaders are not necessarily rewarded for doing what works; rather, they get paid to get things done. Organizations, including hospitals, often do not systematically assess the outcomes of a project or a decision. You will be hard pressed to find an organization that takes a baseline measure in order to evaluate the effectivity of a project or decision. Managers do a great job in understanding and managing power and politics, but they are less trained in the use of evidence in making decisions.

Academics are the suppliers of evidence-based practice: They produce the research outcomes we need to make evidence-based decisions. But the problem is that most of these research findings are behind the paywalls of big, multinational firms. As a result, most practitioners don't have access to research findings, unless they are affiliated with universities. Healthcare managers and hospital administrators may have access to a medical database such as PubMed, but they may not have access to social science and organizational behavior databases. The Gates Foundation has taken an enlightened approach to this problem by saying they won't fund studies unless there is open access to the research findings. In addition, the European Union, in a dramatic statement, has called for open access to all scientific papers by 2020.

Evidence summaries, such as those provided by the Cochrane and Campbell Collaboration, are a possible solution to this problem. Unfortunately, such an initiative does not exist in management yet. In fact, many academics are somewhat ambivalent toward the value of management research, and they often lack incentives to get involved in practice. Primary research on "exciting and new" phenomena is more highly valued than replication studies or meta-analyses.

What is the role of business schools in all this?

Rob Briner, the scientific director of the Center for Evidence-Based Management, has pointed out that there is a difference between the espoused and the implicit goals of business schools. The espoused goals include teaching students to think critically, to challenge assumptions, and to think for themselves. The implicit goals are students feeling successful and being fed selected bits of knowledge, management facts, and models. Students want the grade. They want entertaining narratives such as those they find in *Good to Great*, the 7S model, *Blue Ocean Strategy*, and Lean management.

I think Briner is right. We should not forget that business schools are big business. According to the National Center for Education Statistics, 20 percent of all bachelor's degrees and 25 percent of all master's degrees in the United States are degrees in business. So it's just a simple matter of supply and demand. Why would a top-ranked business school that makes millions of dollars from tuition fees and that receives high grades for student satisfaction by teaching management fads introduce evidence-based practice in its curriculum? Jeffrey Pfeffer, professor at Stanford Business School, once said that business schools are in the entertainment industry rather than the educational business. I'm afraid he is right.

What practical recommendations would you have for a CEO in a large firm who wants to use evidence-based management?

There is a lot of research out there indicating that the right organizational climate promotes asking critical questions. This happens in teaching hospitals, where it is important to ask questions regardless of whether some of the doctors around the table think the answer is obvious. The medical chief sets the example and asks questions—critical questions. Likewise, administrators and management executives must ask and be asked: "How do you know this will work? How much of a problem do we really have?" Evidence-based practice starts with an inquisitive mind-set. But asking questions can only blossom where this is cherished.

Please comment on the politics in getting firms to adopt evidence-based practice and getting junior managers to raise critical questions on-site.

After they graduate, former students working in firms are often not appreciated when they ask critical questions. It is up to senior managers to allow for the questions and demonstrate their importance, as medical chiefs do in teaching hospitals. "Is this your opinion based on your clinical experience, or is there any scientific evidence for it?" You may be surprised to learn how much uncertainty really exists regarding the practices organizations use. But of course, evidence-based practice thrives in a questioning culture—not a cocky one. So questions should be asked respectfully, in a polite way; juniors must be trained to do this. Moreover, students must understand how power works. We seek open, positive discussion. So the question is not so much "Will this work?" but "Given the target group, the problem, and the context involved, what are the main factors determining success or failure that need to be taken into account?"

Juniors must learn how to critically question rather than criticize their seniors. They are up against generations that are not accustomed to evidence-based thinking. David Sackett and Gordon Guyatt, the founders of evidence-based medicine, referred to this as a new paradigm being born. To us it may be common sense, but for many persons, it is completely new.

If someone were to give you $10 million to advance evidence-based practice, how would you choose to spend the money?
First, develop a freely accessible online database with summaries of critically appraised scientific evidence, preferably in plain English, like the Cochrane Reviews. Second, we should work to get evidence-based practice in the curricula of universities and business schools. We should not forget that evidence-based medicine started as a teaching method at McMaster University's medical school. In this age of the Internet and big data, managers are bombarded with information, and, in order to cope with this overload, their brains naturally filter out information that does not confirm their existing beliefs. By teaching evidence-based practice skills, we can help them distinguish trustworthy from less trustworthy information. But this is even more important for young people. So maybe some of the funds should be spent on a demonstration program that schools can use for free. Evidence-based practice takes minutes, as the saying goes, to learn but a lifetime to master, so let young people get an early start by teaching them the basic principles early in their professional life, maybe even at primary school.

PERSPECTIVE ON HOSPITAL PERFORMANCE

INTERVIEW WITH QUINT STUDER, STUDER GROUP, PENSACOLA, FLORIDA

This interview was conducted in June 2015.

What do you consider *evidence*?
Evidence consists of the tools, techniques, and practices put in place long enough so you can evaluate whether they improve performance and achieve desired outcomes. "Long enough" is very variable—depending on the intervention and the context, this could be under a month or over a year. For example, how often should the nurse visit the patient? Research on visit time intervals finds that if she visits every 90 minutes, there is no impact; same with every 2 hours. If she rounds every 60 minutes, patient falls decrease by 50 percent. When people see the impact of the change in behavior or process, the behavior is sustained.

If not all scientific evidence is created equal, where does the critical appraisal fit in?
It depends on what the objective measure is. There is a science and an art to leadership. The key is the direct supervisor. Research shows that workers often leave their job because they don't like their boss, who does not give them adequate consideration as an individual. Or because they don't have the tools to do the job. Gallup has the evidence to show that people leave their boss more than their job. This turnover causes major operational issues.

In healthcare, the Voluntary Hospitals of America has evidence correlating staff turnover and mortality of patients. Hospitals with turnover above a certain number show more patients dying who should be surviving. After seeing the evidence that staff turnover hurts clinical quality, the organization becomes more willing to invest in leadership development.

What does Studer expect from healthcare managers in the way of evidence-based management? Should they be able to search for evidence

in research databases themselves? Critically appraise the evidence themselves? Hire a consulting firm to do it for them?

Evidence comes to managers now. It's out there. Organizations need to bring the data to the manager, because managers are so focused on day-to-day operations that many times they don't have time to search out all the data. After helping the manager see what change is needed for better results, a system to scale the changes within the department and organization comes next.

Employees must understand the "why." The reasons should include (1) the new behavior improves life; (2) it makes the job easier, even if the effect is not immediate (for instance, changes that lead to less turnover mean the manager doesn't need to keep training new coworkers so frequently); and (3) it connects with the individual's own value system. Some of the behavior change takes time. The manager must implement systems to make sure the new behaviors are being carried out. For some people, you must carry out the behaviors with them and show them the results before they will understand the "why." Consistency is a must. Think back to when seatbelts were optional. We forced the new behavior when it became more difficult to drive without fastening. People have now gotten so used to seatbelts—and they are so clear on why seatbelts are worn—that it is uncomfortable not to buckle up. High priority should be given to helping managers understand how to best get employees to comply with change.

What are the barriers that prevent healthcare organizations from using the best available evidence in making important management decisions?
There is a lack of professional development or skill building. Most people in healthcare organizations are promoted from within—in a sense, learning to drive while driving through traffic—so managers are not clear on outcomes or priorities.

For example, in the emergency department (ED), door-to-doctor time is important for patients. A good score on this measure leads to better patient outcomes and satisfaction, so the CEO would like the scores to improve. However, the emergency department leader gets a good evaluation even though his door-to-doctor time isn't so good. If the leader is getting good evaluations despite not fixing the most important issue, the CEO, in effect, reinforces the current behavior. If the accountability is not there, behavior often does not change.

There is a certain conflict of interest between the CEO and the board of trustees. The CEO is most knowledgeable about operations, whereas many people on the board have no experience in managing hospitals. The CEO wants a good evaluation and good compensation, and there is no incentive for the CEO to give the board difficult goals for himself and make it harder for himself to get a bonus. It takes a courageous CEO to achieve desired outcomes for the organization.

How does the Studer Group's own work result in better organizational outcomes through evidence-based practice?

Clients who reach out to Studer Group already are looking to improve performance. There are three areas needed for high performance: (1) align goals, (2) align behavior, and (3) align processes. Usually, aligning processes receives the most attention. However, while some improvement for a better process will be achieved, unless the desired outcome is integrated into the evaluation tool, the gain will not hold.

For example, say the CEO has "physician engagement" measured by an outside consultant, and the scores aren't high. Or, say the scores on "patient experience" are not what the CEO wants personally or what he wants the public to see. Why would the CEO put raising these scores into his own evaluation? Commonly, hospital CEOs get 30 to 40 percent of their compensation in performance bonuses while the rest of the top leadership gets 25 to 35 percent. I suggest that the board set certain outcome measures as "door openers," and if the organization doesn't hit these measures, no bonuses are paid. Make patient experience (or physician engagement) one of your door openers for executive compensation. If you don't hit the standards, no one gets any incentive. Otherwise, the organization is wasting a lot of time and money on executive performance bonus plans.

People get hung up on the CEO needing perfect evidence, but it's not evidence that counts so much as accountability. CEOs will find the evidence. If leaders want to believe something, they don't need a lot of evidence. If there are 500 studies and 400 say better quality improves cost performance, 99 say it's inconclusive, and one says higher quality outcomes increase costs, some doc will point to the study they want to believe.

EVIDENCE-BASED MANAGEMENT: WHERE DO WE GO FROM HERE?

by Anthony R. Kovner and Thomas D'Aunno

This chapter aims to identify key questions about the future of evidence-based management (EBMgmt) that we believe are important for stakeholders to address. The questions and discussion are organized around the four sources of evidence that provided the structure for this book. Key questions and "subquestions" are shown in exhibit 27.1.

How Do We Identify the Field of Evidence-Based Management?

Evidence-based management at present lacks definitional clarity. To address this concern, we must communicate what makes evidence-based management distinctive and meaningful for its practitioners.

People commonly hold one of two extreme, opposing views about evidence-based management:

1. *The view that managers already practice evidence-based management but do not call it by that name.* Proponents of this view point out that managers make rational decisions, use evidence, and are already smart and well trained.
2. *The view that evidence-based management is an ideal that cannot be reached because of the limits of human rationality and behavior.* Proponents of this view might point to confirmation bias—the idea that managers tend to make decisions using evidence that confirms their own biases and political preferences rather than pursue the best evidence. In this view, evidence-based management is a hopeless quest.

We argue that there must be a middle ground. Authors throughout this book have insisted that managers can make better decisions based on the highest-quality available evidence. Managers should not be making decisions on faulty grounds; they should use evidence more regularly to inform their decision making.

EXHIBIT 27.1
Evidence-Based
Management:
Key Questions
and
Subquestions

Book Section	Questions	Subquestions
Overview	How do we identify the field of evidence-based management?	• What is and is not evidence-based management? • Why is it important to identify the field? • How can we disseminate a definition of the field that is recognized and validated by stakeholders?
Scientific Evidence—Doing the Work	How can we get teams to work together?	• How can we overcome language, communication, and support difficulties? • What accommodations can be made to alleviate communication difficulties?
Scientific Evidence—Examples of Practice	How can we facilitate organizational ownership of evidence-based management?	• How can we get leadership to step up to ownership responsibility? • Where in the organization should evidence-based management be based?
Organizational Evidence	How can we prepare managers to engage in evidence-based management?	• What competencies do managers have to learn? • How can managers learn these competencies? • What is the relationship between formal competencies and practice?
Experiential Evidence	How can we originate, standardize, and disseminate data on evidence-based management?	• How can we get evidence on current practice? • How can we encourage and disseminate Capstone team results? • How can we share evidence with practitioners and researchers in other countries?
Stakeholder Concerns	How can we get funders and regulators to behave as partners?	• How should we respond to critiques of practice? • How can we get funders involved in evidence-based management? • How can we get funders and regulators to use evidence-based management in their own operating practices?

Research and evidence-based management overlap considerably. The scientific evidence to answer a question is not always available—in fact, some would say it is *usually* not available—and managers often have to initiate research to collect the data they need to respond to organizational challenges. Conducting searches for evidence is costly for managers, and managers tend to dislike uncertainty. Worse, some managers have an appetite for politics and power, and they let these forces rule decision making. Even so, managers should make sure they have the best available evidence, and then they can let the politics begin. Of course, having the data for an appropriately framed and answerable research question can influence the politics of a situation as well.

The strongest argument for using evidence-based management is that it leads to improved organizational performance. Some major healthcare organizations, such as Kaiser Permanente, already appear to be convinced: They use evidence from operations to drive answerable questions and stimulate management innovations.

How Can We Get Teams to Work Together?

Much literature has focused on the difficulties people face working in teams and learning to work well together. Evidence-based management needs to be a team sport, and the effort needs to range all the way from CEOs to workers and associates on the lowest rungs. One person searching for evidence is not a viable mode. To carry out evidence-based management effectively, we need multiple perspectives to frame the question, to search for evidence, to weigh the evidence, and to respond to stakeholder values and concerns. Yes, doing things this way takes longer. But we have learned that people who participate in decisions take more ownership and better facilitate implementation.

Given the unlikelihood of an immediate, widespread, major change in training people to work together, what can be done now to improve the work of interdisciplinary teams? Where are the success stories? What has to happen for interdisciplinary teams to work well or better together? What can managers do? What can researchers do? What can clinicians and people who train clinicians do? What can librarians, professional association leadership, and journal editors and contributors do? How can members of these groups influence their own disciplinary leadership to take ownership of responding to the managerial challenge of working together in teams to better serve the patient? The path is long, and the way is wide.

How Can We Facilitate Organizational Ownership of Evidence-Based Management?

Why should EBMgmt practice and related research be funded by large healthcare organizations when these organizations currently do not see management research as a primary responsibility? What would have to take place for these organizations to step up to this ownership responsibility? We claim that the aim of evidence-based management is to improve organizational and managerial performance rather than to carry out research. At the same time, we believe organizations will step up to an ownership responsibility when they recognize that doing so is in their interest.

First, managers and researchers must show that evidence-based management works. In other words, they need to demonstrate that it results in better decisions. Second, for ownership to develop at the workplace, evidence-based management has to become the responsibility of someone who uses appropriate metrics and has accountability. How does the leadership know what kind of an investment is necessary? What is the accountability of those carrying out evidence-based management, and what are the metrics of performance?

These questions lead to another: What is the appropriate locus in the organization for furtherance and support of evidence-based management and research? Should there be a separate department of evidence-based management or management research? We are sure that lengthy managerial and academic conferences can set out to answer this question with various stakeholders claiming ownership, if only someone else will provide the funds. We also believe that large healthcare organizations will provide the funds—which, after all, are quite modest in the scheme of healthcare system investments—if leaders believe the effort is in the organizations' interest, relative to other investment opportunities.

How Can We Prepare Managers to Engage in Evidence-Based Management?

This question assumes that organizations (or schools) wish to train graduate students, and graduates of master's programs in healthcare management or related fields, in methods of managerial decision making. What competencies do they need to learn, and how should they learn these competencies?

Simply put, we argue that students must learn how to evaluate research and how to work with researchers. For us, learning to do research involves becoming competent in the six steps of the evidence-based management process, as outlined in chapter 1's discussion of basic principles. How does one learn competencies? One approach is by working on real problems for real organizations under the supervision of managers and academics who understand how to apply analytics and manage themselves as members of an interdisciplinary team. Such teams can divide work so that at least one member can master library resources and take time to talk with other members who gather the evidence and who must weigh and apply the evidence.

Unfortunately, few graduate schools of management offer courses in EBMgmt competencies. To help correct this shortcoming, appendix A provides a list of readings used in a seven-week online course on evidence-based management; additional readings are listed in appendix B.

How Can We Originate, Standardize, and Disseminate Data on Evidence-Based Management?

We need more data, including accounts from managers themselves, to understand how leaders try to respond to organizational and management challenges. The healthcare management literature lacks accounts of the thinking processes of managers and leaders in forming answerable questions, in strategizing searches among the four sources of evidence, and in communicating with managers in other similar organizations. Accounts of finding ways to finance an evidence-based process are similarly missing. And how do managers develop champions for evidence-based management in their own organizations, within the ranks of senior executives or clinical leaders or board members?

The lack of these descriptions is one reason that discouragement is common in the practice of evidence-based management. We have often heard such statements as, "There were only one or two valid and reliable studies bearing on our question," or, "Solutions in other organizations could not be adapted in our organization for many good reasons."

Who is going to pay for publishing these accounts, and why would managers and researchers want to disclose what they likely view as private information? This information is likely to include, for example, descriptions of failure. The information may also show the influence of luck in achieving success; important initiatives often depend on timing and circumstances that may not apply to another manager's organization at a later date, facing a different market.

So, who will take ownership of funding and publishing oral history projects, expanding on the work already made available by the American College of Healthcare Executives? Much can be learned from the failures of large organizations and from major change initiatives. Who will carefully review, as historians do, the narratives behind large initiatives that failed because of low-quality data? What are the lessons to be learned from their failures? What must take place among EBMgmt stakeholders to result in desired behaviors from leaders, researchers, and funders?

How Can We Get Funders and Regulators to Behave as Partners?

Evidence-based management is an innovation in the decision-making process—a new way of doing things for managers and organizations. As Adner (2006) points out, an innovation requires a supporting ecology if it is to be sustained and made widespread. The ecology of healthcare organizations consists of many stakeholders, including patients, clinicians, various health workers, managers, researchers, payers, regulators, accreditors, and taxpayers.

How can we get a powerful stakeholder, such as a funder, to become supportive of evidence-based management? Regulators provide the leverage for organizational change, and we need to develop an understanding of how to get their support for evidence-based management.

Epilogue

In 2017 and beyond, major forces impacting evidence-based management include the following:

- The healthcare field is moving from a volume-oriented to an outcome-oriented system of delivery. It is becoming more like markets for other services in the United States, with customers actively shopping, particularly online, for the services they prefer.
- Concern about costs is a priority for all stakeholders, including providers.
- Change is happening in the way customers get their care—for example, in the amount of care provided at urgent care centers, by large retail pharmacies, or online.
- Experimentation is becoming more common. Witness the number of healthcare "start-ups" in the private sector. Experimentation today is more quickly scaled up (or cut short) and varies considerably from state to state and within large states.

Given the pace and importance of these external forces of change, healthcare organizations, if they are to survive, must improve their decision-making processes. In short, they must make better and faster decisions. Responses to these external forces have included the following:

- Organizations are implementing emerging technology and producing new medical solutions, such as the field of personalized medicine.
- Funding and reimbursing agencies are increasingly focusing on paying fixed amounts for taking care of bundles of needs. They are also limiting choices among providers who will be paid or services that will be paid for.
- Healthcare providers are becoming larger and more complex. Health systems provide services formerly provided by independent providers and insurance companies, and large drugstores now offer services previously provided by large health systems.
- Consumers are becoming more deeply involved in healthcare decision making as members of health plans, as insurance policy holders, as members of chronic care organizations that provide multiple levels of services, or as taxpayers, premium payers, and shoppers.

New technology means faster, deeper change. New payment mechanisms mean new decisions and new marketing opportunities for new providers. Larger organizations require better-trained managers who can make better, faster decisions based on the best available evidence. As organizations increase in size, more opportunities emerge for special functions—such as evidence-based management—to be organized into separate centers.

We would not bet against evidence-based management becoming increasingly widespread. After all, evidence-based practice has already grown in medicine and nursing. What will this trend mean for organizations and managers? It will bring about the increasing use of metrics in healthcare to measure performance, the increasing transparency of results, and more focused accountability for performance. The advance of evidence-based management will hinge on the speed at which costs and benefits can be measured and the results of evidence-based management can be tied directly to organizational and management performance. At this time, because of a lack of high-quality evidence, we cannot make a stronger, more positive, better justified prediction for EBMgmt's prospects. This book is evidence that we still believe. We can always change our mind in the face of new and better evidence.

Reference

Adner, R. 2006. "Match Your Innovation Strategy to Your Innovation Ecosystem." *Harvard Business Review* 84 (4): 98–107.

APPENDIX A
A COURSE REFERENCE GUIDE ON
EVIDENCE-BASED MANAGEMENT

by Eric Barends

This appendix provides a guide to the references I suggested to my students in a seven-week blended online course on evidence-based management at New York University's Robert F. Wagner Graduate School of Public Service in spring of 2016. The course was not specifically about healthcare, although a number health students took the course and completed rapid evidence assessments on healthcare topics. Many of the supplemental readings listed here are perfectly appropriate for healthcare management students because they describe a process that can be applied to any subject matter. Please note, however, that the resources listed in this appendix are mostly just starting points; you will still need to conduct your own searches for relevant material.

The readings have been arranged in sections under various headings, but these headings are for guidance only. Many of the resources could appear under more than one heading, and the chapters from *The Oxford Handbook of Evidence-Based Management* would be appropriate in almost every section.

General Evidence-Based Management Books

Latham, G. P. 2009. *Becoming the Evidence-Based Manager: Making the Science of Management Work for You.* Boston: Davies-Black.
Locke, E. A. 2009. *Handbook of Principles of Organizational Behavior: Indispensable Knowledge for Evidence-Based Management.* New York: Wiley.
Pearce, J. L. 2009. *Organizational Behavior: Real Research for Real Managers,* 2nd ed. Irvine, CA: Melvin Leigh.

Pfeffer, J., and Sutton, R. I. 2006. *Hard Facts, Dangerous Half-Truths and Total Nonsense: Profiting from Evidence-Based Management*. Boston: Harvard Business School Press.

Rousseau, D. M. (ed.). 2012. *The Oxford Handbook of Evidence-Based Management*. New York: Oxford University Press.

Principles of Evidence-Based Management

Briner, R. B. 2007. *Is HRM Evidence-Based and Does It Matter?* Institute for Employment Studies. Available at www.cebma.org/wp-content/uploads/Briner-Is-HRM-evidence-based-and-does-it-matter.pdf.

———. 2000. "Evidence-Based Human Resource Management." In *Evidence-Based Practice: A Critical Appraisal*, edited by L. Trinder and S. Reynolds, 184–211. London: Blackwell Science.

Briner, R. B., D. Denyer, and D. M. Rousseau. 2009. "Evidence-Based Management: Construct Cleanup Time?" *Academy of Management Perspectives* 23 (4): 19–32.

Briner, R. B., and D. M. Rousseau. 2011. "Evidence-Based I-O Psychology: Not There Yet." *Industrial and Organizational Psychology* 4 (1): 3–22.

———. 2011. "Evidence-Based I-O Psychology: Not There Yet but Now a Little Nearer?" *Industrial and Organizational Psychology* 4 (1): 76–82.

Pfeffer, J., and R. I. Sutton. 2006. "Management Half-Truths and Nonsense: How to Practice Evidence-Based Management." *California Management Review* 48 (3): 77–100.

Rousseau, D. M. 2006. "Is There Such a Thing as Evidence-Based Management?" *Academy of Management Review* 31 (2): 256–69.

Rousseau, D. M., and E. Barends. 2011. "Becoming an Evidence-Based HR Practitioner." *Human Resource Management Journal* 21 (3): 221–35.

Relationships Between Academic and Practitioner Knowledge and Action

Anderson, N., P. Herriot, and G. P. Hodgkinson. 2001. "The Practitioner–Researcher Divide in Industrial, Work and Organizational (IWO) Psychology: Where Are We Now and Where Do We Go from Here?" *Journal of Occupational and Organizational Psychology* 74 (4): 391–411.

Bansal, T., S. Bertels, T. Ewart, P. MacConnachie, and J. O'Brien. 2012. "Bridging the Research–Practice Gap." *Academy of Management Perspectives* 26 (1): 73–92.

Bartunek, J. M. 2007. "Academic–Practitioner Collaboration Need Not Require Joint or Relevant Research: Towards a Relational Scholarship of Integration." *Academy of Management Journal* 50 (6): 1323–33.

Bartunek, J. M., and S. L. Rynes. 2010. "The Construction and Contributions of Implications for Practice: What's in Them and What Might They Offer?" *Academy of Management Learning & Education* 9 (1): 100–117.

Cascio, W. F. 2007. "Evidence-Based Management and the Marketplace for Ideas." *Academy of Management Journal* 50 (5): 1009–12.

Cohen, D. J. 2007. "The Very Separate Worlds of Academic and Practitioner Publications in Human Resource Management: Reasons for the Divide and Concrete Solutions for Bridging the Gap." *Academy of Management Journal* 50 (5): 1013–19.

Hodgkinson, G. P., and D. M. Rousseau. 2009. "Bridging the Rigour–Relevance Gap in Management Research: It's Already Happening." *Journal of Management Studies* 46 (3): 534–46.

Lawler, E. 2007. "Why HR Practices Are Not Evidence-Based." *Academy of Management Journal* 50 (5): 1033–36.

Rynes, S. L., J. M. Bartunek, and R. L. Daft. 2001. "Across the Great Divide: Knowledge Creation and Transfer Between Practitioners and Academics." *Academy of Management Journal* 44 (2): 340–56.

Rynes, S. L., K. G. Brown, and A. E. Colbert. 2002. "Seven Common Misconceptions About Human Resource Practices: Research Findings Versus Practitioner Beliefs." *Academy of Management Executive* 16 (3): 92–103.

Rynes, S. L., A. E. Colbert, and K. G. Brown. 2002. "HR Professionals' Beliefs About Effective Human Resource Practices: Correspondence Between Research and Practice." *Human Resource Management* 41 (2): 149–74.

Rynes, S. L., T. L. Giluk, and K. G. Brown. 2007. "The Very Separate Worlds of Academic and Practitioner Periodicals in Human Resource Management: Implications for Evidence-Based Management." *Academy of Management Journal* 50 (5): 987–1008.

Sanders, K., M. van Riemsdijk, and B. Groen. 2008. "The Gap Between Research and Practice: A Replication Study of HR Professionals' Beliefs About Effective Human Resource Practices." *International Journal of Human Resource Management* 19 (10): 1976–88.

Shapiro, D. L., B. L. Kirkman, and H. G. Courtney. 2007. "Perceived Causes and Solutions of the Translation Problem in Management Research." *Academy of Management Journal* 50 (2): 249–66.

Teaching and Training in Evidence-Based Management

Barends, E. G., and R. B. Briner. 2014. "Teaching Evidence-Based Practice: Lessons From the Pioneers—An Interview with Amanda Burls and Gordon Guyatt." *Academy of Management Learning & Education* 13 (3): 476–83.

Briner, R. B., and N. D. Walshe. 2014. "From Passively Received Wisdom to Actively Constructed Knowledge: Teaching Systematic Review Skills as a Foundation of Evidence-Based Management." *Academy of Management Learning & Education* 13 (3): 415–32.

Burke, L. A., and B. Rau. 2010. "The Research–Teaching Gap in Management." *Academy of Management Learning & Education* 9 (1): 132–43.

Charlier, S., K. Brown, and S. Rynes. 2011. "Teaching Evidence-Based Management in MBA Programs: What Evidence Is There?" *Academy of Management Learning & Education* 10 (2): 222–36.

Graen, G. B. 2009. "Educating New Management Specialists from an Evidence-Based Perspective: A Proposal." *Academy of Management Learning & Education* 8 (2): 255–58.

Rousseau, D. M., and S. McCarthy. 2007. "Educating Managers from an Evidence-Based Perspective." *Academy of Management Learning & Education* 6 (1): 84–101.

Rynes, S. L., D. M. Rousseau, and E. Barends. 2014. "From the Guest Editors: Change the World: Teach Evidence-Based Practice!" *Academy of Management Learning & Education* 13 (3): 305–21.

Critiques of Evidence-Based Management

Learmonth, M. 2008. "Evidence-Based Management: A Backlash Against Pluralism in Organizational Studies." *Organization* 15 (2): 283–91.

Morrell, K. 2008. "The Narrative of 'Evidence Based Management': A Polemic." *Journal of Management Studies* 45 (3): 613–35.

Reay, T., W. Berta, and M. K. Kohn. 2009. "What's the Evidence on Evidence-Based Management?" *Academy of Management Perspectives* 23 (4): 5–18.

Tourish, D. 2012. "'Evidence Based Management' or 'Evidence Oriented Organizing'? A Critical Realist Perspective." *Organization* 20 (2): 173–92.

Rapid Evidence Assessments (REAs), Systematic Reviews, and Research Syntheses

Briner, R. B., and D. Denyer. 2012. "Systematic Review and Evidence Synthesis as a Practice and Scholarship Tool." In *The Oxford Handbook of Evidence-Based Management*, edited by D. M. Rousseau, 112–29. New York: Oxford University Press.

Denyer, D., and D. Tranfield. 2009. "Producing a Systematic Review." In *The SAGE Handbook of Organizational Research Methods*, edited by D. A. Buchanan and A. Bryman, 671–89. London: Sage Publications.

Gough, D., S. Oliver, and J. Thomas. 2012. *An Introduction to Systematic Reviews*. London: Sage.

Littell, J. H., J. Corcoran, and V. Pillai. 2008. *Systematic Reviews and Meta-Analysis.* New York: Oxford University Press.

Pawson, R. 2006. *Evidence-Based Policy: A Realist Perspective.* London: Sage.

Petticrew, M., and H. Roberts. 2006. *Systematic Reviews in the Social Sciences: A Practical Guide.* Oxford, UK: Blackwell Publishing.

Rousseau, D., J. Manning, and D. Denyer. 2008. "Evidence in Management and Organization Science: Assembling the Field's Full Weight of Scientific Knowledge Through Syntheses." *Academy of Management Annals* 2 (1): 475–515.

Tranfield, D., D. Denyer, and P. Smart. 2003. "Toward a Methodology for Developing Evidence-Informed Management Knowledge by Means of Systematic Review." *British Journal of Management* 14: 207–22.

Evidence-Based Practice, REAs, and Systematic Reviews in Healthcare

Glasziou, P., L. Irwig, C. Bain, and G. Colditz. 2001. *Systematic Reviews in Health Care: A Practical Guide.* Cambridge, UK: Cambridge University Press.

Hemingway, P., and N. Brereton. 2009. "What Is a Systematic Review?" Hayward Medical Communications. Published April. www.medicine.ox.ac.uk/bandolier /painres/download/whatis/syst-review.pdf.

Higgins, J. P. T., and S. Green (eds.). 2011. *Cochrane Handbook for Systematic Reviews of Interventions.* Updated March. http://handbook.cochrane.org.

Khan, K. S., R. Kunz, J. Kleijnen, and G. Antes. 2003. "Five Steps to Conducting a Systematic Review." *Journal of the Royal Society of Medicine* 96 (3): 118–21.

Kovner, A. R., D. J. Fine, and R. D'Aquila. 2009. *Evidence-Based Management in Healthcare.* Chicago: Health Administration Press.

Sackett, D. L., S. E. Straus, W. S. Richardson, W. Rosenberg, and R. B. Haynes. 2000. *Evidence-Based Medicine: How to Practice and Teach EBM.* New York: Churchill Livingstone.

Examples of Systematic Reviews and REAs Relevant to Human Resources Management

Bamberger, S. G., A. L. Vinding, A. Larsen, P. Nielsen, K. Fonager, R. N. Nielsen, P. Ryom, and Ø. Ormand. 2012. "Impact of Organisational Change on Mental Health: A Systematic Review." *Occupational and Environmental Medicine* 69 (8): 592–98.

Carr, S. C., M. MacLachlan, M. Clarke, T. S. Papola, C. Normand, S. Thomas, E. McAuliffe, and C. Leggatt-Cook. 2010. *What Is the Evidence of the Impact of Increasing Salaries on Improving the Performance of Public Servants,*

Including Teachers, Nurses, and Judges? Palmerston North, New Zealand: Massey University.

Cho, Y., and T. M. Egan. 2009. "Action Learning Research: A Systematic Review and Conceptual Framework." *Human Resource Development Review* 8 (4): 431–62.

Egan, M., C. Bambra, S. Thomas, M. Petticrew, M. Whitehead, and H. Thomson. 2007. "The Psychosocial and Health Effects of Workplace Reorganisation 1: A Systematic Review of Organisational-Level Interventions That Aim to Increase Employee Control." *Journal of Epidemiology and Community Health* 61 (11): 945–54.

Joyce, K., R. Pabayo, J. A. Critchley, and C. Bambra. 2010. "Flexible Working Conditions and Their Effects on Employee Health and Wellbeing." Cochrane Library. Published February 17. www.cochrane.org/CD008009/PUBHLTH _flexible-working-conditions-and-their-effects-on-employee-health-and -wellbeing.

Patterson, M., J. Rick, S. Wood, C. Carroll, S. Balain, and A. Booth. 2010. "Systematic Review of the Links Between Human Resource Management Practices and Performance." *Health Technology Assessment* 14 (51): 1–334.

Skakon, J., K. Nielsen, V. Borg, and J. Guzman. 2010. "Are Leaders' Well-Being Behaviours and Style Associated with the Affective Well-Being of Their Employees? A Systematic Review of Three Decades of Research." *Work and Stress* 24 (2): 107–39.

How to Read Research Articles

Durbin, C. G. Jr. "How to Read a Scientific Research Paper." *Respiratory Care* 54 (10): 1366–71.

Jordan, C. H., and M. P. Zanna. 1999. "How to Read a Journal Article in Social Psychology." University of Waterloo. Accessed August 18, 2016. http://arts .uwaterloo.ca/~sspencer/psych253/readart.html.

Keshav, S. 2016. "How to Read a Paper." Research paper, University of Waterloo. Published February 17. http://blizzard.cs.uwaterloo.ca/keshav/home /Papers/data/07/paper-reading.pdf.

Mitzenmacher, M. 2010. "How to Read a Research Paper." Harvard University, John A. Paulson School of Engineering and Applied Sciences. Updated August 26. www.eecs.harvard.edu/~michaelm/CS222/ReadPaper.pdf.

Websites Relevant to Evidence-Based Management

Campbell Collaboration (library of systematic reviews related to education, crime and justice, and social welfare, plus guidance for conducting reviews): www .campbellcollaboration.org

Carnegie Mellon University Libraries page for a course on evidence-based management: http://guides.library.cmu.edu/content.php?pid=149531 sid=1270070

Center for Evidence-Based Management (aimed at practitioners and managers): www.cebma.org

Cochrane Collaboration (database of systematic reviews relevant to healthcare and resources for conducting systematic reviews): www.cochrane.org

Evidence for Policy and Practice Information and Co-ordinating Centre, part of the Social Science Research Unit at the Institute of Education, University of London (library of systematic reviews relevant to education and social policy, with guidance about conducting reviews and systematic review software): http://eppi.ioe.ac.uk/cms

JAMA Evidence (American Medical Association site that provides guides to the systematic consideration of validity, importance, and applicability of claims about the health problems and outcomes of healthcare): www.jamaevidence.com

Presentation by J. Bettany-Saltikov and K. Sanderson (collection of slides about systematic reviews in medicine): www.rcn.org.uk/__data/assets/pdf_file/0008/318968/2010_RCN_research_workshop_5.pdf

Presentations from the Center for Evidence-Based Management (freely downloadable presentations): www.cebma.org/presentations

Research for development outputs, from the British government's Department for International Development (systematic reviews relevant to evidence-based policy): www.dfid.gov.uk/r4d/systematicreviews.aspx

University of British Columbia Master of Rehabilitation Science program, examples of critically appraised topics: www.mrsc.ubc.ca/site_page.asp?pageid=98

APPENDIX B
STARTER SET OF ADDITIONAL READINGS ABOUT EVIDENCE-BASED MANAGEMENT IN HEALTHCARE

by Anthony R. Kovner

Appendix A presented an excellent reference guide prepared by Eric Barends as part of his course syllabus on evidence-based management (EBMgmt). That guide included dozens of useful resources for evidence-based practice (EBP), but only a limited number dealing specifically with evidence-based management in healthcare. To complement that guide, I have compiled a starter set of additional readings for evidence-based management in healthcare. The sources are listed here and presented with annotations. In selecting articles for inclusion, I looked for those that are relatively recent (preferred publication date of 2007 or later), can be easily applied to healthcare, and are of high quality and readability. In addition, the "Inside the Readings" boxes that accompany this appendix provide reflections from several chapter authors about the articles that most powerfully influenced their thinking.

Highlighted Selections

Axelsson, R. 1998. "Towards an Evidence Based Health Care Management." *International Journal of Health Planning and Management* 13 (4): 307–17.

> *The author describes an evidence-based approach to healthcare management and the skills managers will need to have to implement it.*

Barends, E., and R. B. Briner. 2014. "Teaching Evidence-Based Practice: Lessons from the Pioneers—An Interview with Amanda Burls and Gordon Guyatt." *Academy of Management Learning & Education* 13 (3): 476–83.

> *Pioneers in the field offer lessons in teaching evidence-based medicine.*

Barends, E., D. M. Rousseau, and R. B. Briner. 2014. *Evidence-Based Management: The Basic Principles.* Amsterdam, the Netherlands: Center for Evidence-Based Management.

Not focused on healthcare but completely applicable, this is the place to start in reading about EBMgmt. The article has been adapted as chapter 1 of this book.

Damschroder, L. J., D. C. Aron, R. E. Keith, S. R. Kirsh, J. A. Alexander, and J. C. Lowery. 2009. "Fostering Implementation of Health Services Research Findings into Practice: A Consolidated Framework for Advancing Implementation Science." *Implementation Science.* Published August 7. https://implementation science.biomedcentral.com/articles/10.1186/1748-5908-4-50.

The authors present an example of contributions by the implementation science school of management theory, with an impressive list of references.

INSIDE THE READINGS

Thomas Rundall writes:

On the frontispiece of the now famous Institute of Medicine book Crossing the Quality Chasm *is a quote from Goethe: "Knowing is not enough; we must apply. Willing is not enough; we must do." In his foundational article on evidence-based healthcare management,* **Axelsson** *eloquently channels his inner Goethe, critiquing the management research prevalent at the time for its lack of relevance to practicing managers and for leaving managers vulnerable to influence by fashionable models and concepts that are seldom, if ever, put to empirical examination. While acknowledging the limitations of Frederick Taylor's "scientific management" (e.g., human needs were grossly neglected in the designs of organizations) and the challenges to research-based decision making from some academic quarters (e.g., the perspective that organizations are cultural phenomena and the role of research is to understand different aspects of organizational life), Axelsson cogently lays out the basic arguments for and principles of evidence-based management for healthcare organizations, and he implores managers to use the knowledge gained through this approach to improve healthcare for patients.*

Axelsson's vision of evidence-based healthcare management was stimulated by recent developments in evidence-based medicine, but he was acutely aware of the important differences in the nature of the work and in the ways research can be done on the work of these two fields. While taking those differences into consideration, he persuasively argued that some fundamental ideas and approaches from evidence-based medicine can and should be applied to management: "Evidence Based Management means that managers should be encouraged to examine the scientific basis for their practice. They should learn to search and critically appraise empirical evidence from management research as a basis for their decisions. This will raise a lot of questions: What do we know empirically about different aspects of organization and management? What is the scientific state of this knowledge? What is the effectiveness and efficiency of different models of management? What is the experience of these models from different organizations?"

Axelsson concluded: "Such questions will have important implications both for management practice and management research"—a remarkably understated call for fundamental transformations in the way management research is conducted and communicated, the relationships among managers and researchers, and the decision-making processes within healthcare organizations.

Denise M. Rousseau writes:

As an educator in two schools of management at Carnegie Mellon—one business and the other public policy—I have spent the last few years trying to figure out how to teach evidence-based management. I started with some basic ideas about the four sources of evidence relevant to management practice and worked to flesh out ways that students of management, and managers themselves, might learn to ask practice questions and then gather and appraise relevant evidence.

When **Barends and Briner** published their interview with two of the leading lights of evidence-based medicine, Gordon Guyatt and Amanda Burls, some powerful ideas were brought center stage for me. The first is that there is a big difference between helping people appraise the quality of the evidence and enabling them to actually use that evidence well. Guyatt and Burls make the point that practitioners often have to use the evidence they find even if its quality is less than ideal. The upshot of this insight is that translating evidence into practice often involves incorporating doubt and uncertainty into the way a decision is implemented. If considerable uncertainty characterizes the available evidence, the practitioner may need to execute the decision in small, gradual steps, monitoring results at each step to figure out whether and how to proceed. In contrast, if the evidence is strong and *clear, more complex programs of activities might be put in place to be evaluated at their completion.*

A second point involves the importance of basing learning activities around real problems learners face—that is, where learners face anxieties and concerns in addressing an issue, and where evidence quality is likely to be variable. For a manager, the issue may be a business problem; for a student, it might be a problem related to the study group, where the learner has skin in the game and faces real constraints. As Guyatt points out, the model of teaching at McMaster University School of Medicine, where evidence-based medicine began, involves small-group, problem-based, interactive learning.

A third point is that people forget a lot of what we teach them, so we have to inspire them and promote an attitude toward their decisions and professional conduct. It is important that we tell stories that motivate people to engage in evidence-based practice in the future and that we teach skills to a sufficient depth that people grasp the basic principles of evidence-based practice. We need to prepare people to keep learning, because evidence-based practice is a career and not a course.

Anthony R. Kovner writes:

When Evidence-Based Management: The Basic Principles *by **Barends, Rousseau, and Briner** appeared, so many things became clear to me that hadn't been clear before. I understood the basic principles of evidence-based medicine and realized that they could be applied successfully to management. But I had been used to hearing the detractors of evidence-based management, and now suddenly I had answers to all the questions that were answerable.*

The first insight is that evidence-based management does not rely only on the scientific literature. There is more than that to making decisions based on the best evidence.

The second insight is that managers don't usually make decisions based on the best available evidence. The authors explain that personal judgment is highly susceptible to biases that have negative effects on the quality of the decisions we make. In making decisions, managers often seek to confirm existing intuitions rather than get new evidence that suggests other alternatives.

A third insight involves the importance of asking the right question—that is, of translating a management challenge into an answerable question. Managers sometimes rush to solutions without carefully thinking through whether they have asked the right question. For example, "How do we decrease emergency department waiting time?" may be less answerable than "What are the factors that hold up admitting emergency department patients to inpatient beds?"

The authors don't answer all my questions about evidence-based management, nor do they pretend to. In any organization, politics is still involved in making and implementing decisions. The authors do, however, help generate a strong case for showing decision makers that it is in their interest to use an evidence-based process in decision making.

Finally, the article tells us that we need research to determine the benefit from using evidence-based practice relative to the cost of using it. This was a conclusion the authors didn't push but which I came to on my own after reading the article over again (and I have reread the article numerous times since).

Maja Djukic writes:

I experienced the benefits of evidence-based clinical practice while working as a critical care nurse almost ten years ago. The medical director of an intensive care unit in a hospital in Tulsa, Oklahoma, came in one day and announced that, from that day forward, we were to use evidence-based practice protocols to manage the care of critically ill patients for such issues as rapid extubation after open-heart surgery and insulin titration. Implementing these evidence-based protocols gave me, as a registered nurse, great autonomy to manage patients safely and promptly without having to wait for covering physicians to respond and come up with their own treatment preferences. Then, I started working as a travel nurse and quickly noticed great variations in the extent to which hospitals used an EBP approach and negative outcomes for patients in hospitals that had not yet implemented the approach. This observation piqued my interest in why some organizations are able to implement and sustain EBP and others are not.

The reading by **Damschroder and colleagues**, which synthesizes information from different implementation science frameworks, gave me sudden insight into the complexities of EBP implementation and the importance of managers in facilitating the process. I have used the article to guide my work on nurse manager implementation of management-focused EBP to ensure an organizational context that is optimally primed for implementation and sustainability of clinically-focused EBP.

> While many clinicians now routinely use the best available clinical evidence in their practice, getting managers to use the best available evidence for optimally managing the workforce, work environment, and finances, for example, is a challenge yet to be conquered. Marrying management-focused EBP and clinically focused EBP is necessary for achieving optimal patient outcomes.

Additional Selections for Further Reading

Bayer, R., D. M. Johns, and S. Galea. 2012. "Salt and Public Health: Contested Science and the Challenge of Evidence-Based Decision-Making." *Health Affairs* 31 (12): 2738–46.

The authors provide an example of the application of evidence-based practice to public health.

Berwick, D. M. 2008. "The Science of Improvement." *Journal of the American Medical Association* 299 (10): 1182–84.

This commentary shows the importance of adjusting research methods to fit research questions.

———. 2007. "Eating Soup with a Fork." Plenary address to the National Forum on Quality Improvement in Health Care, Orlando, FL, December 11. Reprinted in *Promising Care: How We Can Rescue Health Care by Improving It*, by D. M. Berwick, 104–21. Hoboken, NJ: Jossey-Bass.

Berwick provides an argument in favor of evidence-based practice as a preferred approach for dealing with "messy" problems. The entire book is highly recommended.

Brownson, R. C., J. E. Fielding, and C. M. Maylahn. 2009. "Evidence-Based Public Health: A Fundamental Concept for Public Health Practice." *Annual Review of Public Health* 30: 175–201.

The authors present the best review of concepts for evidence-based public health, with a discussion of challenges to and opportunities for implementation.

Gillam, S., and A. N. Siriwardena. 2014. "Evidence-Based Healthcare and Quality Improvement." *Quality in Primary Care* 22 (3): 125–32.

Evidence-based practice shares process-based intervention approaches with the quality improvement movement. This article explores the relationship between evidence-based healthcare and quality improvement, implementation science, and the translation of evidence to improve healthcare practice and patient outcomes.

Groopman, J. E. 2009. "Diagnosis: What Doctors Are Missing." *New York Review of Books.* Published November 5. www.nybooks.com/articles/2009/11/05/diagnosis-what-doctors-are-missing.

This article discusses the approximately 10 to 15 percent of all patients who either suffer from delays in correct diagnosis or die before a correct diagnosis is made. Managers, too, work with imperfect information.

Harlos, K., J. Tetroe, I. D. Graham, M. Bird, and N. Robinson. 2012. "Mining the Management Literature for Insights into Implementing Evidence-Based Change in Healthcare." *Healthcare Policy* 8 (1): 33–48.

The authors' syntheses of management and health literatures offer insights into the implementation of evidence-based change in healthcare.

Kovner, A. R., J. J. Elton, and J. Billings. 2000. "Evidence-Based Management." *Frontiers of Health Services Management* 16 (4): 3–24.

My first publication on evidence-based management calls for the establishment of EBMgmt cooperatives between health systems and research centers to improve healthcare management practice.

Kovner, A. R., D. J. Fine, and R. D'Aquila. 2009. *Evidence-Based Management in Health Care,* 1st ed. Chicago: Health Administration Press.

Note in particular Sara Mody's suggestions for additional readings in chapter 8, "Look It Up," and the case studies by Philip DeSalvio, Ann Scheck McAlearney, Arthur Webb and Ellen Flaherty, Kenneth R. White and J. Brian Cassel, Jancy Strauman, Megin Wolfman, and Patricia Gail Bray that were not included in this second edition.

Lavis, J. N., H. T. O. Davies, R. L. Gruen, K. Walshe, and C. M. Farquhar. 2006. "Working Within and Beyond the Cochrane Collaboration to Make Systematic Reviews More Useful to Healthcare Management." *Healthcare Policy* 1 (2): 21–33.

Lavis, J. N., A. D. Oxman, S. Lewin, and A. Fretheim. 2009. "Support Tools for Evidence-Informed Health Policymaking." *Health Research Policy and Systems* 7 (Suppl. 1): 1–7.

Lavis and colleagues are leaders in Canadian scholarship focused on evidence-based management. These articles describe (1) ways to make systematic reviews more useful and (2) support technology and assistance for managers seeking to practice evidence-based management.

Parand, A., S. Dopson, A. Renz, and C. Vincent. 2014. "The Role of Hospital Managers in Quality and Patient Safety: A Systematic Review." *BMJ Open* 4 (9): 1–15.

This article focuses on hospital managers' role in quality improvement, with an example of doing a systematic review.

Rousseau, D. M. (ed.). 2012. *The Oxford Handbook of Evidence-Based Management.* New York: Oxford University Press.

This rich collection comprises 23 chapters, many of which are applicable to health-care management and evidence-based medicine. Chapters include "Learning from Other Evidence-Based Practices: The Case of Medicine," "Research Findings Practitioners Resist: Lessons for Management Academics from Evidence-Based Medicine," and "The Politics of Evidence-Based Decision Making."

Rundall, T. G., P. Martelli, L. Arroyo, R. McCurdy, I. Graetz, E. Neuwirth, P. Curtis, J. Schmittdiel, M. Gibson, and J. Hsu. 2007. "The Informed Decisions Toolbox: Tools for Knowledge Transfer and Performance Improvement." *Journal of Healthcare Management* 52 (5): 325–42.

This toolbox provides a guide to assist managers engaged in the six steps of evidence-based management decision making. Four leadership strategies are suggested to build an organizational environment conducive to EBMgmt.

Shortell, S. M., T. G. Rundall, and J. Hsu. 2007. "Improving Patient Care by Linking Evidence-Based Medicine and Evidence-Based Management." *Journal of the American Medical Association* 298 (6): 673–76.

This article suggests that, until practitioners identify the best content (as in evidence-based medicine) and apply it within effective organizational contexts (as in evidence-based management), consistent, sustainable improvement in the quality of care received in the United States is unlikely to occur.

White, K. R., S. Thompson, and J. R. Griffith. 2011. "Transforming the Dominant Logic of Hospitals." *Advances in Health Care Management* 11: 133–45.

This article suggests moving toward a more transformational style of problem analysis and decision making. Recommendations include visioning, sense making, process questioning, getting the right people together, rewarding innovation, and overcoming risk aversion.

Woten, M. 2015. "National Patient Safety Goals: The Joint Commission." EBSCO Information Services. Published March 20. www.ebscohost.com/images -nursing/assets/national-patient-safety-goals-the-joint-commission-2015.pdf.

This document provides context for EBMgmt from The Joint Commission's accreditation point of view, with aims to improve patient safety.

INDEX

Note: Italicized page locators refer to figures or tables in exhibits.

AAFP. *See* American Academy of Family Physicians (AAFP)

AAP. *See* American Academy of Pediatrics (AAP)

ABI/INFORM, 93

Ability to practice, 123–27; foundational competencies, 123–24; functional competencies, 123, 124–27

Abstracts, 89, 90, 98

Academic literature, searching. *See* Literature searches

Academic medical centers: Canadian, perioperative services, nursing productivity, and patient flow at, 288–92; evidence-based healthcare management at Yale New Haven, 317–23

Academics, as suppliers of evidence-based practice, 344

Accountability, 348, 357; better organizational outcomes and, 349; as impetus for evidence-based healthcare management, 293; organizational ownership of evidence-based management and, 354

Accountable care models: cancer care and, 333

Accountable care organizations: growing percentage of physicians in, 214

Accreditation Council for Graduate Medical Education, 49

ACHE. *See* American College of Healthcare Executives (ACHE)

ACL Analytics, 240

ACP. *See* American College of Physicians (ACP)

Acquiring step, in EBP, 4; Capstone teams and, 270; develop phase in Carpedia project delivery and, 285, 286–87; in evidence-based management, 85, 86; filtering with limits, 95, 97; integrated chronic care management of depression and, 203, 206; at Lyndon B. Johnson General Hospital, 237; preformulated searches and summaries and, 97–98; sources of evidence and, 7; systematically searching for/retrieving evidence, 92–98; translating focused question into search strategy, 93, 95

Acquisition of research evidence: for block scheduling for operating room use, 289–90; functional competencies and, 125; for HT Program in Late Stage Kidney Disease, 153–58; iterative nature of, 88, *89*

Action OI data, 239, 241, 242

Active management: micromanagement *vs.*, 285

Acute myocardial infarction (AMI): organizational evidence example, 70–71

Advanced Workplace Associates (AWA), 24

Index

389

Intervention: scoping search and, 85

Interviews with healthcare managers: experiential evidence example, 74–75

IOM. *See* Institute of Medicine (IOM)

IS. *See* Information sharing (IS)

Job satisfaction: organizational evidence example, 73

Job-shadowing employees: consultants engaged in observation and, 280–81

Johns Hopkins University: Business in Government (BIG) Initiative at, 131–33

Joint Commission, The: disaster planning recommendations, 181, 193

Journal of Healthcare Management, 67

Junior managers: critical questioning by, 346

"Just culture": at Hill Country Memorial, 54

Kahneman, Daniel, 344

Kaiser Foundation Health Plan (KFHP), 217

Kaiser Permanente, 59, 78, 213–31, 353; engineering the care delivery system, 213, 215–19; on the horizon: evidence leading to excellence, 229–30; introduction, 213–14; Northern California Appointment and Advice Call Center, 217–19; OpQ project: evidence leading to excellence, 224–29; scope and scale of care at, *216*; Southern California Regional Outpatient SureNet: evidence leading to excellence, 220–24; system-level care engineering and high-level healthcare at, 230–31; Vioxx case and, 341

Kaiser Permanente Northern California (KPNC), 217

Kaiser Permanente Northern California Appointment and Advice Call Center (AACC): scale demands design at, 217–19

Kaiser Permanente Southern California Regional Outpatient SureNet, 230; abnormal diagnostic test monitoring and, 222; chronic kidney disease detection/treatment and, 220, 222; evidence leading to excellence and, 220–24; goal of, 220; medication safety and, 222, *223*; SMES (subject matter experts and stakeholders) panel, 223; tracking effectiveness of, 224

KDOQI. *See* Kidney Disease Outcomes Quality Initiative (KDOQI)

Kelvin, William, 305

Key performance indicators (KPIs), 300; benchmarks, 302; planning-related problems and, 283

KFHP. *See* Kaiser Foundation Health Plan (KFHP)

Kidney disease, late stage. *See* Northwell Health, Healthy Transitions (HT) Program in Late Stage Kidney Disease

Kidney Disease Outcomes Quality Initiative (KDOQI), 156

Knowledge practices: overview of, 99–102

Knowledge transfer between disciplines: practitioner skills and, 126–27

Knowledge work: assessing level of, 27; definitions of, elements in, 26–27

Knowledge workers: definitions of, elements in, 26–27; rapid evidence assessment of performance of, 23, 24–40

Kovner, Anthony R., 299; "Inside the Readings" reflection by, 370–71

KPIs. *See* Key performance indicators

ABOUT THE EDITORS

Anthony R. Kovner, PhD, is a professor at the Robert F. Wagner Graduate School of Public Service, New York University (NYU), and was director of its health policy and management program for 16 years. He was the fourth recipient on the Filerman Prize for Educational Leadership from the Association of Programs in Health Administration. At NYU, he developed the health program Capstone course and the executive master of public administration program for nurse leaders. He has written 11 books, mostly coedited, and more than 90 peer-reviewed articles, many of them case studies. Kovner has been a senior manager at two hospitals, a nursing home, a group practice, and a neighborhood health center, as well as a senior healthcare consultant for a large industrial union. He has been a leader in the evidence-based management movement and served as a founding member of the Academic Council of the Center for Evidence-Based Management.

Thomas D'Aunno, PhD, is the faculty director of the health policy and management program in the Robert F. Wagner Graduate School of Public Service at New York University. D'Aunno's research and teaching focus on the organization and management of healthcare services. He has a particular interest in organizational change and the diffusion and adoption of evidence-based management and clinical practices. He has examined these issues in a variety of national studies funded by the National Institutes of Health and the Agency for Healthcare Research and Quality. He has served as a faculty member at Columbia University, the University of Chicago, and the University of Michigan, as well as at INSEAD (the European Institute of Business Administration), where he held the Novartis Chair in Healthcare Management. In 2014, he became the editor-in-chief of *Medical Care Research and Review*. He also is a past chairman of the Academy of Management Division of Health Care Management and a recipient of the division's award for career distinguished service.

ABOUT THE CONTRIBUTORS

Sofia Agoritsas, FACHE, is a Fellow of the American College of Healthcare Executives who has multiple years of executive-level health system experience. She has served as the senior administrative director for nephrology and dialysis at Northwell Health since 2012. She was responsible for developing and implementing the Healthy Transitions Program in Late Stage Kidney Disease at Northwell Health.

Eric Barends, PhD, is the managing director of the Center for Evidence-Based Management. He has 20 years of management experience—15 years at the senior management level, including 5 years as an executive. He advises and coaches managers, senior leaders, and executive boards of large and medium-sized companies and nonprofit organizations on evidence-based decision making. In addition, he frequently runs training courses on the topic and serves as a visiting lecturer at universities and business schools.

Ethan Basch, MD, is a practicing medical oncologist at the University of North Carolina, where he is professor of medicine and public health and director of the Cancer Outcomes Research Program. He serves on the Board of Scientific Advisors of the National Cancer Institute, on the Methodology Committee of the Patient-Centered Outcomes Research Institute, and as an associate editor for the *Journal of the American Medical Association.* Dr. Basch's research focuses on bringing the patient voice into cancer clinical care and research.

John Billings, JD, is professor of health policy and public service at the Robert F. Wagner Graduate School of Public Service at New York University. He has been involved in numerous projects to assess the performance of the safety net for vulnerable populations and to understand barriers to optimal health. A founding member of the Foundation for Informed Decision Making, Billings works to provide patients with a clearer mechanism for making decisions about a variety of available treatments. Billings received his JD from the University of California, Berkeley.

Rob B. Briner, PhD, is professor of organizational psychology at the University of Bath's School of Management and a founding member of the Center for Evidence-Based Management. His main research interests for more than 25 years center on the reciprocal links between work conditions, psychological well-being, and various behaviors (e.g., engagement, job crafting). Dr. Briner was ranked as the third most influential British thinker in *HR Magazine*'s "Most Influential" list.

Peter W. Butler has most recently been president of Rush University Medical Center, as well as professor and chairman of the Department of Health Systems Management at Rush University. Prior to serving at Rush, he was president and CEO of the Methodist Hospital System in Houston (now Houston Methodist). He previously served as senior vice president and chief administrative officer at Henry Ford Health System in Detroit. Butler is on the National Center for Healthcare Leadership board and has served as its chairman. He also has been active in national health policy. He served on the Medicare Payment Advisory Commission for two three-year terms.

W. Jeffrey Canar, PhD, is an assistant professor and director of faculty development and operations in the Department of Health Systems Management at Rush University. Prior to joining Rush, he worked for 13 years at the Edward Hines Jr. VA Medical Center on the spinal cord injury service. He also served as the integrated ethics program officer for Hines VA Medical Center. Dr. Canar received his PhD in clinical psychology from the Illinois Institute of Technology.

Kim Carlin, PhD, is the president of Carpedia Healthcare Ltd., based in New York City. Carpedia Healthcare is a tactical consulting resource used by high-performance healthcare organizations interested in step-change performance improvement. Dr. Carlin has worked with more than 200 client organizations across five continents. She holds an honors BA in sociology from the University of Guelph, an MBA in international business and strategy from McGill University, and a PhD in organizational leadership from Capella University.

Bryce Clark, RN, CPHQ, is a process improvement lead at Children's Hospital Colorado, where he manages projects that aim to reduce preventable harm to pediatric patients. He received an executive master in public administration degree with a focus on nursing leadership from the Robert F. Wagner Graduate School of Public Service at New York University.

Patrick Courneya, MD, is the executive vice president of hospitals, quality, and care delivery excellence and chief medical officer of Medicare Advantage, 1876 Cost, and Part D Pharmacy plans at Kaiser Foundation Hospitals and Health Plan, Inc., in Oakland, California. In this role, Dr. Courneya oversees Kaiser Permanente's national quality agenda, helps ensure that the organization's members and communities receive the best quality and service Kaiser Permanente offers, and advocates for the advancement of evidence-based medicine and proven innovation for the industry.

Richard D'Aquila, FACHE, is the president at Yale New Haven Hospital and executive vice president of Yale New Haven Health System in New Haven, Connecticut. He is responsible for all day-to-day operations of the hospital and all aspects of its performance as a destination medical center. He is a member of lecturing faculty at Yale University School of Medicine's Department of Epidemiology and Public Health. He has led the hospital team during an unprecedented period of growth and development, which now includes the successful integration of the Hospital of St. Raphael to make Yale New Haven one of the largest hospitals in the United States.

Maja Djukic, PhD, RN, is an assistant professor at Rory Meyers College of Nursing at New York University. She studies workforce determinants of healthcare quality and teaches quality improvement and evidence-based practice to doctoral students. Her research, published in more than 25 data-based, peer-reviewed publications, is funded by the Robert Wood Johnson Foundation, the Josiah Macy Jr. Foundation, the American Organization of Nursing Executives, and the National Council of State Boards of Nursing Center for Regulatory Excellence. She serves on the editorial board of *Health Care Management Review* and holds a leadership role at the Academy Health Interdisciplinary Research Group on Nursing Issues.

John Donnellan, FACHE, is adjunct professor of public and health administration at the Robert F. Wagner Graduate School of Public Service at New York University. Professor Donnellan joined the faculty at NYU Wagner in June 2009 following a 40-year career in federal service, including 37 years serving veterans in the Department of Veterans Affairs healthcare system. From 1991 until 2009, he was director/CEO of the VA Medical Center New York and later the consolidated New York City VA New York Harbor Healthcare System.

Michael Dowling is president and chief executive officer of Northwell Health. Prior to becoming president and CEO in 2002, Dowling was the health system's executive vice president and chief operating officer. Before joining Northwell in 1995, he was a senior vice president at Empire Blue Cross / Blue Shield. Dowling served in New York state government for 12 years, including 7 years as state director of health, education, and human services and deputy secretary to the governor. Before his public service career, he was a professor of social policy and assistant dean at the Fordham University Graduate School of Social Services, as well as director of the Fordham campus in Westchester County.

David Fine, PhD, FACHE, is president and CEO of the Catholic Health Initiatives Institute for Research and Innovation in Englewood, Colorado. Fine has enjoyed a 40-year career in the management of hospitals, health systems, medical groups, and HMOs. He has held tenured, graduate teaching positions at Tulane University, where he was regents professor and chair of the Department of Health Systems Management; the University of Alabama at Birmingham; and, most recently, Baylor College of Medicine. In 2007, he was recognized by the University of Southern Mississippi by conferral of a doctor of philosophy degree, honoris causa. He is the author or coauthor of four books and 60 scholarly publications.

Steven Fishbane, MD, is chief of the division of nephrology at Hofstra Northwell Health School of Medicine. He is also vice president for dialysis services at Northwell Health.

Andrew N. Garman, PsyD, is professor and associate chair of external relations in the Health Systems Management Department at Rush University. Dr. Garman also serves as CEO of the National Center for Healthcare Leadership and as executive director of the US Cooperative for International Patient Programs.

Kyle L. Grazier is the Richard Carl Jelinek Professor and chair of the Department of Health Management and Policy in the School of Public Health and professor of psychiatry in the School of Medicine at the University of Michigan. Her research, funded by the National Institutes of Health and foundations, focuses on the structural and process impacts of healthcare financing, particularly in behavioral health, on health status and quality of care. She serves on the board of trustees of the Health Research and Educational Trust; on the board of directors of Indiana University Health System, where she chairs the patient safety and quality committee; and on the Technical Measurement Advisory Board of the National Committee for Quality Assurance. She has also served as a director of the Commission on Accreditation of Health Management Education and as treasurer of the Association of

University Programs in Health Administration. She has also contributed to committees on quality and efficiency for the Institute of Medicine. She was editor of the *Journal of Healthcare Management* from 2000 to 2010. Prior to joining the University of Michigan, she was on the faculties of the Yale School of Medicine, the University of California at Berkeley, and Cornell University.

John R. Griffith, LFACHE, professor emeritus at the University of Michigan, is the original author of *The Well-Managed Healthcare Organization*, which is now in its eighth edition with coauthor Kenneth R. White (Health Administration Press, 2015). Griffith has published widely on the management of healthcare delivery organizations, and he has received a number of awards from the American College of Healthcare Executives. He is a member of the *Modern Healthcare* Hall of Fame.

Brian C. Gunia, PhD, is an assistant professor at Johns Hopkins University. His research focuses on negotiation, ethical decision making, and sleep and has been published in a number of academic journals, including the *Academy of Management Journal*, the *Journal of Applied Psychology*, the *Annual Review of Psychology*, and *Personality and Social Psychology Bulletin*. Dr. Gunia's work has also been featured in popular media outlets such as the *Economist*, the *Wall Street Journal*, and *Forbes*, and it has received several awards, including the International Association of Conflict Management's 2013 Best Paper Award.

Candice Halinski, NP-C, is the director of the service line in the clinical division of nephrology of Northwell Health, where she coordinates, supervises, develops, and assesses quality management, existing services, new programs, clinical implementation, geographic program expansion, and regulatory requirements. She has more than 15 years of clinical nephrology experience. Halinski has direct clinical oversight and supervision of a $2.5 million Centers for Medicare & Medicaid Services innovation grant for chronic kidney disease patients, which focuses on the preparation, education, and transition to renal replacement therapy for patients with late-stage kidney disease.

Tricia J. Johnson, PhD, is professor and associate chair for research and education in the Health Systems Management Department at Rush University. In this role, she also leads the Masters Project Program.

Susan Kaplan Jacobs, BSN, serves as health sciences librarian (curator) at New York University's Elmer Holmes Bobst Library. She provides instruction, collection development, faculty liaison services, and reference assistance for students and faculty at the Rory Meyers College of Nursing and the Steinhardt School departments of communicative sciences and disorders, occupational therapy, and physical therapy. She also serves as adjunct assistant professor of public administration in NYU's Robert F. Wagner Graduate School of Public Service.

Chien-Ching Li, PhD, is an assistant professor and a health services researcher in the Department of Health Systems Management at Rush University.

Andrew Mawson, managing director of Advanced Workplace Associates (AWA), is a leading pioneer, thinker, and speaker on matters "work and place." In his consulting work, he has led workplace change programs with such clients as Invesco, the United Nations Children's Emergency Fund, Willis, Direct Line Group, National Rail, the Royal Bank of Scotland, and Merrill Lynch. In 2014, he worked as an adviser with the United Kingdom Cabinet Office, participating in a review of 13 government departments' efforts to implement agile working as part of the government's civil service reform program. AWA's latest research project looked at how businesses can create the conditions that help each individual's brain be as effective as it can be.

K. Joanne McGlown, PhD, RN, FACHE, is the CEO of McGlown-Self Consulting, LLC, a healthcare management firm specializing in operations, nursing, risk, emergency, and disaster management. Dr. McGlown has more than 40 years of experience in the healthcare field, with broad teaching, consulting, and leadership experience, and she has filled leadership roles domestically and globally. She is an adjunct faculty member at the University of Alabama in Birmingham and a master's-level instructor at the Department of Homeland Security / Federal Emergency Management Agency's Noble Training Facility.

Lynn McVey is head of operations at the New Jersey Innovation Institute. McVey is passionate about healthcare and believes that "traditional" healthcare management is no longer a viable model. Her goal is to provide managers with evidence-based management tools and coach them to consistently monitor and improve their outcomes. Her clinical background and business curiosity provide a unique and successful management approach.

Stephen J. O'Connor, PhD, FACHE, is a professor in the Department of Health Services Administration at the University of Alabama at Birmingham.

Terese Otte-Trojel, PhD, is a healthcare information technology consultant at NNIT's public and healthcare advisory department, in Copenhagen, Denmark.

Her recent publications focus on the development and implementation of patient portals in both integrated and fragmented healthcare delivery systems.

Karen Plum is a business studies graduate currently serving as director of research and development at Advanced Workplace Associates, a United Kingdom–based workplace management consultancy. As leader of AWA's Performance Innovation Network, she designs and delivers workshops, events, and training courses to help organizations deliver and sustain advanced/agile ways of working. She also leads AWA's research program, which uses an evidence-based approach to answer questions of interest to AWA and its sponsors.

Lawrence Prybil, PhD, FACHE, received his master's and doctorate degrees from the University of Iowa's College of Medicine. He held senior executive positions in two of the nation's largest nonprofit health systems for nearly 20 years, with 10 years as CEO of a six-state division of the Daughters of Charity National Health System. He has also served in faculty and administrative roles at Virginia Commonwealth University, the University of Iowa, and the University of Kentucky and has led several national studies about healthcare governance and partnerships.

Denise M. Rousseau, PhD, is the H. J. Heinz II University Professor of Organizational Behavior and Public Policy at Carnegie Mellon University's Heinz College and the Tepper School of Business. She is the faculty director of the Institute for Social Innovation and chair of the healthcare policy and management program. In 2007, Dr. Rousseau founded the Evidence-Based Management Collaborative, a network of scholars, consultants, and practicing managers working to promote evidence-informed organizational practices and managerial decision making. Her teaching and research focus on evidence-based management and positive organizational practices in managing people and change.

Thomas Rundall, PhD, is the Henry J. Kaiser Professor of Organized Health Systems, Emeritus, at the University of California, Berkeley. Professor Rundall has published extensively across a broad array of topics, including evidence-based management, integration of healthcare services, hospital–physician relationships, health information technology, and quality improvement. He currently is codirector of the Center for Lean Engagement and Research and serves on the boards of directors for On Lok, a program of all-inclusive care for the elderly, and John Muir Health, an integrated healthcare delivery system.

Shital C. Shah, PhD, is the director of program development and assessment and assistant professor in the Department of Health Systems Management at Rush University. Dr. Shah completed his PhD degree in industrial engineering at the University of Iowa in 2005. He has assisted numerous applied learning projects that evaluate various clinical, operations, and management issues in healthcare.

Richard M. Shewchuk, PhD, is professor emeritus in the Department of Health Services Administration at the University of Alabama at Birmingham.

Eric Slotsve, analyst at McKinsey Solutions (Healthcare Analytics), is a graduate of New York University's Robert F. Wagner Graduate School of Public Service, where he studied under Anthony R. Kovner and Thomas D'Aunno. Passionate about problem solving and optimization, Slotsve started his journey into healthcare by studying various healthcare practices around Europe. To him, problem solving is a matter of analyzing the situation at hand and applying it to existing paradigms from other organizations and countries.

Michael Slubowski, FACHE, FACMPE, serves as president/CEO of Sisters of Charity of Leavenworth Health System (SCL Health). He provides executive leadership to SCL Health's healthcare ministry, which includes ten acute care hospitals, an adolescent mental health facility, and numerous ambulatory facilities, home care agencies, senior service facilities, safety net clinics, and physician practices in Colorado, Montana, and Kansas. Slubowski holds fellowships from both the American College of Healthcare Executives and the American College of Medical Practice Executives. He currently serves on the boards of directors of the Catholic Health Association (CHA), the Denver Metro Chamber of Commerce, and the Catholic CEO Healthcare Connection, and he sits on CHA's Advocacy and Public Policy Committee and Governance Committee.

Quint Studer founded Studer Group in 2000 after years of working in healthcare operations, including serving in a hospital president role. Studer Group was a 2010 recipient of the Malcolm Baldrige National Quality Award. Studer has written and contributed to a number of books, including *A Culture of High Performance* (2013); *Results That Last* (2007), a *Wall Street Journal* best seller; and *Hardwiring Excellence* (2004), one of the most widely read leadership books ever written for healthcare.

Jessie L. Tucker III, PhD, FACHE, is the chief operating officer of Robert Wood Johnson University Hospital (RWJUH) in New Brunswick, New Jersey. He is an Academy of Management Health Care Management Division board member (practitioner-at-large), a former Commission on Accreditation of Healthcare Management Education commissioner, and a former American College of Healthcare Executives Regent. Dr. Tucker retired from the Army Medical Department in 2009 and served as the administrator of Lyndon B. Johnson General Hospital in Houston, Texas, prior to joining the RWJUH team. For more than 25 years, he has leveraged research, evidence, and the many talents of his teams in the pursuit of cost-efficient quality.

Jed Weissberg, MD, served the members of Kaiser Permanente for 30 years as a clinician, physician executive, and health plan leader. He now is a senior fellow with the Institute for Clinical and Economic Review, based in Boston.